Diagnosis and Treatment of Liver Cancer in China

Xiaoping Chen
Editor

Diagnosis and Treatment of Liver Cancer in China

Past, Present and Prospects

Springer
PMPH
PEOPLE'S MEDICAL PUBLISHING HOUSE

Editor
Xiaoping Chen
Tongji Hospital Affiliated to Tongji Medical College,
Huazhong University of Science & Technology
Wuhan, China

ISBN 978-981-97-7968-0 ISBN 978-981-97-7969-7 (eBook)
https://doi.org/10.1007/978-981-97-7969-7

Jointly published with People's Medical Publishing House, PR of China.

This Springer imprint is published by the registered company Springer Nature Singapore Pte Ltd.
The registered company address is: 152 Beach Road, #21-01/04 Gateway East, Singapore 189721, Singapore

Contents

Part I

Overview of Liver Cancer Diagnosis and Treatment in China

Epidemiology of Liver Cancer in China

1

Yinghao Shen, Yan Li, Huichuan Sun, and Jian Zhou

1.1 Characteristic Onset and Epidemiology of Liver Cancer in China

1.1.1 Epidemiological Characteristics

Liver cancer is a common malignancy in China, accounting for 85–90% of all liver tumors. According to the archival data at the China National Cancer Center and the Chinese Center for Disease Control and Prevention (CCDC), China's yearly numbers of newly diagnosed cases of liver cancer and deaths related to liver cancer have been stabilized in the past 15 years. However, the incidence of liver cancer remains high. The International Agency for Research on Cancer (IARC) reported in 2018 that although China's incidence of liver cancer ranks ninth in the world, China has the largest number of liver cancer patients due to the huge population base in China. It is estimated that China has about seven million patients with liver cirrhosis. The yearly number of newly diagnosed patients with liver cancer is about 460,000, and the 5-year survival is only 12.1%. Among the common cancers, liver cancer ranks fifth in terms of overall incidence and second in terms of mortality. Liver cancer is second only to pancreatic cancer in terms of M/I ratio. Among all cancers in males, liver cancer ranks fourth in terms of incidence and second in terms of mortality. Among all cancers in females, liver cancer ranks seventh in terms of incidence but second in terms of mortality. Liver cancer is the second most common cause of cancer-related deaths in both urban and rural regions. Liver cancer is more common in males than in females, with a male-to-female ratio of approximately 3.5:1.

Y. Shen · Y. Li · H. Sun · J. Zhou (✉)
ZhongShan Hospital Fudan University, Shanghai, China
e-mail: zhou.jian@zs-hospital.sh.cn

1.1.2 Etiological Characteristics

The etiology and pathogenesis of liver cancer still remain largely unknown. A combination of factors may work together to result in the development of liver cancer. Chronic liver diseases caused by any factor may play important roles in the occurrence and development of liver cancer. According to an estimate, more than 1/5 of the Chinese population is affected by certain types of liver disease, especially infections caused by hepatitis B virus (HBV) and hepatitis C virus (HCV). Other risk factors for liver cancer include liver cirrhosis, hepatic adenoma, prolonged consumption of aflatoxin, smoking, nonalcoholic fatty liver disease (NAFLD), alcoholic liver disease (ALD), and drug-induced liver injury (DILD).

X. Chen (ed.), *Diagnosis and Treatment of Liver Cancer in China*,
https://doi.org/10.1007/978-981-97-7969-7_1

Viral hepatitis is still the leading cause of liver cancer in China. In China, about 90% of liver cancer patients have a history of HBV infection. The overall prevalence of HBV is 6.52% and that of HCV is 0.72%. Chronic hepatitis B (CHB) and chronic hepatitis C (CHC) affect 90 million and 10 million people in China, respectively. HBV infection can cause a significant number of deaths among liver cancer patients (63.9%, 65.9% among male patients and 58.4% among female patients). The overall mortality related to HCV among liver cancer patients is 27.7% (27.3% among male patients and 28.6% among female patients), which is lower than that of HBV. However, HCV causes more deaths than aflatoxin exposure (25.0%), alcohol consumption (15.7%), and smoking (13.9%). China began to implement the National Immunization Plan for Hepatitis B in 1992 and has been providing free hepatitis B vaccination for all newborns since 2005. Because of these measures, China's HBV infection rate and HBV-related mortality have been steadily declining over the years. But surprisingly, China's annual incidence of HCV infection rose abruptly almost tenfold from 2003 to 2017.

Viral hepatitis remains the main cause of liver cancer in China. But in the meantime, the incidence of metabolic liver disease has been rising steadily. For example, NAFLD (affecting 173–338 million people) and ALD (affecting about 62 million people) make a profound contribution to the increase in liver cancer patients. Statistics on the incidence and distribution of hospitalized patients with different liver diseases at 11 major tertiary public hospitals in China have revealed the following: The number of hospitalized patients due to liver diseases has dramatically increased in the past few years (from 24,375 in 2009 to 62,711 in 2017). Although viral hepatitis is still one of the most important liver diseases, the number of hospitalized patients due to NAFLD surpassed that of patients requiring inpatient treatment for chronic viral hepatitis from 2009 to 2016. Liver fibrosis, cirrhosis, and liver/bile duct cancer are also among the leading causes of hospitalization due to liver-related diseases. Hospitalized patients due to other common liver diseases, such as acute hepatitis, ALD, drug/toxin-induced liver diseases, and autoimmune hepatitis (AIH), account for smaller percentages.

1.2 Development of Hepatectomy for Liver Cancer and Postoperative Survival in the Past Decade

Hepatectomy remains the most important treatment for achieving long-term survival of patients with liver cancer, especially those diagnosed at an early stage. For some with intermediate and locally advanced liver cancer, surgical resection may result in better efficacy than other treatments.

In recent years, China has achieved a significant increase in the 5-year survival rate after hepatectomy, which reaches 30–50% on the whole. The 5-year survival rate after hepatectomy for small liver cancer (<2 cm) reaches up to 90%. It was about 75% for liver cancer (2–5 cm), 40% for large liver cancer (>5 cm and ≤10 cm), and 30% for giant liver cancer (>10 cm). As for hepatectomy among liver cancer patients meeting the Milan criteria, the postoperative 5-year survival rate reported by Queen Mary Hospital has increased from 62.7% in the past to 72.5% in the present day. The postoperative 5-year survival rate reported at other centers in China has also reached 70%. According to similar overseas reports, the postoperative 5-year survival rate has increased from 36% to 61%. The increase in postoperative survival rate among liver cancer patients is closely related to the continuous optimization of perioperative management, improvement of hepatic surgery techniques, and development of multi-modality treatment strategies.

Early diagnosis and treatment of liver cancer are crucial for improving surgical efficacy. The Liver Cancer Institute of Fudan University once reported that the postoperative 5-year survival rate after hepatectomy for liver cancer increased from 1958 to 1987 along with the increase in the percentage of patients with small liver cancers.

West China Hospital of Sichuan University reported that the percentage of patients with small liver cancers increased from 7.1% to 19.9% and the postoperative 5-year survival rate increased from 34% to 40.2% before and after 1997. One of the effective measures to achieve early diagnosis of liver cancer is monitoring and screening among high-risk populations. At present, regular screening protocol has not been popularized in China. Besides, the existing screening techniques (ultrasound plus α-fetoprotein) have limited sensitivity. Although computed tomography (CT) and magnetic resonance imaging (MRI) have higher sensitivity and specificity, they are costly, involve complex process, and are therefore not suitable for routine screening. Thus, most liver cancers are diagnosed at the intermediate and advanced stages. Only about 30% of the patients are diagnosed at an early stage. Establishing effective screening mechanisms and protocols for populations at high risk for hepatitis and cirrhosis and developing more sensitive early diagnostic markers or methods are highly important for further improving the early detection rate of liver cancer.

As for surgical indications, large liver cancers above 5 cm, intermediate and advanced multinodular liver cancers combined with tumor thrombus are not usually indicated for hepatectomy according to liver cancer treatment guidelines in western countries. However, most liver centers, including some in western countries, do not completely agree with the above guidelines in clinical practice. According to the opinions from the Group of Hepatic Surgery, Surgical Branch of Chinese Medical Association in 2010 and the Guidelines for Diagnosis and Treatment of Primary Liver Cancer (2017 Edition), surgical resection is still recommended for large or giant liver cancers with a good liver functional reserve and clear margins as long as the surgical safety can be ensured. Radical resection can be performed for multiple liver cancers if they are fewer than three and confined in the hepatic segments or lobes. If the lesions are scatteredly distributed and the FLR (Future liver remnant) is above 40%, the lesions can be locally resected one by one. For those combined with tumor thrombus of the portal vein, resection is still recommended based on preoperative evaluation if the tumors are confined to the hemiliver and the tumor thrombus can be completely removed After the resection, the patients should receive transcatheter arterial chemoembolization (TACE), portal vein chemotherapy, or other systemic treatments. If there are hepatic hilar lymph node metastases, lymph node dissection should be performed simultaneously with tumor resection, followed by postoperative radiotherapy. For those with one metastatic lesion, the primary and metastatic lesions can be resected simultaneously. According to the report by the Eastern Hepatobiliary Surgery Hospital affiliated to the PLA Second Military Medical University (currently the Third Affiliated Hospital of Naval Medical University (Eastern Hepatobiliary Surgery Hospital), hereafter referred to as Shanghai Eastern Hepatobiliary Surgery Hospital), patients of Barcelona clinic liver cancer (BCLC)-stage C accounted for 43.9% among all patients receiving hepatectomy between 2001 and 2007; their 5-year survival rate was 30.5%. In another report, patients of BCLC-stage B and BCLC-stage C accounted for 46.1% and 12.7%, respectively, between 2001 and 2014; the 5-year survival rate was 32.8% and 10.6%, respectively. At the Affiliated Tumor Hospital of Guangxi Medical University, the postoperative 5-year survival rate of patients of BCLC-stage B and BCLC-stage C receiving hepatectomy between 2000 and 2007 was 39%. A 2013 analysis covered hepatectomy data at 10 centers throughout the world between 1990 and 2009. It was found that the patients of BCLC-stage B (including those with one tumor above 5 cm) and BCLC-stage C accounted for 50%. Their postoperative 5-year survival rate was 57% and 38%, respectively. In 2018, another systematic analysis was concerned with hepatectomy data from patients at the middle and advanced stages published between 1999 and 2014. The median postoperative 5-year survival rate was 38.7% in patients of BCLC-stage B, 20% in patients of BCLC-stage C, 33% for liver cancers above 10 cm, and 54% for multinodular liver cancers. Another similar study conducted in China in the same year analyzed the hepatectomy data from

14,808 patients with solitary large liver cancer and multinodular liver cancers worldwide between 2000 and 2017. It was found that the postoperative 5-year survival rate among patients from Asian countries was significantly higher than that among patients from non-Asian countries (42% vs. 32%). Besides, the postoperative overall 5-year survival rate and tumor-free survival rate increased significantly in recent years among these patients:

1. For solitary large liver cancers (>5 cm), several studies have indicated that hepatectomy is still the safe and reliable treatment so long as the patients' general condition or liver function allows them to. At Xiangya Hospital, Central South University, a total of 260 solitary large liver cancers were resected between 1992 and 2002. The median overall survival and tumor-free survival were close to that in patients receiving resection for small liver cancers. In the former, the postoperative 5-year survival rate reached 38.2%. At West China Hospital of Sichuan University, 268 solitary liver cancers were resected between 2009 and 2013. The postoperative 5-year survival rate was 25.4–52.1%.
2. For multiple liver cancers, many studies have confirmed that surgical resection is still the best treatment as long as survival benefits are concerned. It was reported in Japan in 2008 that the postoperative 5-year survival rate after hepatectomy for multiple liver cancers was 58%. Another study analyzed all of the hepatectomy data at eight hospitals in China from 2006 to 2015. The results showed that the patients with ≥3 nodules receiving the hepatectomy accounted for 15%. In these patients, the postoperative 5-year survival rate and tumor-free survival rate were 34.6% and 24.7%, respectively.
3. Liver cancer combined with tumor thrombus was once considered the absolute contraindication for surgery. But in recent years, a growing body of evidence has shown that patients with the combined condition may also benefit from hepatectomy. Tokyo University conducted a nationwide multi-center propensity score matching score matching analysis in liver cancer patients combined with tumor thrombus of portal vein tumor in 2016. The result showed that so long as the main portal vein or its contralateral branch is not invaded. T, the median survival of patients receiving hepatectomy, was significantly longer than those receiving nonsurgical treatment (2.45 years vs. 1.57 years). Shanghai Eastern Hepatobiliary Surgery Hospital reported in 2018 that the median survival of patients combined with tumor thrombus of the portal vein, hepatic vein, and bile duct was 26.4, 30.4, and 37.6 months after hepatectomy, respectively. Tianjin Medical University Cancer Institute and Hospital reported in 2016 that the median survival was 18 months in patients combined with tumor thrombus of the portal vein after hepatectomy. Apparently, different centers vary significantly in the choice and efficacy of treatments for intermediate and advanced liver cancers. An increasing number of studies have been focused on establishing a scoring system or new classification method for the subdivision of such patients, so as to identify the subgroups fit for surgery. Besides, along with the popularization of associating liver partition with portal vein ligation for staged hepatectomy (ALPPS) in liver cancer, many liver cancer patients that are otherwise considered unresectable now may be given the chance for radical resection. Many conditions that were considered contraindications for hepatectomy in the past are no longer so. However, whether intermediate and advanced liver cancers are fit for surgery is still disputable. No uniform treatment protocols or guidelines have been established yet. More high level evidence will be needed for confirmation.

At present, the safety of hepatectomy has already been improved. At many centers, perioperative mortality has been decreased to below 5%, and below 2% at some centers. Such an improvement is mainly attributed to continuous progress in perioperative management and surgical skills in recent years. Preoperative use of modified Child-Pugh scoring system, indocyanine green excretion test, or computer-assisted 3D simulation imaging to precisely evaluate the liver function reserve has attracted growing attention as part of perioperative management. CT imaging has been used to determine the residual liver volume. Microinvasiveness and precision represent the latest trends in surgery methods. Laparoscopic hepatectomy has been increasingly applied in clinics. However, wider applications of this technique rely on building an effective risk evaluation system and a standardized surgical training system. Precision treatment has become the development trend of liver surgery. However, some standardization of key technologies are still the primary concerns.

Effective postoperative adjuvant treatments and sequential or combined use of various treatment modalities after recurrence are highly importance for prolonging patients' survival:

1. Postoperative adjuvant TACE and systematic treatment have been extensively confirmed to prolong the patients' survival and prevent a recurrence, especially for those at high risk for recurrence or combined with microvascular metastases. Recent studies have shown that for patients with microvascular metastases, preoperative TACE has equal efficacy in prolonging postoperative survival.
2. Postoperative antiviral treatment has been confirmed to have a beneficial effect on the prognosis of liver cancer patients in recent years. The research team led by Professor Weiping ZHOU has found recently that even for patients with a low preoperative HBV DNA level, postoperative antiviral treatment can also reduce recurrence and prolong the benefit considerably. One study conducted by the Chinese University of Hong Kong in 2015 showed that the postoperative antiviral treatment could result in improved liver function and offer a better chance for recurrent patients to receive radical treatment. Therefore, normalized implementation of antiviral treatment is an effective pathway to enhancing the efficacy of hepatectomy.
3. Combining traditional Chinese medicine and Western medicine is a unique treatment for liver cancer in China. A Chinese phase IV clinical trial involving 39 centers in 2018 confirmed again that a postoperative treatment with Huaier Granule could significantly prolong the tumor-free survival of liver cancer patients and reduce extrahepatic metastases.
4. Clinical practice has proved that any treatment modality for liver cancer can be applied to liver cancer recurrence. Re-resection is one of the most effective treatments for liver cancer recurrence and has become a mature surgical modality for liver cancer. Affiliated Tumor Hospital of Guangxi Medical University reported that the postoperative 5-year survival rate was 35% after re-resection for recurrent liver cancer patients between 1998 and 2008. At Shanghai Eastern Hepatobiliary Surgery Hospital, the 5-year survival rate after re-resection was 51% between 2007 and 2011. One study has shown that the efficacy of re-resection for early recurrence (within 2 years) is much worse than that for late recurrence (after 2 years). This finding indicates the need to strictly determine the indications for re-resection and identify those fit for re-resection. In recent years, some effective drugs for systematic treatment (e.g., sorafenib, lenvatinib, and regorafenib) have successively entered clinical trials. Some of them have become the first- and second-line drugs for middle and advanced liver cancers. The combined use of immunotherapy (e.g., immune checkpoint inhibitors) and other treatments has become the new research hotspot.

Recurrence and metastasis are the biggest obstacles to prolonged postoperative survival in liver cancer patients. However, many basic and clinical studies have been conducted over treatments against recurrence and metastasis. At present, there are still no widely accepted treatments with definite efficacy in reducing postoperative recurrence. The postoperative 5-year recurrence remains as high as 60–70%. The 5-year recurrence rate also reaches 50% in patients with small liver cancer. The majority of postoperative anti-recurrence treatments are intended for prolonging the patients' survival. Reducing the recurrence rate is hardly possible without deep understanding and revelation of the biological mechanism of tumor recurrence or the development of therapeutic targets.

1.3 Concluding Remarks

Promoting regular screening and monitoring for high-risk populations and developing more sensitive early diagnostic markers are the prerequisites for improving the early diagnostic rate of liver cancer. Currently, hepatectomy can be applied to treat most liver cancers. However, no uniform treatment specification has been established for intermediate and advanced liver cancer. More high level of evidence is needed for this purpose. Treatments against the recurrence and metastasis of liver cancer are still the primary concerns and difficulties following surgeries. Further explorations into the biological mechanism of tumor recurrence and metastasis are urgent. Postoperative adjuvant treatment, regular recurrence monitoring, and multi-modality treatment strategies are considered effective pathways to prolong survival of the patients.

Suggested Reading

1. Wang FS, Fan JG, Zhang Z, et al. The global burden of liver disease: the major impact of China. Hepatology. 2014;60(6):2099–108.
2. Zhou J, Sun HC, Wang Z, et al. Guidelines for diagnosis and treatment of primary liver cancer in China (2017 edition). Liver Cancer. 2018;7(3):235–60.
3. Bray F, Ferlay J, Soerjomataram I, et al. Global cancer statistics 2018: GLOBOCAN estimates of incidence and mortality worldwide for 36 cancers in 185 countries. CA Cancer J Clin. 2018;68(6):394–424.
4. Wu J, Yang S, Xu K, et al. Patterns and trends of liver cancer incidence rates in eastern and southeastern Asian countries (1983-2007) and predictions to 2030. Gastroenterology. 2018;154(6):1719–28.
5. Pan R, Zhu M, Yu C, et al. Cancer incidence and mortality: a cohort study in China, 2008–2013. Int J Cancer. 2017;141(7):1315–23.
6. Chen WQ. Strategies of primary prevention of liver cancer in China: expert consensus (2018). J Clin Hepatol. 2018;34(10):2090–7.
7. Chen W, Zheng R, Baade PD, et al. Cancer statistics in China, 2015. CA Cancer J Clin. 2016;66(2):115–32.
8. Chen JG. Trends in the incidence of liver cancer and its primary prevention in China. J Clin Hepatol. 2012;28(4):256–60.
9. Sangwangmu G, Zhongfei C, Yalu D, Yunqi L, Yaxin L, Modi L. An analysis on the epidemiological characteristics of primary liver cancer at our hospital from 2001 to 2017. Chin J Interv Radiol. 2019;7(3):206–10.
10. Xiao J, Wang F, Wong NK, et al. Global liver disease burdens and research trends: analysis from a Chinese perspective. J Hepatol. 2019;71(1):212–21.
11. Prevention of Infection Related Cancer Group. Strategies of primary prevention of liver cancer in China: expert consensus (2018). Zhonghua Yu Fang Yi Xue Za Zhi. 2019;53(1):36–44.
12. Kowdley KV, Wang C, Welch S, et al. Prevalence of chronic hepatitis B among foreign born persons living in the United States by country of origin. Hepatology. 2012;56(2):422–33.
13. Liu G, Dibonaventura MD, Yuan Y, et al. The burden of illness for patients with viral hepatitis C: evidence from a national survey in Japan. Value Health. 2012;15(1 Suppl):S65–71.
14. Edlin BR, Eckhardt BJ, Shu MA, et al. Toward a more accurate estimate of the prevalence of hepatitis C in the United States. Hepatology. 2015;62(5):1353–63.
15. Zhu RX, Seto WK, Lai CL, et al. Epidemiology of hepatocellular carcinoma in the Asia pacific region. Gut Liver. 2016;10(3):332–9.
16. Rao H, Wei L, Lopez Talavera JC, et al. Distribution and clinical correlates of viral and host genotypes in Chinese patients with chronic hepatitis C virus infection. J Gastroenterol Hepatol. 2014;29(3):545–53.
17. Feng RN, Du S, Wang C, et al. Lean non-alcoholic fatty liver disease increases risk for metabolic disorders in a normal weight Chinese population. World J Gastroenterol. 2014;20(47):17932–40.
18. Fan JG. Epidemiology of alcoholic and nonalcoholic fatty liver disease in China. J Gastroenterol Hepatol. 2013;28(Suppl 1):11–7.
19. Mao YL. Liver cancer: questions and answers. Beijing: Scientific and Technical Documentation Press; 2018.
20. Fan ST, Mau LOC, Poon RT, et al. Continuous improvement of survival outcomes of resection of hepatocellular carcinoma: a 20 year experience. Ann Surg. 2011;253(4):745–58.
21. Zhang SC. A retrospective study on the influence of preoperative adjuvant TACE on the long-term survival of patients meeting Milan Criteria after hepatectomy for hepatitis B-related liver cancer. Shanghai: Naval Medical University; 2018.
22. Chen X, Li C, Wen TF, et al. An analysis on the prognostic factors for hepatectomy for hepatocellular carcinoma meeting Milan criteria. Chin J Bases Clin Gen Surg. 2015;22(10):1175–8.
23. Krenzien F, Schmelzle M, Struecker B, et al. Liver transplantation and liver resection for cirrhotic patients

with hepatocellular carcinoma: comparison of long term survivals. J Gastrointest Surg. 2018;22(5):840–8.
24. Tang ZY, Yu YQ, Lin ZY, et al. Efforts in improving the long-term efficacy for primary liver cancer in the past thirty years. Chin J Cancer. 1987;6(3):187–91.
25. Yan LN. Surgical treatment of primary liver cancer (with a report of 1038 cases). Beijing: The 2000 National Tumor Symposium; 2000.
26. Qian XJ, Qu CF, Lu FM. Early detection of hepatocellular carcinoma-expanding the utility of circulating tumor markers. Chin Hepatol. 2019;24(8):851–3.
27. Yarchoan M, Agarwal P, Villanueva A, et al. Recent developments and therapeutic strategies against hepatocellular carcinoma. Cancer Res. 2019;79(17):4326–30.
28. Bureau of Medical Administration, National Health and Family Planning Commission of the PRC. Guidelines for diagnosis and treatment of primary liver cancer (2017 edition). Chin J Dig Surg. 2017;16(7):635–47.
29. Yang T, Lin C, Zhai J, et al. Surgical resection for advanced hepatocellular carcinoma according to Barcelona clinic liver cancer (BCLC) staging. J Cancer Res Clin Oncol. 2012;138(7):1121–9.
30. Li J, Huang L, Yan J, et al. Liver resection for hepatocellular carcinoma: personal experiences in a series of 1330 consecutive cases in China. ANZ J Surg. 2018;88(10):E713–7.
31. Chen J. Survival benefit analysis of hepatectomy for patients with BCLC stage B/C hepatocellular carcinoma and analysis of the prognostic factors. Nanning: Guangxi Medical University; 2014.
32. Torzilli G, Belghiti J, Kokudo N, et al. A snapshot of the effective indications and results of surgery for hepatocellular carcinoma in tertiary referral centers: is it adherent to the EASL/AASLD recommendations: an observational study of the HCC East West study group. Ann Surg. 2013;257(5):929–37.
33. Koh YX, Tan HL, Lye WK, et al. Systematic review of the outcomes of surgical resection for intermediate and advanced Barcelona Clinic Liver Cancer stage hepatocellular carcinoma: a critical appraisal of the evidence. World J Hepatol. 2018;10(6):433–47.
34. Liu L. Restaging of BCLC stage B HCC from the perspective of hepatectomy. Nanning: Guangxi Medical University; 2018.
35. Yang LY, Fang F, Ou DP, et al. Solitary large hepatocellular carcinoma: a specific subtype of hepatocellular carcinoma with good outcome after hepatic resection. Ann Surg. 2009;249(1):118–23.
36. Shen JY, Li C, Wen TF, et al. Establishment of prognostic scoring system for single large hepatocellular carcinoma after hepatectomy. Chin J Hepatic Surg, Electron Ed. 2018;7(3):197–201.
37. Ishizawa T, Hasegawa K, Aoki T, et al. Neither multiple tumors nor portal hypertension are surgical contraindications for hepatocellular carcinoma. Gastroenterology. 2008;134(7):1908–16.
38. Li ZL, Yu J, Guo JW, et al. Liver resection is justified for multinodular hepatocellular carcinoma in selected patients with cirrhosis: a multicenter analysis of 1,066 patients. Eur J Surg Oncol. 2019;45(5):800–7.
39. Kokudo T, Hasegawa K, Matsuyama Y, et al. Survival benefit of liver resection for hepatocellular carcinoma associated with portal vein invasion. J Hepatol. 2016;65(5):938–43.
40. Cui YL, Li Q, Zhang T, et al. Influencing factors for prognosis of patients with hepatocellular carcinoma complicated with portal vein tumor thrombus after surgical treatment. Chin J Hepatic Surg, Electron Ed. 2016;5(4):249–53.
41. Kokudo T, Hasegawa K, Matsuyama Y, et al. A prognostic scoring system for patients with multiple hepatocellular carcinomas treated by hepatectomy. Ann Surg Oncol. 2015;22(3):826–33.
42. Kokudo T, Hasegawa K, Matsuyama Y, et al. Development of Hong Kong liver cancer staging system with treatment stratification for patients with hepatocellular carcinoma. Gastroenterology. 2014;146(7):1691–700.e3.
43. Li Q, Hao XS. Progress in surgical treatment of primary liver cancer. Chin J Surg Integr Tradit West Med. 2010;16(2):130–3.
44. Lu SD, Li L, Liang XM, et al. Updates and advancements in the management of hepatocellular carcinoma patients after hepatectomy. Expert Rev Gastroenterol Hepatol. 2019;13(11):1077–88.
45. Zhong JH, Ma L, Li LQ. Postoperative therapy options for hepatocellular carcinoma. Scand J Gastroenterol. 2014;49(6):649–61.
46. Huang G, Li P, Lau WY, et al. Antiviral therapy reduces hepatocellular carcinoma recurrence in patients with low HBV DNA levels: a randomized controlled trial. Ann Surg. 2018;268(6):943–54.
47. Chong C, Wong GL, Wong VW, et al. Antiviral therapy improves post hepatectomy survival in patients with hepatitis B virus related hepatocellular carcinoma: a prospective retrospective study. Aliment Pharmacol Ther. 2015;41(2):199–208.
48. Chen Q, Shu C, Laurence AD, et al. Effect of Huaier granule on recurrence after curative resection of HCC: a multicentre, randomised clinical trial. Gut. 2018;67(11):2006–16.
49. Xiang BD, Li LQ, Zhao YN, et al. Prognostic factors of patients with recurrent hepatocellular carcinoma after re-excision. Chin J Clin Oncol. 2010;37(17):994–7.
50. Xu Y, Shen Q, Wang N, et al. A study on the efficacy of secondary surgical resection after recurrence following the resection of hepatocellular carcinoma. Chin J Pract Surg. 2016;36(6):652–5.
51. Xu JF, Dai J, Guo T, et al. Repeated hepatectomy for recurrent liver cancer: efficacy and prognostic factors. Chin J Gen Surg. 2014;23(7):873–7.
52. Forner A, Reig M, Bruix J. Hepatocellular carcinoma. Lancet. 2018;391(10127):1301–14.
53. Motoyama H, Kobayashi A, Yokoyama T, et al. Impact of advanced age on the short and long term outcomes in patients undergoing hepatectomy for hepatocellular carcinoma: a single center analysis over a 20 year period. Am J Surg. 2015;209(4):733–41.

2 Exploration and Technological Innovations in Early Diagnosis, Recurrence, and Metastasis Mechanism of Liver Cancer

Qiang Gao, Bo Hu, Jie Hu, Yunfan Sun, Jiabin Cai, Peiyun Zhou, Shuangjian Qiu, and Jian Zhou

Early detection is the most important means to improve liver cancer prognosis. In the 1970s, a large number of patients with early stage liver cancer were detected by the alpha-fetoprotein (AFP) test in Shanghai, Jiangsu, and other territories across China. In the 1990s, Professor Yang Bing et al. pointed out that patients aged above 40 and positive for hepatitis B surface antigen (HBsAg) or with chronic hepatitis are high-risk populations for liver cancer. The detection rate of liver cancer in the above populations was 34.5-fold higher than that in the general population. Two AFP tests per year plus B-ultrasound were thus recommended for these populations. Recent years have witnessed the rapid development of medical imaging like magnetic resonance imaging (MRI). In the meantime, a series of early diagnostic molecular markers for liver cancer have been widely accepted, including alpha-fetoprotein alloplasm 3 (AFP-L3), des-γ-carboxy prothrombin (DCP/PIVKA II), and Golgi protein 73 (GP73). Liquid biopsy techniques, such as detections of circulating tumor cells (CTCs), circulating microRNAs (miRNAs), and circulating tumor DNA (ctDNA), have undergone rapid development. The early diagnosis of liver cancer has taken a great leap forward because of these novel techniques.

Recurrence and metastasis of liver cancer are the most important barriers to improving the treatment efficacy of liver cancer. Thus, tremendous efforts have been made to understand the mechanism underlying them. A wide range of new technologies, such as the patient-derived xenograft mouse model, have been applied. Relevant studies have promoted the understanding of liver cancer recurrence and metastasis.

It could be expected that in the near future, the clinical management and prognosis of liver cancer will be dramatically improved with the continuous improvement of the early diagnosis and the deepening understanding of the mechanism of recurrence and metastasis. An increasing number of patients will benefit from such progress and achieve better treatment efficacy.

2.1 High-Risk Population and Early Detection of Liver Cancer

As reported by the National Cancer Center, the number of newly diagnosed cases of liver cancer in China was about 367,700 in 2012. The morbidity was 26.04/100,000 (ranking the fourth), and the mortality was 22.42/100,000 (ranking the second). The risk of liver cancer in males is 2–3 times higher than that in females.

Q. Gao · B. Hu · J. Hu · Y. Sun · J. Cai · P. Zhou
S. Qiu · J. Zhou (✉)
ZhongShan Hospital Fudan University,
Shanghai, China
e-mail: zhou.jian@zs-hospital.sh.cn

X. Chen (ed.), *Diagnosis and Treatment of Liver Cancer in China*,
https://doi.org/10.1007/978-981-97-7969-7_2

Liver cancer can be mainly divided into hepatocellular carcinoma (HCC), intrahepatic cholangiocarcinoma (ICC), and combined hepatocellular and cholangiocarcinoma (cHCC-CC). HCC accounts for 75–85% of all primary liver cancers.

The risk factors for HCC include chronic hepatitis B and C virus (HBV, HCV) infection, aflatoxin, cirrhosis caused by various reasons, autoimmune liver disease, nonalcoholic steatohepatitis, obesity, type 2 diabetes, excessive ethanol intake, smoking, and family history of liver cancer. The risk factors for ICC mainly include intrahepatic bile duct stone, repeated biliary tract infections, primary sclerosing cholangitis, congenital abnormalities of the biliary tract, parasitic infections, and there is also a certain relationship between hepatitis virus infections and cholangiocarcinoma.

Regular monitoring of high-risk populations of liver cancer is particularly necessary given the fact that early diagnosis and treatment of liver cancer are crucial for improving the survival. Patients may have the chance for radical surgery if diagnosed at an early stage, which further reduces mortality and prolongs survival. Generally, patients with the above risk factors are collectively known as the high-risk population of liver cancer and should receive regular examinations. Hematological tests [e.g., routine blood test, liver function test, AFP, carbohydrate antigen 19-9 (CA19-9), des-γ-carboxy prothrombin (DCP), AFP-L3] and ultrasound diagnosis are the primary screening means for liver cancer. For an unconfirmed diagnosis, computed tomography (CT), MRI, digital subtraction angiography (DSA), and nuclear medicine imaging are usually used to determine the nature of the lesion. Evidence has shown that screening once every 6 months for the high-risk population can effectively diagnose liver cancer at an early stage, and thus plays a crucial role in the early diagnosis and treatment of liver cancer. Further efforts should be made to develop more sensitivity and specificity early screening methods for liver cancer, which enable a early treatment and improve patient's over all survival.

2.2 Dissecting the Mechanism of and Control Strategies to Recurrence and Metastasis

Surgery remains the most effective treatment for liver cancer. However, even after radical resection, the 5-year recurrence and metastasis rate is still as high as 60–70%, leading to a dismal outcome. Postoperative recurrence and metastasis are thus the bottleneck to the long-term survival of patients. It is urgent to explore the molecular mechanism of and propose new strategies against liver cancer recurrence and metastasis.

Liver cancer recurrence and metastasis are a multistep, multilevel, and complex process. Currently, the following mechanisms have been proposed: alterations in cancer genes and surface structures, enhancement of angiogenesis, increased cell adhesion capacity, tumorhypoxia and alterations in metabolic function, interactions between cancer cells and local immune and inflammatory cells, and extracellular matrix. Generally, recurrence and metastasis are not only related to the biological characteristics of cancer cells themselves, such as invasive and metastatic abilities. The tumor microenvironment also plays an important promoting role during these processes. It is noteworthy that systematic and in-depth studies have shown that CTCs and cancer stem cells (CSCs) are "seed cells" playing extremely important roles in liver cancer recurrence and metastasis.

This section focuses on the mechanism of liver cancer recurrence and metastasis. As for individualized treatment of liver cancer, the preliminary exploration was carried out based on the two major technologies, that is high-throughput omics like next-generation sequencing and novel tumor models like patient-derived xenograft (PDX) or organoid (PDO) for anticancer drugs screening.

2.2.1 Immune Microenvironment and Liver Cancer Recurrence and Metastasis

In 2011, *Cell* expanded the previous six hallmarks of cancer to ten, with the acknowledgment of tumor microenvironment. There is even an argument that tumor is a "microenvironment-related disease." Since then, the concept of and study on tumor microenvironment has been further highlighted. Liver cancer is closely related to microenvironment-related factors, including chronic hepatitis and cirrhosis. It is considered the most typical microenvironment-related tumor. The invasive and migration abilities of liver cancer not only depend on the cancer cells but, more importantly, also on the interactions among the host, local microenvironment, and cancer cells. The immune and inflammatory cells in the microenvironment, such as Treg cells, Th17 cells, macrophages, neutrophils, fibroblasts, and endothelial cells, along with various soluble molecules and extracellular matrix, have been well known for their roles in promoting liver cancer occurrence and development. With the advances in flow cytometry and single-cell sequencing, the identification and classification of immune cell subsets in the microenvironment have become more accurate. One single-cell sequencing study has indicated the unprecedented heterogeneity and plasticity of T-cells in the liver cancer microenvironment, which defines at least 11 T-cell subsets. Many studies have reported significant intertumoral and intratumor heterogeneity of the immune microenvironment in liver cancer: (1) cancer cells are able to dynamically edit and remodel immune cells through various mechanisms, leading to local immunosuppression. (2) Chemotactic factor and their receptor expression profiles determine the type, density, and spatial distribution of immune cells in the microenvironment, which may even have an impact on clinical outcome.

About 80–90% of postoperative recurrence and metastasis of liver cancer are intrahepatic. Apart from cancer cell intrinsic features, the diseased liver itself is the soil for such recurrence. Its special physicochemical properties, tissue structure, and immune and inflammatory profiles may play crucial roles in directional metastasis of cancer cells toward the diseased liver. Studies have confirmed that the immune and inflammatory status of the diseased liver can influence the intrahepatic spread of liver cancer. Besides, cancer cells can specifically induce the cancer-promoting traits and abnormal activation of hepatic stellate cells and inflammatory cells in the diseased liver tissues. According to the "pre-metastatic niche" theory proposed by Kaplan et al., liver cancer cells may exert a certain regulatory effect on the liver microenvironment. Most of the existing studies on the "pre-metastatic niche" focus upon lung metastasis of tumors. A well-designed experiment is usually needed to determine the changes in the cellular components and protein expressions of the "pre-metastatic sites" such as the liver tissue. Such experiments are prerequisite for confirming the pre-metastatic hypothesis of intrahepatic spread of liver cancer. The technological advances in cancer models and extensive applications of single-cell analysis will bring new breakthroughs for understanding the heterogeneity, plasticity, and cancer-promoting effect of liver cancer microenvironment.

2.2.2 CTCs, Cancer Stem Cells, and Liver Cancer Recurrence and Metastasis

Recurrence and metastasis are the fundamental causes of the poor prognosis of liver cancer, representing the major barrier to improve treatment efficacy. CSCs and CTCs are considered "seed cells" of liver cancer recurrence and metastasis. Molecular and cell biology have undergone dramatic development in recent years. There has been a shift from the conventional single-gene and single-molecule studies to more profound and systematic studies on these recurrence- and metastasis-initiating cells.

At present, Chinese scholars have identified a variety of liver cancer CSC subsets, including side population cells, CD133+, CD90+, OV6+, CD24+, and ICAM+ liver cancer CSCs. Although CSCs account for no more than 5% of the entire liver cancer cell population, they are highly carcinogenic and strongly self-renewable, with multidirectional differentiation, migration, and invasive capacities. The composition of CSC subsets is highly heterogeneous from one liver cancer patient to another. The expressions of the molecular markers of CSC can be used as independent predictors of liver cancer recurrence and metastasis. The following achievements have been made by the authors' institute: (1) Molecular markers that can be used to predict the prognosis of patients with liver cancer are identified. (2) The Hedgehog pathway inhibitor NanoHHI or the calcium channel-targeting monoclonal antibody 1B50-1 are found to inhibit the self-renewal, differentiation, proliferation, invasion and metastasis, and the tumor-forming ability of liver cancer CSCs in mice. (3) CTCs with stem cell-like features are successfully isolated from patients with liver cancer, and their high tumorigenicity is confirmed. The CTC count in the preoperative peripheral blood of patients with liver cancer is an independent prognostic predictor of early recurrence after radical resection. (4) The systemic immune and inflammatory status is conducive to CTC spread and metastasis. Besides, a patent has been granted to the CTC detection kit recently developed by the authors' institute (ZL201410081508.9), which can enrich heterogeneous CTCs in the circulation. The preliminary results of 1000 cases showed its ability in predicting liver cancer recurrence and metastasis after surgical resection, transcatheter arterial chemoembolization (TACE), and radiotherapy. It should be noted that the heterogeneity of CTC remains an important issue. New enrichment techniques, such as aptamer nanoarray, nanomagnetic heads, and microfluidic antibody array, have opened up new pathways for high-efficiency CTC sorting of liver cancer.

2.2.3 Patient-Derived Liver Cancer Models and Its Application

Despite the encouraging antitumor efficacy in animal or in vitro models, over 90% of the new drugs did not reach the primary endpoints in phase III clinical trials. This failure points to the need in new model systems mimicking cancer biological features for development of new drugs against liver cancer. The existing cell line-derived xenografts (CDX) cannot meet the above need for the following reasons: (1) CDX cannot fully represent the interindividual diversity of patients. (2) Long-term in vitro treatment and passage may lead to dramatic alterations in the organizational and genetic features of cell lines. (3) The cell lines cannot reflect the intratumor heterogeneity and microenvironmental features.

PDX model is constructed by inoculating the patient-derived tumor tissues collected by surgery or biopsy to immunodeficient mice. In early 2016, the National Cancer Institute (NCI) announced the use of PDX in place of the NCI-60 cell line for cancer study, which testifies for the advantages of PDX. First of all, PDX can maximally preserve the biological features and tumor heterogeneity without the need of in vitro culture, and especially it partially retains the interactions between tumor cells and their microenvironment. Second, PDX model can accurately reflect clinical efficacy of anticancer drugs. A case-control study using the PDX model and corresponding patients has reported a 90% agreement in the efficacy between them. Finally, PDX model can reproduce the tumor clonal evolution dynamics, thus representing as a suitable object for studying cancer recurrence and metastasis. However, PDX model has its defects, such as low throughput, high expense, and prolonged time for drug susceptibility test. Since PDX model does not incorporate a human-derived immune system, it cannot be used for the basic and clinical studies of immune-related drugs.

The authors' institute has conducted a series of studies on PDX. A standardized construction protocol for PDX model of liver cancer is developed innovatively (patent No.: ZL201410100264.4), which dramatically increases the xenograft formation. Besides, an optimal freezing medium is determined, yielding the resuscitation rate after cryopreservation of >98%. The above model and the information on PDX for liver cancer accessible from the PubMed database have been input into a database, which is the largest PDX database for liver cancer accessible so far. It contains data on the clinicopathologic information, drug susceptibility, gene expression, somatic mutation, and copy number variation in 116 liver cancer patients. It offers an effective search and analysis tool for researchers focusing on PDX and drug research and development at home and abroad. For an example, it can be used to predict susceptibility to sorafenib. Using the PDX model, the authors' institute and team of professor He Fuchu have jointly demonstrated the antitumor effect of avasimibe, a small-molecular inhibitor of sterol O-acyltransferase 1 (SOAT1), which has been published in *Nature* in 2019.

2.3 Research, Development, and Exploration of Early Diagnostic Techniques for HCC

Early diagnosis and treatment are crucial for survival of patients with HCC. Early diagnosis of HCC primarily relies on radiologic examination, AFP blood test, and histological detection. However, the specificity and sensitivity of these early diagnostic approaches remain to be improved. At present, China's research in early diagnosis of HCC mainly focuses on imaging examination and molecular marker.

Imaging examinations for early diagnosis of HCC include ultrasound examination, MRI, and CT. Ultrasound examination is easy to perform and noninvasive. It is the most commonly used method to screen HCC clinically. MRI and CT have higher accuracy than ultrasound in differentiating between benign and malignant liver tumors. The integrated application of imaging examinations can significantly increase the detection rate of early stage HCC.

In recent years, substantial progress has been made in the molecular markers for early diagnosis of HCC, especially liquid biopsy. Liquid biopsy is convenient and allows for dynamic monitoring and screening. Especially, cfDNA methylation/hydroxymethylation (5hmC) and microribonucleic acid are considered superior to AFP for the early diagnosis of HCC. They have higher specificity and sensitivity and therefore are promising for HCC screening and early diagnosis.

Up to now, AFP is still one of the most important markers for screening HCC. There are many other promising markers for early diagnosis of HCC, AFP-L3, des-γ-carboxy prothrombin DCP and Golgi glycoprotein 73 (GP73), whose diagnostic sensitivity or specificity even surpasses that of AFP.

AFP-L3 is a glycoprotein specific to hepatocellular carcinoma. The percentage of AFP-L3 in total AFP is usually used as a marker for early HCC diagnosis. In patients with HCC, the percentage of AFP-L3 in total AFP is usually above 20%, while it is lower in those with benign liver disease. In some Asian countries (e.g., Japan, South Korea, and India), DCP is used as a routine molecular marker for HCC diagnosis.

GP73 expression in normal liver cells is extremely low or even absent. But it is significantly higher in the serum of patients with HCC. Professor Mao Yilei conducted a multicenter study involving a large sample size ($n = 4217$) and found that the diagnostic sensitivity and specificity of GP73 for HCC were 74.6% and 97.4%, respectively. This result indicated the potential of GP73 as a diagnostic molecular marker for early stage HCC.

Heat shock protein 90α (Hsp90α) level in the peripheral blood of patients with HCC is significantly increased. It is positively correlated to the malignant and metastatic ability of tumors. In a multicenter clinical trial with a large sample size ($n = 1647$), professor Luo Yongzhang found that the diagnostic sensitivity and specificity of plasma Hsp90α for early stage HCC were 92.4% and 90.3%, respectively, which were higher than AFP. It is noteworthy that GP73 and Hsp90α are pan-cancer markers and their levels will also increase in patients with other types of cancer.

Dickkopf-1 (DKK1) is a secretory protein, which is expressed specifically and highly in many cancers, including HCC. Professor Qin Wenxin has shown that the overall diagnostic sensitivity of the serum DKK1 protein for HCC was 69.1% and the specificity was 90.6%. Its sensitivity for early stage HCC (BCLC 0+A) and small tumor (<2 cm) reached 70.9% and 58.5%, with specificity of 90.5% and 84.7%, respectively. Thus, DKK1 is a promising molecular marker for the early diagnosis of HCC.

A large number of studies have shown that miRNAs are widely involved in tumor occurrence, development, recurrence, and metastasis. miRNAs can resist degradation mediated by the RNA enzymes in the blood. Therefore, miRNAs are highly stable in peripheral blood and serve as ideal molecular biomarkers. Professor Jia Fan from Zhongshan Hospital of Fudan University used a high-throughput array to identify seven liver cancer-related miRNAs from the plasma in a multicenter study with large sample size. They further built a model for early diagnosis of HCC, with sensitivity and specificity both over 80%. At present, patents of invention have been granted to the miRNA-based HCC screening kit derived from the above model in several countries and districts. It is the first NMPA-approved miRNA-based in vitro detection kit for HCC in China.

ctDNA exists in a very low level in the blood, only about 20 ng per milliliter. By detecting the methylation level of specific sites in ctDNA, we can increase the diagnostic sensitivity for early stage HCC from 60% to 84.9% and predict the prognosis of patients based on the methylation level. The 5hmC-targeted technologies have been advanced rapidly in liquid biopsy-based biomarker discovery recently and show a potential of outstanding performance in clinical applications. The 5hmC levels are known to reflect cancer type and clinical stage. A more accurate 5hmC profiling can be achieved by high-throughput sequencing. It is expected to overcome the limitations of other liquid biopsy-based approaches such as CTC and ctDNA mutations, which generally have inadequate sensitivity and specificity. Academicians Fan Jia and Wang Hongyang collaboratively built the 5hmC model trained in cfDNA samples derived from blood, which can accurately distinguish early-stage HCC from healthy controls. Professor Xu Ruihua completed a study on liver cancer diagnosis based on ctDNA methylation, finding 10 loci for to accurate early diagnosis of HCC. Circulating markers for HCC have been extended from traditional protein markers to nucleic acid markers. At present, many new molecular markers have been approved by NMPA for clinical use. These markers are expected to improve the early diagnosis and treatment efficacy of HCC, thereby further improving patient prognosis.

Suggested Reading

1. Yang BH, Ren ZG. Progress of liver cancer research in China. China Cancer. 1993;2(9):23–5.
2. Yang BH, Liu KD, Yang ZY. Preliminary research on liver cancer screening in the high-risk population. Tumor. 1987;7(2):82–3.
3. Yang BH, Tang ZY. Current situation and defects of China's liver cancer screening. Cancer Res Prev Treat. 1991;18(4):199–201.
4. Zheng RS, Sun KX, Zhang SW, et al. An analysis of the prevalence of cancers in China in 2015. Chin J Oncol. 2019;41(1):19–28.
5. Siegel RL, Miller KD, Jemal A. Cancer statistics, 2019. CA Cancer J Clin. 2019;69(1):7–34.
6. European Association for the Study of the Liver. EASL clinical practice guidelines: management of hepatocellular carcinoma. J Hepatol. 2018;69(1):182–236.
7. Bruix J, Reig M, Sherman M. Evidence based diagnosis, staging, and treatment of patients with hepatocellular carcinoma. Gastroenterology. 2016;150(4):835–53.
8. Zhang H, Shen F, Han J, et al. Epidemiology and surgical management of intrahepatic cholangiocarcinoma. Hepat Oncol. 2016;3(1):83–91.
9. Rizvi S, Gores GJ. Pathogenesis, diagnosis, and management of cholangiocarcinoma. Gastroenterology. 2013;145(6):1215–29.
10. Hanahan D, Weinberg RA. Hallmarks of cancer: the next generation. Cell. 2011;144(5):646–74.
11. Qiu SJ, Fan J. An inspiration from liver cancer microenvironment studies for liver cancer diagnosis and treatment. Med Philos. 2011;32(12):16–8.
12. Zheng C, Zheng L, Yoo JK, et al. Landscape of infiltrating T cells in liver cancer revealed by single cell sequencing. Cell. 2017;169(7):1342–56.
13. Duan M, Goswami S, Shi JY, et al. Activated and exhausted MAIT cells foster disease progression and indicate poor outcome in hepatocellular carcinoma. Clin Cancer Res. 2019;25(11):3304–16.
14. Ma LJ, Feng FL, Dong LQ, et al. Clinical significance of PD 1/PD ls gene amplification and overexpression in patients with hepatocellular carcinoma. Theranostics. 2018;8(20):5690–702.

15. Gao Q, Qiu SJ, Fan J, et al. Intratumoral balance of regulatory and cytotoxic T cells is associated with prognosis of hepatocellular carcinoma after resection. J Clin Oncol. 2007;25(18):2586–93.
16. Gao Q, Zhao YJ, Wang XY, et al. CXCR6 upregulation contributes to a proinflammatory tumor microenvironment that drives metastasis and poor patient outcomes in hepatocellular carcinoma. Cancer Res. 2012;72(14):3546–56.
17. Liu LZ, Zhang Z, Zheng BH, et al. CCL15 recruits suppressive monocytes to facilitate immune escape and disease progression in hepatocellular carcinoma. Hepatology. 2019;69(1):143–59.
18. Zhou SL, Dai Z, Zhou ZJ, et al. Overexpression of CXCL5 mediates neutrophil infiltration and indicates poor prognosis for hepatocellular carcinoma. Hepatology. 2012;56(6):2242–54.
19. Zhu XD, Zhang JB, Zhuang PY, et al. High expression of macrophage colony stimulating factor inperitumoral liver tissue is associated with poor survival after curative resection of hepatocellular carcinoma. J Clin Oncol. 2008;26(16):2707–16.
20. Shi JY, Yang LX, Wang ZC, et al. CC chemokine receptor like 1 functions as a tumour suppressor by impairing CCR7 related chemotaxis in hepatocellular carcinoma. J Pathol. 2015;235(4):546–58.
21. Chen DP, Ning WR, Li XF, et al. Peritumoral monocytes induce cancer cell autophagy to facilitate the progression of human hepatocellular carcinoma. Autophagy. 2018;14(8):1335–46.
22. Chen DP, Ning WR, Jiang Z, et al. Glycolytic activation of peritumoral monocytes fosters immune privilege via the PFKFB3 PD L1 axis in human hepatocellular carcinoma. J Hepatol. 2019;71(2):333–43.
23. Kaplan RN, Rafii S, Lyden D. Preparing the "soil": the premetastatic niche. Cancer Res. 2006;66(23):11089–93.
24. Shi GM, Xu Y, Fan J, et al. Identification of side population cells in human hepatocellular carcinoma cell lines with stepwise metastatic potentials. J Cancer Res Clin Oncol. 2008;134(11):1155–63.
25. Zhu Z, Hao X, Yan M, et al. Cancer stem/progenitor cells are highly enriched in CD133+CD44+ population in hepatocellular carcinoma. Int J Cancer. 2010;126(9):2067–78.
26. Yang ZF, Ho DW, Ng MN, et al. Significance of CD90+ cancer stem cells in human liver cancer. Cancer Cell. 2008;13(2):153–66.
27. Yang W, Wang C, Lin Y, et al. OV6(+) tumor initiating cells contribute to tumor progression and invasion in human hepatocellular carcinoma. J Hepatol. 2012;57(3):613–20.
28. Lee TK, Castilho A, Cheung VC, et al. CD24(+) liver tumor initiating cells drive self renewal and tumor initiation through STAT3 mediated NANOG regulation. Cell Stem Cell. 2011;9(1):50–63.
29. Liu S, Li N, Yu X, et al. Expression of intercellular adhesion molecule 1 by hepatocellular carcinoma stem cells and circulating tumor cells. Gastroenterology. 2013;144(5):1031–41. e10
30. Yang XR, Xu Y, Yu B, et al. High expression levels of putative hepatic stem/progenitor cell biomarkers related to tumour angiogenesis and poor prognosis of hepatocellular carcinoma. Gut. 2010;59(7):953–62.
31. Xu Y, Chenna V, Hu C, et al. Polymeric nanoparticle encapsulated hedgehog pathway inhibitor HPI 1(NanoHHI) inhibits systemic metastases in an orthotopic model of human hepatocellular carcinoma. Clin Cancer Res. 2012;18(5):1291–302.
32. Zhao W, Wang L, Han H, et al. 1B50 1, a mAb raised against recurrent tumor cells, targets liver tumor initiating cells by binding to the calcium channel alpha2delta1 subunit. Cancer Cell. 2013;23(4):541–56.
33. Sun YF, Xu Y, Yang XR, et al. Circulating stem cell like epithelial cell adhesion molecule positive tumor cells indicate poor prognosis of hepatocellular carcinoma after curative resection. Hepatology. 2013;57(4):1458–68.
34. Yang ZF, Ngai P, Ho DW, et al. Identification of local and circulating cancer stem cells in human liver cancer. Hepatology. 2008;47(3):919–28.
35. Fan ST, Yang ZF, Ho DW, et al. Prediction of posthepatectomy recurrence of hepatocellular carcinoma by circulating cancer stem cells: a prospective study. Ann Surg. 2011;254(4):569–76.
36. Qi LN, Xiang BD, Wu FX, et al. Circulating tumor cells undergoing EMT provide a metric for diagnosis and prognosis of patients with hepatocellular carcinoma. Cancer Res. 2018;78(16):4731–44.
37. Hu B, Yang XR, Xu Y, et al. Systemic immune inflammation index predicts prognosis of patients after curative resection for hepatocellular carcinoma. Clin Cancer Res. 2014;20(23):6212–22.
38. Guo W, Yang XR, Sun YF, et al. Clinical significance of EpCAM mRNA positive circulating tumor cells in hepatocellular carcinoma by an optimized negative enrichment and qRT PCR based platform. Clin Cancer Res. 2014;20(18):4794–805.
39. Guo W, Sun YF, Shen MN, et al. Circulating tumor cells with stem like phenotypes for diagnosis, prognosis, and therapeutic response evaluation in hepatocellular carcinoma. Clin Cancer Res. 2018;24(9):2203–13.
40. Wang S, Zhang C, Wang G, et al. Aptamer mediated transparent biocompatible nanostructured surfaces for hepotocellular circulating tumor cells enrichment. Theranostics. 2016;6(11):1877–86.
41. Chen L, Wu L, Zhang ZL, et al. Biofunctionalized magnetic nanospheres based cell sorting strategy for efficient isolation, detection and subtype analyses of heterogeneous circulating hepatocellular carcinoma cells. Biosens Bioelectron. 2016;85:633–40.
42. Roberts TG, Goulart BH, Squitieri L, et al. Trends in the risks and benefits to patients with cancer participating in phase 1 clinical trials. JAMA. 2004;292(17):2130–40.
43. Reichert JM, Wenger JB. Development trends for new cancer therapeutics and vaccines. Drug Discov Today. 2008;13(1-2):30–7.

44. Siolas D, Hannon GJ. Patient derived tumor xenografts: transforming clinical samples into mouse models. Cancer Res. 2013;73(17):5315–9.
45. Tentler J, Tan AC, Weekes CD, et al. Patient derived tumour xenografts as models for oncology drug development. Nat Rev Clin Oncol. 2012;9(6):338–50.
46. Byrne AT, Alferez DG, Amant F, et al. Interrogating open issues in cancer precision medicine with patient derived xenografts. Nat Rev Cancer. 2017;17(4):254–68.
47. Izumchenko E, Meir J, Bedi A, et al. Patient derived xenografts as tools in pharmaceutical development. Clin Pharmacol Ther. 2016;99(6):612–21.
48. Khor TO, Zvi IB, Katz A, et al. Abstract 3219: a patient centric repository of PDX models for translational oncology research. Cancer Res. 2015;75(Suppl 15):3219.
49. Aparicio S, Hidalgo M, Kung AL. Examining the utility of patient derived xenograft mouse models. Nat Rev Cancer. 2015;15(5):311–6.
50. Kato S, Kurzrock R. An avatar for precision cancer therapy. Nat Biotechnol. 2018;36(11):1053–5.
51. Hu B, Li H, Guo W, et al. Establishment of a hepatocellular carcinoma patient derived xenograft platform and its application in biomarker identification. Int J Cancer. 2020;146(6):1606–17.
52. He S, Hu B, Li C, et al. PDXliver: a database of liver cancer patient derived xenograft mouse models. BMC Cancer. 2018;18(1):550.
53. Jiang Y, Sun A, Zhao Y, et al. Proteomics identifies new therapeutic targets of early stage hepatocellular carcinoma. Nature. 2019;567(7747):257–61.
54. Crowley E, Di Nicolantonio F, Loupakis F, et al. Liquid biopsy: monitoring cancer genetics in the blood. Nat Rev Clin Oncol. 2013;10(8):472–84.
55. Mao Y, Yang H, Xu H, et al. Golgi protein 73 (GOLPH2) is a valuable serum marker for hepatocellular carcinoma. Gut. 2010;59(12):1687–93.
56. Fu Y, Xu X, Huang D, et al. Plasma heat shock protein 90alpha as a biomarker for the diagnosis of liver cancer: an official, large scale, and multicenter clinical trial. EBioMedicine. 2017;24:56–63.
57. Shen Q, Fan J, Yang XR, et al. Serum DKK1 as a protein biomarker for the diagnosis of hepatocellular carcinoma: a large scale, multicentre study. Lancet Oncol. 2012;13(8):817–26.
58. Zhou J, Yu L, Gao X, et al. Plasma microRNA panel to diagnose hepatitis B virus related hepatocellular carcinoma. J Clin Oncol. 2011;29(36):4781–8.
59. Song CX, Szulwach KE, Fu Y, et al. Selective chemical labeling reveals the genome wide distribution of 5 hydroxymethylcytosine. Nat Biotechnol. 2011;29(1):68–72.
60. Song CX, Clark TA, Lu XY, et al. Sensitive and specific single molecule sequencing of 5 hydroxymethylcytosine. Nat Methods. 2011;9(1):75–7.
61. Cai J, Chen L, Zhang Z, et al. Genome wide mapping of 5 hydroxymethylcytosines in circulating cell free DNA as a non-invasive approach for early detection of hepatocellular carcinoma. Gut. 2019;68(12):2195–205.
62. Xu RH, Wei W, Krawczyk M, et al. Circulating tumour DNA methylation markers for diagnosis and prognosis of hepatocellular carcinoma. Nat Mater. 2017;16(11):1155–61.

3 Multimodality Treatment for Liver Cancer in China

Jian Zhou, Xiaoying Wang, and Kai Zhu

Modern liver surgical techniques can be dated back to the early twentieth century. But in the 1960s, hepatectomy was still a daunting procedure that carried a high risk of death in China. In those days, few surgeons had the skills and courage to perform it and the surgical outcome was unpredictable. Nowadays, liver resection has become a safe, plannable procedure. All of these revolutions and developments would not have been possible without the advent of antibiotics, the application of blood transfusion, the improvement of anesthetic techniques, and the efforts of generations of surgeons. Thanks to a better understanding of the anatomy and biology of the liver, the mechanism of liver hyperplasia, and the improvement of the hemostatic equipment, liver surgery has been developing rapidly. The late 1980s witnessed the rapid progress of liver transplantation, which enabled liver surgeons and anesthesiologists to push the field of liver surgery forward. What was once considered technically impossible has already become possible. Many surgeries that were previously difficult have become conventional. Besides, the advent of minimally invasive surgery has replaced the need for long incisions, and keyhole surgeries are the new paradigm. Laparoscopic or robotic surgeries have been performed as conventional surgeries at healthcare centers throughout the world.

J. Zhou (✉) · X. Wang · K. Zhu
ZhongShan Hospital Fudan University, Shanghai, China
e-mail: zhou.jian@zs-hospital.sh.cn

3.1 Surgical Resection

China's liver surgery was first started in the 1950s. After over 60 years of development and relentless efforts, China's liver surgery is among the best in the world.

In the 1950s, China surgeons represented by Professor Wang Cheng'en from Guangzhou and Professor Zeng Xianjiu from Beijing had already performed hepatectomy for over 50 patients. In the same time period, Professor Wu Mengchao, Academician from the Chinese Academy of Sciences, first created the classical liver anatomy theory of "five lobes and four segments," which laid the foundation for China's segmental anatomy of the liver and liver surgery. His contribution pushed forward the progress of liver surgery to the stage of selective lobar and segmental resection of the liver based on the distribution of intrahepatic vessels.

Liver surgery developed rapidly in China in the 1960s. At this stage, China could not only perform local hepatectomy but also right trisegmentectomy, a much more difficult procedure. In 1962, Xia et al. proposed the viewpoint of three hepatic hila, which was then widely accepted and applied clinically. In 1963, the team led by Wu Mengchao was the first to describe hepatectomy

X. Chen (ed.), *Diagnosis and Treatment of Liver Cancer in China*,
https://doi.org/10.1007/978-981-97-7969-7_3

with intermittent hepatic hilus occlusion under room temperature. They were also the first to successfully complete the surgery in the middle lobe of the liver, which represented a major breakthrough in liver surgery. Since then, the surgical indications for hepatectomy have been greatly expanded. Besides, the surgical efficacy for liver cancer and other liver diseases has been substantially improved.

In the 1970s, Professor Tang Zhaoyou from Zhongshan Hospital, Fudan University, Academician of the Chinese Academy of Engineering, was the first to promote the clinical use of alpha feto-protein (AFP) for early diagnosis of liver cancer. The concept of "subclinical liver cancer" was proposed for the first time. Tang advocated local resection of small liver cancer with cirrhosis to replace lobectomy. Re-resection of subclinical recurrence was recommended to further improve the efficacy. He also proposed "resection following shrinkage of the previously unresectable liver cancer" so as to prolong the survival in some patients with unresectable liver cancer and achieve a radical cure in a small fraction of patients. The concept of "subclinical liver cancer" is considered "a landmark in the understanding and treatment of liver cancer" according to Hans Popper, the founding father of hepatology. At this stage, the emergence of two important viewpoints, namely, re-resection for liver cancer recurrence and surgery following downstaging of liver cancer, made the surgical treatment of intermediate and advanced liver cancer possible.

Professor Chen Xiaoping, Academician of the Chinese Academy of Sciences, reported for the first time in China that ultrasound-guided hepatectomy could achieve a more precise tumor resection. Chen later reported China's first case of systematic hepatic segmentectomy in 1989 and put forward the innovative idea of no contraindicated areas for surgery in the liver. In the late 1980s, the idea of blocking liver blood inflow at room temperature for 20–60 min was first described, which completely broke the previous idea of "safe duration" of 15–20 min. Thus, a theoretical basis was laid for more complex liver surgeries. The establishment of bloodless hepatectomy, re-resection for liver cancer recurrence, and two-stage hepatectomy procedures at room temperature has improved the surgical success rate and prolonged the survival of patients with middle and advanced liver cancer.

In the 1990s, Professor Chen Xiaoping was the first to report the planned resection of giant liver cancers in China. He was also the first to suggest that tumor size was not the only criterion for evaluating whether surgical resection could be performed, bringing new hopes for many patients with giant liver cancers. The two-stage hepatectomy procedure, which can turn unresectable large liver cancers into smaller ones through various means, has further improved the overall efficacy of surgical treatment of liver cancer. Laparoscopic techniques have already gained international recognition due to their minimal invasiveness and fast postoperative recovery. In 1994, the team led by Professor Zhou Weipipng at Eastern Hepatobiliary Surgery Hospital completed the first case of laparoscopic hepatectomy in China. Since then, laparoscopic hepatectomy was soon popularized and conducted throughout China.

In the twenty-first century, breakthroughs in liver surgery largely are more about surgical treatments for those who were previously not indicated for surgery and the development and popularization of minimally invasive techniques for liver cancer. Associating liver partition and portal vein ligation for staged hepatectomy (ALPPS) brings hope for patients who are otherwise contraindicated for surgery due to large volume of liver cancer, small volume of residual liver, and multiple intrahepatic metastases of the tumor. In 2013, Zhou Jian et al. from Zhongshan Hospital, Fudan University reported the first case of ALPPS in Asia, which greatly promotes the rapid development of ALPPS in China. As for minimally invasive hepatectomy, the indications for laparoscopic hepatectomy have been gradually expanded along with the advancement of laparoscopic technology and equipment. Laparoscopic hepatectomy has overcome nearly every bottleneck in hepatectomy, with the history of its applications traced as follows: It was initially applied to local resection of peripheral lesions, then to left lateral segment liver resection, left and right hemihepatectomy, and to caudate lobectomy, and then to anatomical hepatectomy, or even laparoscopic ALPPS. Professor Dong Jiahong, Academician of the Chinese Academy of Engineering, further standardized and refined the concept and principle of precise hepatectomy. His achievements have facilitated the transition from conventional experience-based surgical treatment to precise surgical treatment. The constant emergence of new technologies has contributed to the gradual popularization of precise hepatectomy. In recent years, preoperative 3D visualization and indocyanine green (ICG)-guided anatomical hepatectomy have been gradually used at various stages of laparoscopic hepatectomy, including preoperative diagnosis, surgical planning, and intraoperative navigation. These techniques can achieve a more radical removal of lesions, thus ensuring the certainty and predictability of precise hepatectomy. Liver surgery will soon enter the age of digital surgery along with the developments of computer technology, surgical techniques, and equipment.

3.2 Liver Transplantation

Liver transplantation is one of the most effective treatments for liver cancer, especially for those meeting the Milan criteria. For the latter, the postoperative 5-year survival rate approaches that in patients with benign liver diseases. Liver transplantation was not started in China until the 1970s. After decades of hard work and hardships, liver transplantation in China has gone through the initial stage of explorations and has become an effective clinical treatment for end-stage liver diseases in China. Both the number and quality of liver transplantations performed in China have reached the international leading level in the past 20 years through continuous clinical explorations and technological innovation. In 2010, the Ministry of Health (currently the National Health Commission) and the Red Cross Society of China joined hands in promoting organ donation after death among Chinese citizens. Such efforts have contributed considerably to the healthy development of China's liver transplantation cause.

In the early 1970s, Professor Xia Huisheng, Professor Wu Zaide, and Professor Qiu Fazu were among the first to conduct liver transplantation tests in animals. They founded the *Chinese Journal of Organ Transplantation* in 1980, laying the groundwork for the development of China's liver transplantation. In October 1977, the team led by Professor Lin Yanzhen completed the first case of orthotopic liver transplantation in China, blazing a new path for China's liver transplantation. Theirs is also Asia's first human liver transplantation. From 1977 to 1983, China successively completed 57 cases of liver transplantation. However due to various technical limitations, 90% of patients died within 3 months after surgery. Besides, the shortage of organ donors and other factors led to the stagnation of China's liver transplantation from 1984 to 1990.

As liver transplantation technology becomes increasingly mature in western countries, a large number of young and middle-aged scholars return to China after studying overseas. They summed up the experience and lessons of their predecessors and learned from the latest technology abroad, ushering in a veritable boom of liver transplantation in China. In April 1993, the First Affiliated Hospital of Sun Yat-sen University conducted China's first case of liver transplantation under in vitro venous bypass. In the same year, Professor Fan Shangda at Queen Mary Hospital, Academician of the Chinese Academy of Sciences, successfully performed living donor liver transplantation. In January 1995, Professor Wang Xuehao from the First Affiliated Hospital of Nanjing Medical University, Academician of the Chinese Academy of Engineering, successfully completed the first case of living donor liver transplantation in China. In the late 1990s, China entered a period of fast development of liver transplantation. The team led by Professor Shen Zhongyang at the Oriental Organ Transplantation Center of the Tianjin First Central Hospital completed China's first case of secondary liver transplantation, reduced-size liver transplantation, and domino liver transplantation in 1999, 2000, and

2005, respectively. Furthermore, they made the world record of performing over 600 cases of liver transplantation within a year from 2005 to 2006. In 2005, Professor Wang Jiefu et al. reported China's first case of stereoscopic hepatectomy plus auto liver transplantation. In 2008, Professor Chen Xiaoping reported China's first case of living donor liver transplantation between relatives. The emergence of laparoscopic and robotic techniques has stimulated the development of liver transplantation. In 2014, Professor Fan Jia from Zhongshan Hospital, Fudan University, Academician of the Chinese Academy of Sciences, carried out robot-assisted living donor hepatectomy. It was China's first case of completely minimally invasive living donor hepatectomy. In China, liver transplantation has entered the stage of an ever-growing number of clinical applications. To be specific, the number of patients receiving liver transplantation nearly doubles every year. Liver transplantation has been widely performed in China. Postoperative survival is the same as international results. Moreover, China has made fruitful explorations in the expansion of surgical indications, innovation of surgical skills, and standardization of postoperative management.

3.3 Radiation Therapy

China's first attempt at radiation therapy for liver cancer started in the 1960s. At that time, extensive radiotherapy covering half of the liver or the entire liver was generally performed, resulting in poor efficacy. This was mainly due to imprecise radiotherapy dose estimation given the underdeveloped skills and equipment and poor understanding of the liver's radiation tolerability. The above limitations posed obstacles to the application of radiotherapy in liver cancer. In the past decade, three-dimensional conformal radiotherapy and intensity-modulated radiotherapy have appeared thanks to the highly developed computer technology and its application in the medical field. The local tumor control rate has been greatly improved, while the complications are reduced in large number. The goals of tumor control, prolonging patients' survival, and reducing the side effects of radiotherapy have been largely met.

3.4 Transcatheter Arterial Chemoembolization

Since the application of transcatheter arterial chemoembolization (TACE) to treat liver cancer was first reported by Goldstein et al. in 1976, TACE has been considered a preferred minimally invasive treatment with high safety, effectiveness, and repeatability for unresectable liver cancers. China's interventional radiology started a little later, but developed rapidly. Selective arteriography via percutaneous puncture was first introduced in China in the early 1970s. Lin et al. were the first to conduct the experimental study of transcatheter arterial embolization (TAE) agents in the early 1980s. They were also the first to report the results of the clinical application of TAE in liver cancer. In 1985, Yan and Feng et al. prepared a TAE agent using brucea javanica oil microcapsules. They further established a new method that combined traditional Chinese medicine and western medicine. Hu et al. were among the first to perform the implantation of an indwelling arterial perfusion catheter and infusion pump via the percutaneous femoral artery approach. At present, superselective TACE has been widely accepted as a liver cancer treatment in the world and has been increasingly applied in hospitals. Since 2012, several clinical guidelines have recommended TACE as the first-line therapy for intermediate liver cancer. Along with the invention of new materials, such as drug-carrying microspheres and radioactive microspheres, TACE is evolving toward standardization.

3.5 Radiofrequency Ablation or Percutaneous Radiofrequency Ablation

In 1995, Rossi et al. reported the first use of radiofrequency ablation (RFA) to treat liver cancer, thereby opening up a new pathway for nonsurgical palliative treatment of liver cancer. Recently, RFA has been widely used to treat liver cancer due to its high effectiveness, minimal invasiveness, and safety. RFA is currently a representative local treatment for liver cancer. For a very long time, however, clinicians have been highly concerned about which is the better treatment for liver cancer, surgical resection or RFA. Patients even receiving the more advanced minimally invasive laparoscopic surgery will need a long time to recover due to the trauma caused by the resection. By contrast, RFA is much less invasive and has a shorter treatment time. The patients recover more rapidly after RFA. As for the treatment of small liver cancers, the Hepatobiliary Department of the Sun Yat-sen University Cancer Center was the first to report comparable efficacy of surgical resection and RFA in small liver cancers. In China, Academicians Wu Mengchao and Tang Zhaoyou have given their favorable appraisals of RFA.

3.6 Cryoablation

Cryoablation involves the use of a cryoprobe that goes deep into the tumor to kill the tumor cells with alternate freezing and thawing. It is most commonly used for patients with unresectable HCC found during surgery. In 1973, the Liver Cancer Institute of Shanghai Medical University (currently Shanghai Medical College of Fudan University) carried out experimental and clinical studies of cryotherapy for liver cancer. Cryotherapy has become an important treatment for unresectable liver cancers. Compared with other treatments, cryotherapy can reduce damage to normal tissues, delivering a safe treatment for liver cancers near major vessels.

3.7 Microwave Ablation

The first clinical application of microwave technology dates back to the 1970s. But given the immature design of microwave antennas at that time, only a few people chose it as a means of treatment. At an earlier stage, microwave ablation was mainly used for the laparotomy treatment of liver cancer. Chinese scholar Gao Youbi was the first to use microwave ablation to treat liver cancer in 1987. In the late twentieth century, the development of microwave technology was dramatically propelled by the progress in percutaneous microwave ablation for liver cancer at the time of rapid advances in biomedical engineering. In 1996, Dong et al. at the General Hospital of the People's Liberation Army improved the ultrasound-guided implantable microwave coagulation therapy apparatus and radiation electrode. Later, many efforts have been made by scholars to enlarge the scope of microwave ablation so as to increase the radical ablation rate of liver cancer and improve the long-term efficacy. Professor Chen Xiaoping was the first to apply microwave ablation to laparoscopic hepatectomy, which successfully overcame the problem of intraoperative bleeding during the surgery, and made an enormous contribution to the promotion of laparoscopic hepatectomy.

3.8 Percutaneous Ethanol Ablation or Acetic Acid Ablation

Similar to RFA, percutaneous ethanol injection (PEI) is often considered applicable to patients unfit for hepatectomy due to small HCC lesions with poor liver function reserve. Before the appearance of RFA, PEI was once the most widely accepted minimally invasive treatment for the above-described patient population. PEI is featured by low cost, less need for equipment, and good clinical outcomes. However, RFA is considered to be more effective and has already replaced PEI at many institutions.

3.9 Systemic Treatment

3.9.1 Cytotoxic Chemotherapy

Systemic chemotherapy was used to treat primary HCC as early as the 1950s. Most conventional chemotherapeutic drugs including doxorubicin, fluorouracil, cisplatin, and mitomycin had been used to treat liver cancer, though the effective rate was low, the repeatability was poor and the toxic effects of the drugs were significant with any monotherapy. Besides, the above drugs used in monotherapy failed to prolong the survival. For these reasons, the application of chemotherapy to treat liver cancer has been stagnating over the years. So far, there have been no established chemotherapeutic drugs or regimens for liver cancer.

As for the multi-drug combination, the FOLFOX4 regimen consisting of oxaliplatin has shown a better overall response rate, disease control rate, progression-free survival, and overall survival compared with the conventional chemotherapeutic drug doxorubicin. Besides, the tolerance and safety are more favorable. Due to the above benefits, oxaliplatin has been approved in China to treat locally advanced and metastatic liver cancers that are unfit for surgical resection or local treatment.

3.9.2 Targeted Drugs

Targeted drugs provide another sharp sword for the integrated treatment of liver cancer. The favorable results from the SHARP and Oriental trials have established sorafenib as the standard first-line treatment for advanced liver cancer. Sorafenib was approved for the treatment of advanced hepatocellular carcinoma (HCC) by Food and Drug Administration (FDA) in 2007 and China Food and Drug Administration (CFDA; currently National Medical Products Administration (NMPA)) in 2008. In March 2018, lenvatinib was first approved in Japan as the first-line therapy for HCC. On September 4, 2018, China also approved lenvatinib for use in this indication. In 2016, the RESORCE clinical study on regorafenib as the second-line therapy for advanced liver cancer achieved success. This study showed that the median overall survival with sorafenib followed by regorafenib was 26 months. The FDA and CFDA (currently NMPA) have successively approved regorafenib for patients with advanced liver cancer who had progression or drug resistance after sorafenib treatment. A number of drugs developed by domestic pharmaceutical companies for Chinese HCC patients have also gained indications for liver cancer treatment in China, including Donafenib, Sintilimab in combination with Bevacizumab analogs, and Apatinib in combination with Camrelizumab. A number of second-line treatment options, including Regorafenib, Apatinib, Pembrolizumab, Camrelizumab, and Tislelizumab treatments, all of which were clinically studied in patients who failed Sorafenib treatment (partly because of failure of systemic chemotherapy), have gained indications for second-line treatment of advanced HCC in China, and thus have been recommended by domestic guidelines. These drugs are expected to bring hope to patients with liver cancer in the near future.

3.10 Multidisciplinary Integrated Treatment

3.10.1 From a Simple Local Treatment to the Combination of Several Local Treatments

Clinical practice has demonstrated that a multimodal approach consisting of several of the above treatments is the preferred choice to improve the clinical efficacy for treatment of liver cancer. In the early 1990s, some Chinese centers commenced exploring the combination of several local treatments as one multimodal approach. In 1991, Professor Yu Yeqin at the Liver Cancer Institute of Zhongshan Hospital, Fudan University reported 27 patients who received surgical resections after TACE. In 1996, Academician Tang Zhaoyou published the efficacy data collected from 2388 patients within

30 years on the *Chinese Journal of Surgery*. These patients with primary liver cancer received multimodal treatments such as early surgical resection, secondary resection after initial unresectable tumor reduction, re-resection for recurrence, and local freezing of liquid nitrogen. The data confirmed the effectiveness of the combination of several local therapies. In 2000, Academician Wu Mengchao proposed the concept of "multimodal integrated treatment for advanced liver cancer" on the *Chinese Journal of Practical Surgery*.

3.10.2 Combination of Local and Systemic Treatments

Since the approval of sorafenib as the standard first-line treatment for advanced HCC in 2008, multidisciplinary integrated treatment has entered the stage of fast progress of the combination of local and systemic treatments. Studies on the combination of surgeries, TACE, RFA, and liver transplantation plus targeted drugs have been published in an increasing number. As a result, the overall survival of patients with liver cancer has been improved dramatically.

In the past decade, a consensus has been reached over the multidisciplinary diagnosis and treatment mode for liver cancer in China. There has been a gradual transition from the conventional "one-to-one" mode to the "many-to-one" mode. The patients are placed at the center, and multiple therapies are scientifically and reasonably selected and used in combination through a multidisciplinary approach. This new mode is expected to achieve the goals of improving the patients' prognosis and life quality.

Suggested Reading

1. Wang CE, Li GC. Surgical treatment for primary liver cancer. Proceedings of the Zhongshan School of Medicine; 1962. p. 1–23.
2. Zhou WP, Sun ZH, Wu MC, et al. Laparoscopic hepalobectomy: the first case report. J Hepatobiliary Surg. 1994;2(2):82.
3. Zhou J, Wang Z, Sun J, et al. Associating liver partition and portal vein ligation for staged hepatectomy. Chin J Dig Surg. 2013;12(7):485–9.
4. Wang XY, Gao Q, Zhu XD, et al. Application of laparoscopic ultrasound plus 3D visualization-guided portal vein puncture with indocyanine green fluorescence staining in accurate anatomical segmentectomy. Chin J Dig Surg. 2018;17(5):452–8.
5. Wu J, Zheng S. Liver transplantation in China: problems and their solutions. Hepatobiliary Pancreat Dis Int. 2004;3(2):170–4.
6. Chen GH. Liver transplantation in China: retrospect and prospect. Chin Med J (Engl). 2009;122(19):2229–30.
7. Goldstein HM, Wallace S, Anderson JH, et al. Transcatheter occlusion of abdominal tumors. Radiology. 1976;120(3):539–45.
8. Rossi S, Di Stasi M, Buscarini E, et al. Percutaneous radiofrequency interstitial thermal ablation in the treatment of small hepatocellular carcinoma. Cancer J Sci Am. 1995;1(1):73–81.
9. Gao BY, Chen DZ, Yang SZ. Microwave coagulation therapy in 11 cases of liver cancer. Sichuan Med J. 1988;9(1):8–9.
10. Llovet JM, Ricci S, Mazzaferro V, et al. Sorafenib in advanced hepatocellular carcinoma. N Engl J Med. 2008;359(4):378–90.
11. Cheng AL, Kang YK, Chen Z, et al. Efficacy and safety of sorafenib in patients in the Asia Pacific region with advanced hepatocellular carcinoma: a phase III randomised, double blind, placebo controlled trial. Lancet Oncol. 2009;10(1):25–34.
12. Bruix J, Qin S, Merle P, et al. Regorafenib for patients with hepatocellular carcinoma who progressed on sorafenib treatment (RESORCE): a randomised, double blind, placebo controlled, phase 3 trial. Lancet. 2017;389(10064):56–66.
13. Chen XP, Zhang ZW. Setting and working of multidisciplinary team for liver cancer. Chin J Pract Surg. 2014;34(8):685–7.
14. Yu YQ, Xu DB, Zhou XD, et al. Analysis of liver cancer resection after TACE in 27 cases. Chin J Pract Surg. 1991;11(5):247–8.
15. Zhou XD, Tang ZY, Yu YQ, et al. Long-term efficacy of multimodal treatment of liver cancer. Chin J Surg. 1996;34(9):7–10.
16. Wu BW, Pan ZY, Wu MC. Multimodal integrated treatment of advanced liver cancer. Chin J Pract Surg. 2000;20(10):19–22.
17. Kudo M. Proposal of primary endpoints for TACE combination trials with systemic therapy: lessons learned from 5 negative trials and the positive TACTICS trial. Liver Cancer. 2018;7(3):225–34.
18. Jia WD. Adjuvant sorafenib after radical liver resection for the treatment of hepatocellular carcinoma: recent research advances. World Chin J Digestol. 2012;20(22):2019–23.

4 Standardized Diagnosis and Treatment Process for Liver Cancer

Jia Fan, Jian Zhou, and Yinghong Shi

4.1 Preparation and Revision History of Chinese Guidelines for Diagnosis and Treatment of Liver Cancer

Tumor staging has a major bearing on the prognosis and development of treatment regimens. China's earliest liver cancer staging can be dated back to the 1970s. The National Collaborative Meeting on the Research of Liver Cancer Prevention and Treatment held in Shanghai in 1977 developed the diagnosis, classification, and staging criteria for primary liver cancer. According to this system, liver cancer is divided into three stages: Liver cancer of stage I is usually asymptomatic; liver cancer of stage II is intermediate between those of stage I and III; liver cancer of stage III is usually combined with any of the following conditions: jaundice, ascites, cachexia, and extrahepatic metastases. In 1997, the Sichuan Liver Cancer Committee made a revision of the 1977 staging system. That is, by further dividing liver cancer of stage II into four substages. The updated staging system not only included patients' clinical conditions but also tumor size and the modified Child-Pugh score. In 1999, the Chinese Society of Liver Cancer further revised the 1977 staging system by subdividing stage II into substages IIa and IIb (Table 4.1). This new staging system also considered tumor thrombus in the portal vein, hepatic vein, inferior vena cava, and bile duct and liver function apart from the T, N, and M classification in scheme of Union for International Cancer Control (UICC). However, the earlier staging systems did not incorporate treatment guidelines or treatment recommendations. Nevertheless, all of them represented active explorations in liver cancer staging and laid a foundation for the subsequent development of China's guidelines for liver cancer diagnosis and treatment.

In 2011, the guidelines for the diagnosis and treatment of liver cancer were revised by several Chinese institutes and liver cancer experts as organized by Zhongshan Hospital, Fudan University under the leadership of the Bureau of Medical Administration, National Health Commission. The revised edition incorporated the multidisciplinary treatment mode for liver cancer (Fig. 4.1). One major innovation was that specific treatment recommendations were made for different disease situations, thus offering substantial clinical value. In 2017, the editorial committee recommended the following staging system for liver cancer based on China's practice of liver cancer diagnosis and treatment and relevant evidence, which was a modification of the *Guidelines for Diagnosis and Treatment of*

J. Fan (✉) · J. Zhou · Y. Shi
ZhongShan Hospital Fudan University, Shanghai, China
e-mail: fan.jia@zs-hospital.sh.cn

X. Chen (ed.), *Diagnosis and Treatment of Liver Cancer in China*,
https://doi.org/10.1007/978-981-97-7969-7_4

Table 4.1 China liver cancer staging (1999)

Staging	Neoplasm	Cancer thrombus (portal vein, hepatic vein, inferior vena cava, bile duct)	Lymph node metastases (hepatic hila, abdominal cavity)	Distant metastasis	Liver function (modified Child-Pugh score)
I	One or two tumors, each with a diameter ≤5 cm, in the same lobe	None	None	None	A
IIa	One or two tumors, each with a diameter >5 cm and ≤10 cm in the same lobe; or one or two tumors, each with a diameter ≤5 cm, in the two lobes	None	None	None	A or B
IIb	One or two tumors, each with a diameter >10 cm, or three tumors, each with a diameter ≤10 cm, in the same lobe; or one or two tumors, each with a diameter >5 cm, in two lobes	No tumors in the stem or having tumors in the branches		None	A or B
III	Any	Having tumors in the stem	Or having tumors	Or having tumors	C

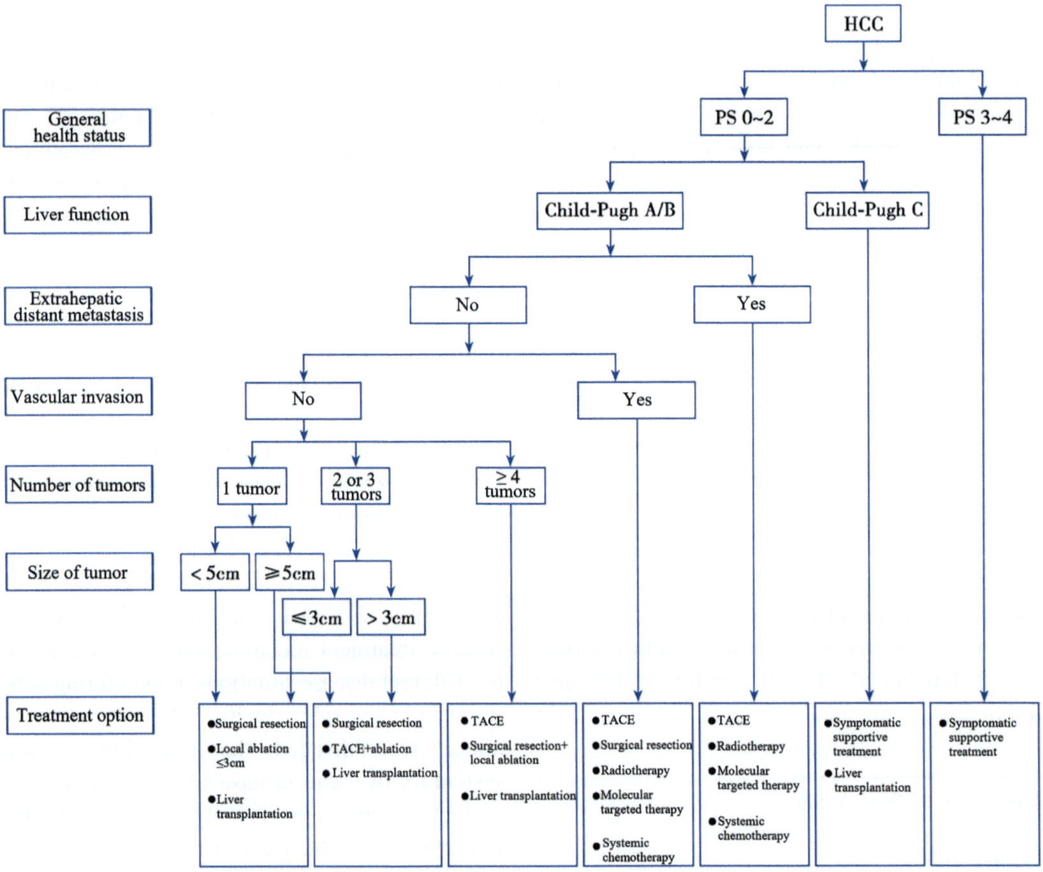

Fig. 4.1 Guidelines for diagnosis and treatment of primary liver cancer (2011 edition)

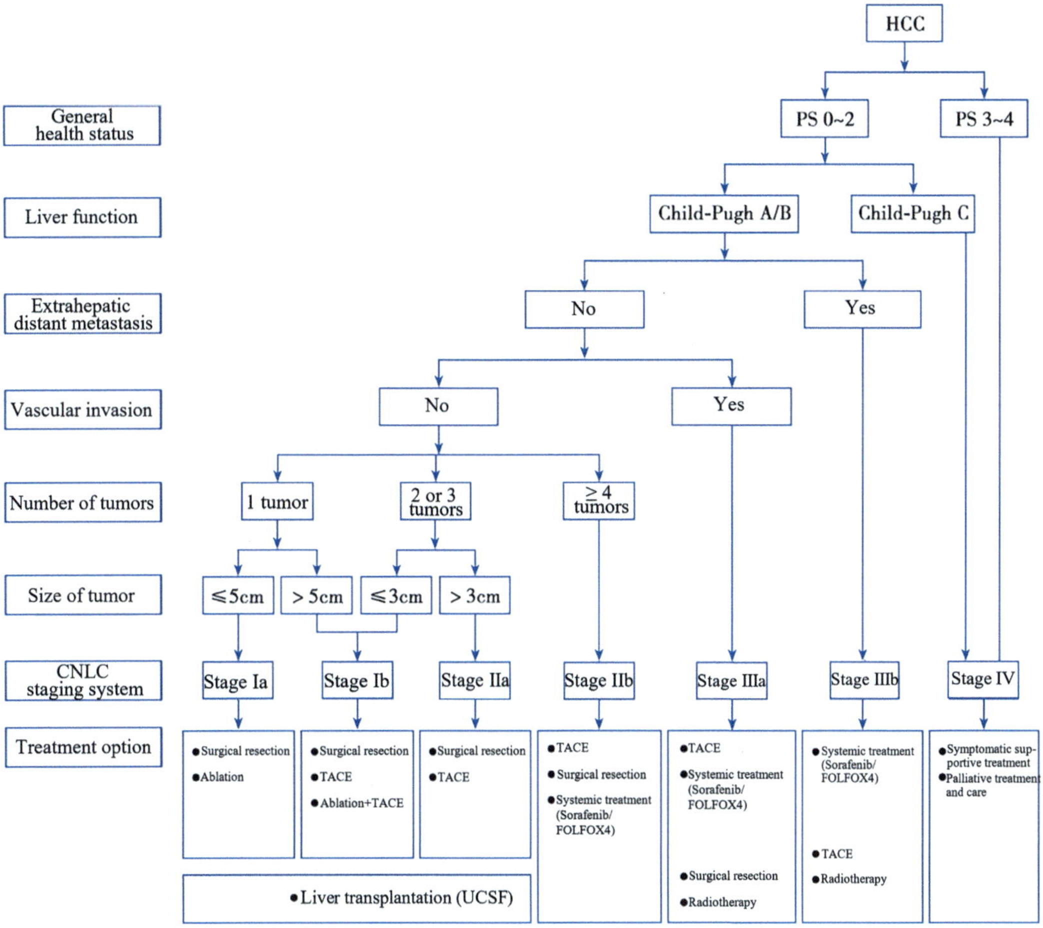

Fig. 4.2 Guidelines for diagnosis and treatment of primary liver cancer (2017 edition)

Primary Liver Cancer (2011 edition): Stage Ia, stage Ib, stage IIa, stage IIb, stage IIIa, stage IIIb, and stage IV. More details about this staging system can be found in the following figure (Fig. 4.2). The new staging system expanded the surgical indications for hepatectomy and offered the following benefits: enhancing the diversity of treatments for liver cancer combined with vascular invasion, establishing the value of radiation therapy for liver cancer metastases, expanding the indications of liver transplantation, and highlighting psychological intervention for patients with advanced liver cancer. Therefore, this staging system is more adapted to China's national conditions. The updated version published in 2019 and 2022 includes more optimal clinical evidence and new therapies based on the existing staging system. Some typical treatments include targeted therapy, immunotherapy, and traditional Chinese medicine (Fig. 4.3).

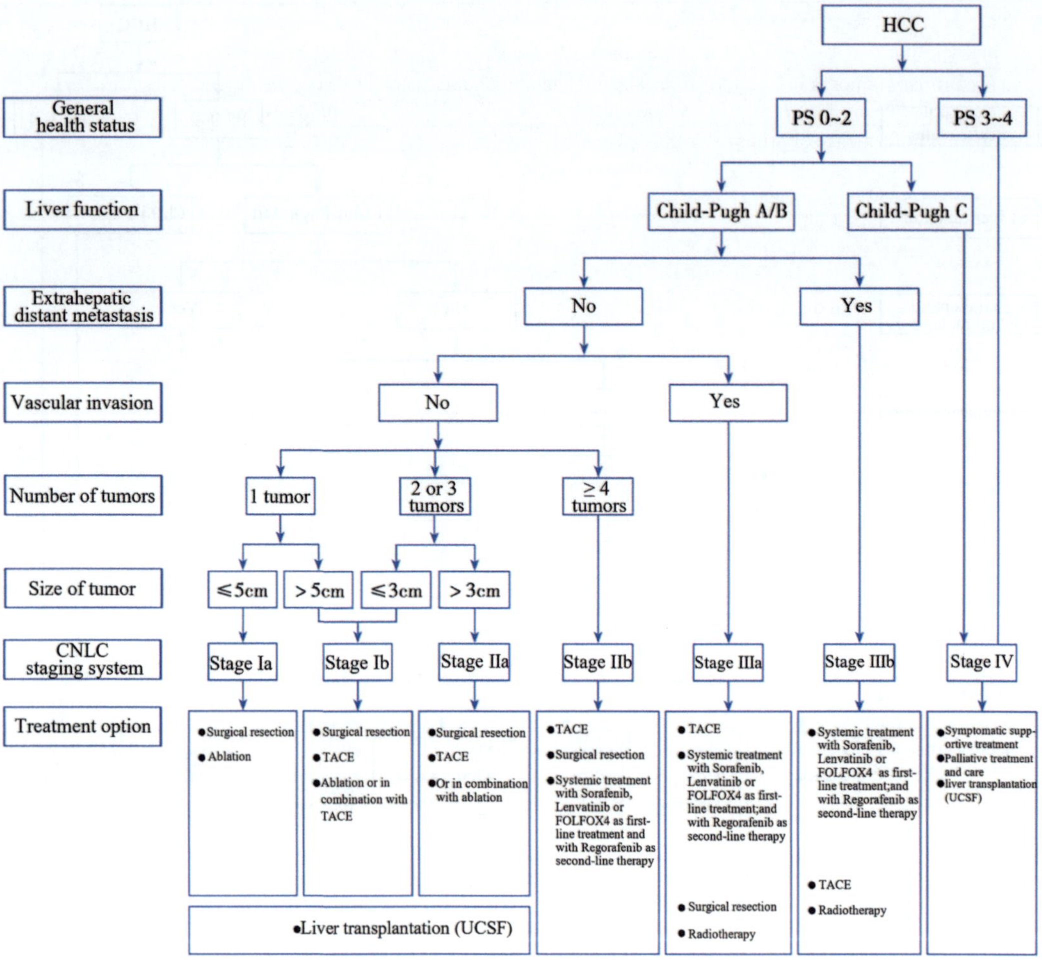

Fig. 4.3 Guidelines for diagnosis and treatment of primary liver cancer (2019 edition)

4.2 Guidelines with Chinese Characteristics Go Global

In addition to the guidelines for the diagnosis and treatment of liver cancer developed in China, several academic organizations or study centers have proposed their respective guidelines/criteria. Some more famous ones are the following: Barcelona Clinic Liver Cancer (BCLC), clinical practice guidelines of the Asian Pacific Association for the Study of the Liver (APASL), and the National Comprehensive Cancer Network (NCCN) guidelines for the treatment of liver cancer. Hong Kong China, Japan, and South Korea have also published their respective guidelines for the staging, diagnosis, and treatment of liver cancer. However, there are some disagreements between the guidelines by the American Association for the Study of Liver Diseases (AASLD), American College of Surgeons (ACS), and NCCN. Each has its own priorities and highlights.

NCCN recommends the TNM staging (AJCC eighth edition) (Table 4.2). Compared with the seventh edition, the AJCC eighth edition contains varying degrees of refinement and revision. Some key points include the following: (1) Stage T1 is further divided into T1a and T1b, depending on tumor size and presence or absence of vascular invasion.

T1a means there is a solitary tumor with diameter ≤2 cm, regardless of whether there is a vas-

Table 4.2 TNM staging for hepatocellular carcinoma (AJCC eighth edition)

T-primary lesion	N-regional lymph nodes	M-distant metastases
Tx: The primary tumor is unmeasurable	Nx: The regional lymph nodes are unmeasurable	Mx: The distant metastases are unmeasurable
T0: There is no evidence of primary tumor	N0: There is no lymph node metastasis	M0: There is no distant metastasis
T1: Single tumor with diameter ≤2 cm, or single tumor with diameter >2 cm without vascular invasion	N1: There is regional lymph nodes metastasis	M1: There is distant metastasis
T1a: Single tumor with diameter ≤2 cm		
T1b: Single tumor with diameter >2 cm without vascular invasion; N1: Regional lymph node metastases; M1: There are no distant metastases		
T2: Single tumor with diameter >2 cm with vascular invasion, or multiple tumors, with the largest one diameter ≤5 cm		
T3: Multiple tumors, with diameter >5 cm		
T4: With the vascular invasion of the portal vein or main branches of the hepatic vein regardless of the tumor size; or tumor directly invading organs other than peritoneum or gallbladder		
TNM staging		
Stage IA: T1aN0M0		
Stage IB: T1bN0M0		
Stage II: T2N0M0		
Stage IIIA: T3N0M0		
Stage IIIB: T4N0M0		
Stage IVA: Any T, N1M0		
Stage IVB: Any T, any N, M1		

cular invasion or not; T1b means there is a solitary tumor with diameter >2 cm without vascular invasion. A solitary tumor with diameter >2 cm with vascular invasion is classified as T2; (2) T3a in the previous edition is T3 in the new edition. T3b and T4 are combined into T4 in the new edition. Liver cancers directly invading the gallbladder or other organs outside the peritoneum are classified as T4. The NCCN staging system is the most standardized, though it has only gained a low level of recognition, probably due to the following reasons: (1) It is usually difficult to accurately assess vascular invasion before treatment (especially before surgery), which has a decisive impact on the treatment and prognosis of liver cancer. (2) Functional compensation of the liver is prioritized in liver cancer treatment, but the TNM staging system does not consider the functional status of the liver. (3) The criteria of TNM staging vary considerably across the editions, thus making the comparison difficult.

The AASLD guidelines adopt the BCLC staging system and treatment strategies (Table 4.3). The guidelines comprehensively consider the tumor, liver function, and systematic conditions, which, in turn, are supported by high-level evidence. The BCLC staging system is based on evidence and establishes treatment principles for liver cancers with different stages. At present, the

Table 4.3 Barcelona clinic liver cancer (BCLC) staging system (2018 edition)

Stage	PS score	Tumor status Number of tumors	Tumor size	Liver function status
Stage 0	0	Individual	≤2 cm	Not combined with portal hypertension
Stage A	0	Individual Within three	Any other ≤3 cm	Child-Pugh A-B Child-Pugh A-B
Stage B	0	Multinodular tumor	Any other	Child-Pugh A-B
Stage C	1–2	Portal vein invasion or N1, M1	Any other	Child-Pugh A-B
Stage D	3–4	Any other	Any other	Child-Pugh C

BCLC staging system has been widely accepted throughout the world, though the scope of surgical indications is narrow among liver cancer patients under this system. Some controversies centering around this system include the following: (1) According to this staging system, indications for resection and liver transplantation are confined to a narrow scope. That is, only liver cancer patients with a solitary tumor and meeting the Milan criteria are suitable for surgical treatment. Therefore, some patients may miss a chance of a radical cure and hence an opportunity for long-term survival. (2) The BCLC staging system recommends sorafenib for liver cancer patients combined with tumor thrombus of the portal vein. But in clinical practice, integrated treatment modality based on surgery has dramatically improved survival and reduced postoperative metastasis and recurrence rates. (3) The BCLC staging system completely denies the value of radiation therapy. (4) The BCLC staging system only relies on the clinical and pathological factors to assess prognosis and select the treatment regimen.

The Okuda staging system, which was once widely used in the twentieth century, includes the following parameters: tumor diameter, ascites, bilirubin, and albumin. Thus, liver cancer is divided into stage I (0 point), stage II (1–2 points), and stage III (3–4 points). This system has a good staging value for progressive/symptomatic liver cancers. The Cancer of the Liver Italian Program (CLIP) staging system consists of four parameters, namely, tumor morphology, modified Child-Pugh score, AFP, and tumor thrombus of the portal vein. This staging system divides liver cancer into five stages. The Hong Kong liver cancer (HKLC) staging system is based on liver cancer patients from Asian countries. This system divides liver cancer into five stages according to the Eastern Cooperative Oncology Group (ECOG) performance status, modified Child-Pugh score, tumor, and presence or absence of vascular invasion/extrahepatic metastases.

China's liver cancer staging system makes a reference to the existing staging systems developed in oversea countries. But considering the difference in etiology of liver cancer between Chinese and western patients, China's staging system prioritizes the distinctive features of Chinese patients for the purpose of liver cancer staging and treatment. As liver cancer treatment is making new progress, China's new staging system for liver cancer will be further modified. Continuous improvements in China's staging system for liver cancer are necessary to meet the Chinese patients' treatment and prognosis.

Suggested Reading

1. Prospective validation of the CLIP score: a new prognostic system for patients with cirrhosis and hepatocellular carcinoma. The Cancer of the Liver Italian Program (CLIP) Investigators. Hepatology. 2000;31(4):840–5.
2. Yau T, Tang VY, Yao TJ, et al. Development of Hong Kong Liver Cancer staging system with treatment stratification for patients with hepatocellular carcinoma. Gastroenterology. 2014;146:1691–700. e1693.

3. Yang BH, Ren ZG. Studies and recommendations on the clinical staging of primary liver cancer. Chin J Hepatobiliary Surg. 1999;5(1):67.
4. Ministry of Health of the People's Republic of China. Abstract of the guidelines for the diagnosis and treatment of primary liver cancer (2011 edition). Chin J Hepatol. 2012;20(6):419–26.
5. Zhou J, Sun HC, Wang Z, et al. Guidelines for diagnosis and treatment of primary liver cancer in China (2017 edition). Liver Cancer. 2018;7:235–60.
6. National Comprehensive Cancer Network (NCCN). NCCN clinical practice guidelines in oncology [EB/OL]. http://www.nccn.org/professionals/physician_gls/pdf/hepatobiliary.pdf. Accessed 15 Oct 2020.
7. Forner A, Reig M, Bruix J. Hepatocellular carcinoma. Lancet. 2018;391:1301–14.
8. Okuda K, Ohtsuki T, Obata H, et al. Natural history of hepatocellular carcinoma and prognosis in relation to treatment. Study of 850 patients. Cancer. 1985;56:918–28.

Part II

Clinical Diagnosis and Staging of Liver Cancer

5 Clinical and Differential Diagnoses of Liver Cancer

Tian Yang and Feng Shen

The majority of early stage hepatocellular carcinoma (HCC) is asymptomatic without any manifestations. In the past, HCC was found only due to clinical symptoms and signs caused by large tumor size or ruptured tumor nodules, or accidentally during surgery. Thus, many patients with HCC have already been at an advanced stage of disease diagnosis, for which the effective treatment is lacking. Early detection, early diagnosis, and early treatment are critical to improve overall prognosis of HCC patients.

5.1 History of Screening and Surveillance for HCC in China

Abnormity of serum alpha-fetoprotein (AFP) in HCC was discovered over 50 years ago. In the early 1970s, researchers in China improved AFP detection by significantly increasing its diagnostic sensitivity and specificity. Later, Prof. Zhaoyou Tang, from the Liver Cancer Institute of Zhongshan Hospital, affiliated with Fudan University, performed a screening survey in the region with high liver cancer incidence (Qidong city of Jiangsu province). The survey results were verified by surgery and showed that disease screening with AFP increased the percentage of early diagnosis of HCC to 35% and the 3-year survival rate of patients who underwent surgical resection to 38.7%. These findings indicated that AFP screening could significantly improve the early diagnosis and treatment of HCC, and AFP could be used as a biomarker for the early diagnosis of HCC.

In the 1980s, considering the issue of expenses and cost-effectiveness of mass screening, most researchers advocated the change of screening subjects from normal population to high-risk population, and screening examination from AFP alone to AFP in combination with ultrasound. Especially in the mid-1980s, Prof. Yuhua Zhao from Changhai Hospital of Second Military Medical University introduced color Doppler ultrasound and applied this technique in combination with AFP for early screening of HCC. This combined test significantly improved the sensitivity of early diagnosis of HCC. Moreover, the identification and classification of Chinese populations at high risk for HCC considerably facilitated the early diagnosis of HCC through improving disease screening. For example, in the mid-1980s, some epidemic areas of HCC, such as the Qidong city of Jiangsu province, launched a follow-up program with AFP plus ultrasound for retired individuals with chronic hepatitis B and cirrhosis. By the end of the 1980s, Chinese researchers began to conduct regular follow-up visits for individuals aged 30 and above and posi-

T. Yang · F. Shen (✉)
Shanghai Eastern Hepatobiliary Surgery Hospital, Shanghai, China

X. Chen (ed.), *Diagnosis and Treatment of Liver Cancer in China*,
https://doi.org/10.1007/978-981-97-7969-7_5

tive for hepatitis B surface antigen (HBsAg) based on the experience of HCC diagnosis in Chinese population. The time interval between each follow-up visit was set to 6 months.

With the continuous progress in epidemiological studies in China, populations at high risk for HCC mainly included those with hepatitis B virus and/or hepatitis C virus infection, long-term alcohol abuse (alcoholic liver disease), non-alcoholic steatohepatitis, cirrhosis caused by various reasons, long-term consumption of aflatoxin-contaminated foods or drinking of gutter water containing certain microcystins, and family history of HCC in first-degree relatives. Recent studies have shown that diabetes, obesity, and smoking are risk factors for HCC. Individuals at high risk for HCC have been recommended to be closely monitored by disease screening, and an AFP test combined with ultrasound has been recommended once every 3–6 months. At this time, an early screening system for HCC was gradually established in China.

5.2 Diagnosis of HCC

In the 1970s and earlier, the diagnosis of HCC relied mainly on clinical presentation, as well as space-occupying lesions identified by initially established isotopic scans at that time. However, HCC diagnosed by these means was often at an advanced stage. Significant advancements in the diagnostic techniques for HCC have been made since the first clinical application of serum AFP test in the 1970s. The sensitivity and specificity of these techniques are being continuously improved.

5.2.1 Clinical Manifestation

1. Symptoms: most patients with HCC are asymptomatic during the disease's early stage. As the tumors grow in size, patients may present with liver area pain, decreased appetite, abdominal distension, asthenia, emaciation, and diarrhea.
   (a) Liver area pain: liver area pain is the most common chief complaint of patients when seeking medical consultation. The incidence of this symptom is 74–84% among Chinese HCC patients. The manifestation is typically presented as persistent dull, swelling, or stabbing pain, especially at night or after physical exertion, usually caused by increased tension in the liver capsule due to fast tumor growth. The site of pain is closely related to the location of the lesion. If the lesion is located in the right lobe, the patient may suffer from pain in the right hypochondriac region; if it is located in the left lateral lobe, the patient may present stomach discomfort; if the one is located in the diaphragmatic dome, the pain may radiate to the scapula or the lower back.
   (b) Symptoms of the digestive system: primarily presenting with decreased appetite, nausea, and vomiting. Decreased appetite is the most common symptom of the digestive system and becomes more pronounced as the disease condition exacerbates. Some patients may present with diarrhea, which usually occurs after eating but is not accompanied by abdominal pain.
   (c) Systemic symptoms: systemic symptoms are usually not prominent during the early stage. Patients may present with asthenia, emaciation, or even cachexia during the advanced stage. In addition, patients with advanced-stage disease may present with low to moderate-grade fever of unknown cause in the afternoon.
   (d) Special symptoms: sudden severe abdominal pain and acute abdominal syndrome may be associated with tumor spontaneous rupture and abdominal hemorrhage Obstructive jaundice may be caused by a tumor compressing the bile duct. Abdominal distension is possibly due to increased ascites resulting from cancer invading the portal vein. Ostalgia is usually caused by cancer invading the bones, which is even the only symptom in some patients.

2. Signs: most patients with HCC have no associated positive signs, while others may be accompanied by the following signs
   (a) Hepatomegaly: hepatomegaly is the most common positive sign and usually occurs asymmetrically. It is characterized by a local protuberance that moves upward and downward with breathing. The liver surface is smooth or has large hard nodules and is tender upon palpation. HCC located in the left lobe can present as a subxiphoid mass. Tumor located in the lower right liver is characterized by palpable mass below the right costal margin, and tumor developed in the liver near the diaphragmatic dome may present an elevated right diaphragm.
   (b) Ascites: ascites are usually observed in patients with advanced HCC. The leading causes of ascites include portal hypertension and hypoproteinemia due to liver decompensation. Portal hypertension may be associated with tumor invasion into the portal vein or hepatic vein. Malignant ascites may be caused by abdominal colonization and metastasis. Turbid or cheliform ascites may result from tumor metastases and blockage of lymphatic vessels. Intraabdominal fluid should be suspected as tumor spontaneous rupture and bleeding. Identifying the nature of ascites is of particular importance for the subsequent treatment of HCC.
   (c) Jaundice: the leading causes of jaundice include jaundice with increased indirect bilirubin due to impaired hepatic function usually in patients with advanced HCC, and jaundice with increased direct bilirubin due to tumor compressing the intrahepatic bile ducts, swollen lymph nodes at the hepatic hilum compressing the hilar bile ducts or the tumor invading and blocking the bile ducts. The causes of jaundice should be differentiated carefully during clinical practice to guide appropriate treatment approaches.
   (d) Other: patients with hepatic decompensation may present with liver palms, spider nevus, and varicose veins of the abdominal wall. If the patients have recently suffered from cough, hemoptysis, nostalgia, pathological fractures, and enlargement of left supraclavicular lymph nodes, the possibility of distant metastases should be noticed.

5.2.2 Auxiliary Examinations

1. Serological tests: for patients who are suspected to have HCC, changes may be observed in liver function tests such as increased serum alkaline phosphatase, aspartate transaminase, D-lactate dehydrogenase, or bilirubin and decreased albumin levels, as well as in immune parameters such as lymphocyte subsets.
2. Serum tumor markers: tumor markers are a group of substances synthesized and released by tumor cells or generated by host cells in response to tumor cells as the tumors grow and proliferate. Discovery and progress have recently been made in the field of HCC biomarkers, ranging from serum protein markers to genetic materials (e.g., cell-free DNA and miRNA) and proteomics and metabolomics. However, significant challenges remain in the clinical applications of these findings.
   (a) AFP: since the first introduction of serum AFP test in China in the 1970s and the subsequent improvement of this test, AFP has become the most commonly used marker for HCC diagnosis. In healthy people, the level of serum AFP is <20 μg/L. The diagnostic sensitivity of AFP for early HCC is 39–65%, while its specificity is as high as 76–97%. HCC should be highly suspected if serum AFP level is ≥400 μg/L, and other causes of elevated AFP, such as chronic or active hepatitis, cirrhosis, testicular, ovarian or embryonic-derived tumors, and pregnancy are excluded.

(b) α-Fetoprotein heterogeneity L3 (AFP-L3): in the early 1990s, Taketa et al. conducted a binding experiment on serum AFP and different agglutinins, followed by electrophoresis and separation. They found that AFP protein derived from the serum of HCC patients, when bound to exogenous agglutinins (e.g., concanavalin A and lentil lectin), could be separated into three bands, which were, respectively, named AFP-L1, AFP-L2, and AFP-L3 (earlier reports described these as AFP variants). AFP-L1 originates from benign hepatic disease and is the main component of AFP. AFP-L2 usually occurs in pregnant women. AFP-L3 is specific to HCC cells, and its normal level should be less than 10%. An AFP-L3 level above 10% may indicate HCC. Although the sensitivity of AFP-L3 is only 37–60%, its specificity can be as high as 90%. In China, AFP-L3 has been used in clinical research almost contemporaneous with AFP, and the combination of AFP-L3 with AFP has been continuously explored in the diagnosis of early HCC combined.

(c) Des-γ-carboxy-prothrombin (DCP): DCP is an inactive prothrombin precursor synthesized in the liver. DCP is normally converted into its active form by vitamin K via γ-carboxylation. In the case of vitamin K deficiency or vitamin K antagonists, specific glutamate cannot be converted into γ-carboxyglutamic acid and the prothrombin precursor is released. This is known as prothrombin induced by vitamin K absence or antagonist-II (PIVKA-II) or DCP. In 1984, Liebman reported increased DCP levels in 91% of HCC patients for the first time. Numerous subsequent studies indicated that the sensitivity and specificity of DCP for diagnosing early HCC were 48–62% and 81–98%, respectively. The sensitivity of DCP may increase as the tumor grows in size. The sensitivity and specificity of DCP for diagnosing hepatitis-related HCC are higher than those of AFP. The clinical diagnostic cut-off for DCP is usually 40 ng/mL. At this level, the sensitivity and specificity are about 80% and above 90%, respectively. Lo KJ et al. reported the first clinical application of DCP. However, the authors only concluded that DCP had a lower sensitivity than AFP based on the small sample size of 35 patients in the study. The clinical application and study of DCP started late in China. Yang et al. from the Eastern Hepatobiliary Surgery Hospital conducted a meta-analysis to show that DCP had higher diagnostic sensitivity and specificity for HCC than AFP. The team led by Tian Yang and Feng Shen published a China-based large-cohort multicenter study. They constructed a diagnostic model for hepatitis B-related HCC based on age, sex, AFP, and PIVKA-II, named ASAP. This study pointed out that the ASAP model exhibited a good diagnostic efficacy for hepatitis B-related HCC. In the training and validation cohorts, the diagnostic sensitivity for early hepatitis B-related HCC was 76.1% and 73.8%, and the specificity was 90.4% and 90.0%, respectively, which were far higher than AFP or PIVKA-II alone. The researchers believed that compared with conventional imaging studies, the ASAP model integrated the basic clinical data (e.g., age and sex) as well as serum AFP and PIVKA-II achieve rapid, convenient, and objective diagnoses as well as excluding the subjectivity of the operators in experience-based interpretation. The model can serve as a promising screening tool for HCC among patients with chronic hepatitis B and is worthy of wide clinical application.

(d) Glypican-3 (GPC-3): the team led by Prof. Hongyang Wang successfully developed a novel HCC diagnostic kit GPC-3 with independent intellectual property rights in 2014. This kit was mainly used for pathological diagnosis and histological classification, especially for the differential diagnosis of benign and malignant hepatic tumors in complicated cases. This kit is of important application value for guiding personalized treatment of malignant liver tumors and avoiding overtreatment for patients with benign tumors.

(e) Other biomarkers of HCC: given growing in-depth basic and clinical studies on HCC biomarkers in China in recent years, novel tumor biomarkers are continuously being discovered, such as annexin A3, apolipoprotein A1, osteopontin (OPN), Wnt pathway inhibitors (dickkopf-1 and DKK-1), α-1-fucosidase (AFU), Golgi protein-73 (GP-73), and squamous cell carcinoma antigen (SCCA).

(f) Combined application of HCC biomarkers: given a 60–70% sensitivity and moderate specificity of AFP, Chinese researchers have continuously investigated and explored the combined use of different diagnostic biomarkers for HCC since the discovery of AFP variants in the 1990s, such as AFP plus AFP-L3, AFP plus AFU, and AFP plus AFP-L3 and DCP. Various studies have demonstrated that the combined utilization of biomarkers can significantly improve the sensitivity and specificity compared with any biomarker alone. Both the ASAP model and the GALAD model belong to this category of combined biomarker use for diagnostic purposes.

3. Genomics-proteomics and metabolomics: since the launch of the Human Genome Project in 2003, constant progress has been made in gene detection technology. The basic and clinical studies of genetic testing have also undergone continuous development. Chinese researchers have discovered several promising genetic markers for early diagnosis of HCC. For example, Prof. Weiping Zhou used the circular RNA (cirRNA) kit (consisting of hsa_circ_0000976, hsa_circ_0007750, and hsa_circ_0139897) to diagnose hepatitis B-related HCC, with a higher diagnostic accuracy than AFP. Moreover, the kit also exhibited good sensitivity for small or AFP-negative HCC. Prof. Ruihua Xu from the Sun Yat-sen University Cancer Center found that circulating tumor DNA (ctDNA) carries cancer-specific genetic and epigenetic abnormalities, making noninvasive liquid biopsy-based diagnosis and monitoring of cancers possible. Additionally, detection of ctDNA methylation can also be used for early diagnosis of HCC. Prof. Shimei Zhuang from the Third Affiliated Hospital of Sun Yat-sen University identified a miRNA classifier consisting of seven differentially expressed miRNAs (i.e., miR-29a, miR-29c, miR-133a, miR-143, miR-145, miR-192, and miR-505). This classifier was proven feasible for HCC detection, with a higher sensitivity than AFP. Prof. Hongyang Wang investigated the noncoding RNA regulatory network and found that the noncoding regulatory region of cirRNA was altered in HCC, with a potential value for HCC detection. Prof. Yuchen Jiao from the National Cancer Center developed a liquid biopsy method for HCC screening, reporting 100% sensitivity, 94% specificity, and 17% positive predictive value with this method. A team led by Prof. Rong Liu from the General Hospital of the People's Liberation Army discovered the potential value of exosomal miRNAs (miR-30d, miR-140, and miR-29b) in predicting HCC development. In 2019, Prof. Jia Fan published a proteogenomic study of HBV-related HCC by analyzing differential expressions between HCC tissues and paracancerous tissues. His findings had potential clinical application value. As for metabolomics, the team led by Prof. Tian Yang characterized the metabolic profile of HCC using liquid chromatography-mass spectrometry and identified candidate biomarkers for HCC diagnosis and prognostic prediction from metabolites in the liver tissues and serum. The study found that retinol metabolism-related substances had high diagnostic and predictive value for HCC patients.

4. Other studies on HCC diagnosis: in recent years, Chinese scholars have pursued various avenues in the research of HCC diagnosis. The

team led by Prof. Shusen Zheng from the First Affiliated Hospital of Zhejiang University School of Medicine characterized the gut microbiota in HCC patients for the first time. The authors reported the successful construction of a microbial marker-based diagnostic model for HCC along with cross-regional validation, demonstrating the feasibility of gut microbiota as biomarkers for the noninvasive early diagnosis of HCC. Furthermore, the combined use of several hematological parameters can improve the sensitivity and specificity for early HCC diagnosis. For example, a study by Prof. VW Wong et al. from the Chinese University of Hong Kong reported that the combined utilization of age, bilirubin level, albumin level, HBV DNA level, and cirrhosis could predict the early development of HCC. The results showed that the proposed predictive scoring system was highly accurate in predicting the development of HCC in patients with hepatitis B.

5. Radiological Examination.
   (a) Ultrasonography (US): despite the first introduction of US into China in the 1950s, US was limited in HCC diagnosis in the early application in that US was only able to differentiate solid and cystic space-occupying lesions in the liver. In the 1980s, Prof. Yuhua Zhao was the first to apply Doppler US in HCC screening. Since then, US has been the preferred method of liver examination due to its ease of operation, low cost, real-time, noninvasiveness, and repeatability. Advancements in US, especially the application of 3D US and contrast-enhanced ultrasound (CEUS) in recent years, have significantly improved the resolution, diagnostic sensitivity, and specificity of US, demonstrating important values of US in HCC detection and qualitative diagnosis.
   (b) Computed tomography (CT): early CT had a low detection rate of liver lesions ≤1 cm. CT angiography was first applied clinically in the early 1980s, a technique involving direct injection of contrast agents into the hepatic artery followed by a dynamic scan. CT angiography can yield a distinctive enhancement pattern of the liver lesions primarily supplied by the hepatic artery, which are in stark contrast with the liver parenchyma. The detection rate of liver lesions ≤1 cm is up to 80% using this examination technique. Arterial phase CT angiography was later introduced. This technique involves the insertion of a catheter into the superior mesenteric artery or splenic artery, followed by contrast agent injection. CT scan is performed after the contrast agent returns to the liver via the portal vein. Normal liver tissues are usually enhanced significantly, and its detection rate of liver lesions ≤1 cm is up to 85%. Spiral CT scan was first applied in the clinical setting in the late 1980s. This technique can scan an entire liver in a single breath-hold, avoid missing scans and artifacts caused by respiratory motion, provide dual-phase (arterial phase and portal venous phase) scanning, and detect lesions with different types of blood supply. Lipiodol CT (CT plus hepatic arteriography) can further increase the diagnostic sensitivity for HCC and detect lesions as small as 0.3 cm. However, one major drawback of CT is that diffuse liver lesions and isodense lesions are likely to be missed. In addition, tumors in the left lobe can be misdiagnosed due to artifacts produced by gas in the stomach.
   (c) Magnetic resonance imaging (MRI): MRI is a multi-dimensional, multi-series imaging technique without ionizing radiation and with a high tissue resolution. MRI has a similar diagnostic value as CT. However, MRI is superior to CT and US in visualizing tissues and structures within the liver lesions, such as hemorrhage, necrosis, fatty degeneration, and envelope. MRI can also help differentiate liver cancer nodules; a feature that makes MRI surpass other exam-

inations except for hepatic arteriography. Major progress has been made in contrast agents in recent years. Contrast-enhanced MRI is preferably performed using liver-specific contrast agents (e.g., Gd-EOB-DTPA and Disodium Gadostate Injection). The use of these contrast agents can increase the detection rate of small lesions or even small tumor embolias as well as differentiate posttreatment necrotic foci, hemorrhagic foci, regenerative nodules, and HCC recurrence. MRI is the most widely accepted imaging technique for HCC.

(d) Selective hepatic arteriography: in 1979, China reported the first case of liver cancer diagnosis by hepatic arteriography. As the most sensitive radiological diagnostic technique for HCC, selective hepatic arteriography can be used to detect small liver lesions and their blood supply, applicable to patients who cannot be definitively diagnosed by other examinations. The detection rate of hepatic angiography is over 90%, and its diagnostic accuracy is 88–93%. The diagnostic value of hepatic arteriography depends on whether the liver tumor is rich in blood vessels. In other words, if tumor lacks blood supply, it cannot be differentiated from cholangiocarcinoma by this work-up. Moreover, hepatic arteriography can be performed concurrently with chemotherapy and lipiodol embolism. Given that hepatic arteriography is an invasive examination with the risk of spontaneous bleeding and embolism, certain experience is needed to achieve high selectivity.

(e) Fluorine-18 fluorodeoxyglucose (^{18}F-FDG): positron emission tomography (PET)/CT^{18}F-FDG and ^{18}F-labeled deoxyglucose can be taken up by tumor cells in large quantities and converted to ^{18}FDG-6-P in the presence of hexokinase. However,^{18}FDG-6-P cannot be converted to hexose diphosphate due to deoxygenation. Therefore, ^{18}FDG-6-P is not further metabolized and remains in the tumor cells. PET can clearly visualize the sites with increased FDG uptake in the transverse, coronal, and sagittal views. This is also the oncologic principle by which PET works. PET/CT is a functional molecular imaging system that combines PET and CT. This technique allows for the visualization of the biochemical metabolism of space-occupying lesions in the liver by PET functional imaging and precise anatomical localization of the lesions by CT morphology imaging. Furthermore, PET/CT can be used to assess the patients' overall conditions and metastases through a whole-body scan. This examination allows early lesion detection and provides information on the changes in tumor size and metabolism after treatment. The glucose uptake pattern is unique in HCC cells. Within a high concentration of glucose 6-phosphatase, well-differentiated HCC cells accelerate the metabolism of ^{18}F-FDG. Due to lower ^{18}F-FDG concentration in well-differentiated HCC cells, the cells appear to lack hypermetabolism and PET is usually negative, resulting in false-negative results. PET/CT is not yet popularized in most Chinese centers and its sensitivity and specificity still need further improvements. PET/CT is not a conventional examination for HCC diagnosis, though it can be used to supplement other examinations.

(f) US-guided fine-needle aspiration cytology: one advantage of this examination is that the needle is inserted at a certain orientation and kept away from the large blood vessels and other organs near the target of aspiration. If the tumor is large with irregular necrosis and liquidation at the center, this technique enables selective sampling of tissue components while avoiding degenerative necrosis, which may otherwise lead to a false-negative result. This technique has a >80% diagnostic rate for HCC and provides histological diagnosis for early cancerous nodules.

5.2.3 Diagnostic Strategy for Primary HCC

Figure 5.1 shows the diagnostic strategy for HCC.

5.2.4 Pathological Diagnosis

Pathological diagnosis is the gold standard for HCC diagnosis. However, pathological diagnosis should be performed in conjunction with clinical findings, such as status of HBV/HCV infection, serum AFP and CA19-9 test results, and radiological characteristics of space-occupying lesions of the liver.

1. Tissue sampling: tumor tissues should be sent to the department of pathology for sampling and fixation within 30 min after resection. The pathology samples should be collected using the "seven-point baseline sampling method", which involves collecting samples from the tumor and paracancerous junction at a 1:1 ratio at the 12, 3, 6, and 9 o'clock positions. At least one block of sample should be collected from within the tumor. One block of sample is collected each at ≤1 cm from the tumor margin (near the paracancerous tissues) and at >1 cm from the tumor margin (away from the paracancerous tissues). For a single tumor ≤3 cm, the entire tumor should be sampled for

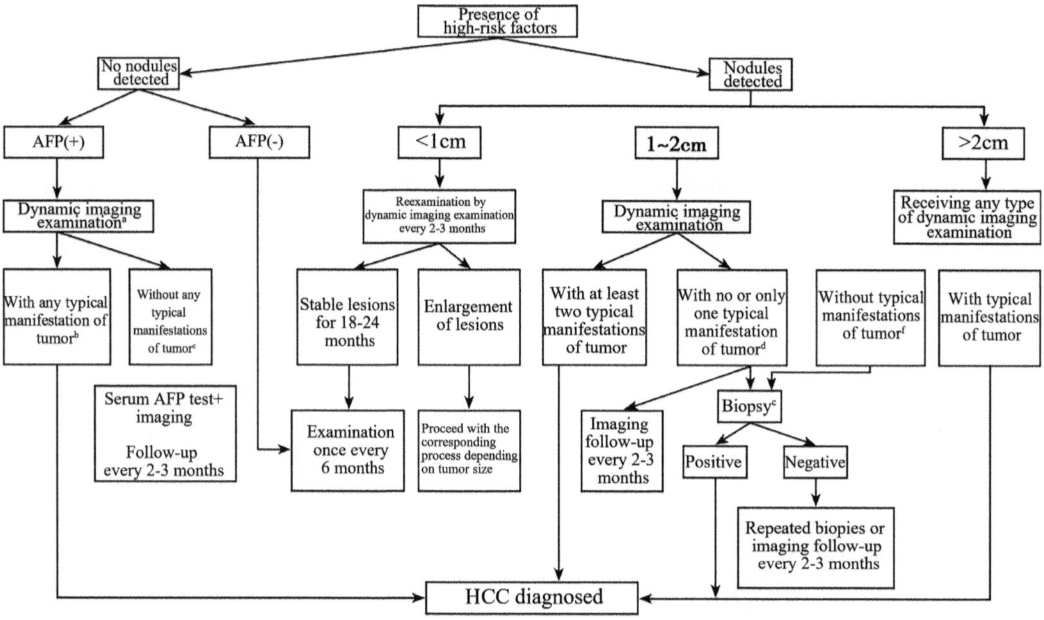

Fig. 5.1 Diagnostic idea for HCC. Note: (a) Mainly includes four radiological modalities: dynamic contrast-enhanced CT scan, dynamic contrast-enhanced MRI, Gd-EOB-DTPA-enhanced MRI, and ultrasound. (b) The clinical diagnosis of HCC can be made if typical characteristics of rapid wash-in and quick wash-out, i.e., significant enhancement of the lesion in the arterial phase and reduced enhancement in the portal venous/or delayed phases, are observed in one of the four radiographic modalities. (c) If no typical characteristics of HCC are observed in the four modalities, close follow-up is recommended. The patients should receive AFP tests plus imaging studies every 2–3 months. If hepatic nodules are detected during the follow-up period, the corresponding handling procedures will be implemented based on the nodule size. (d) The patients should be followed-up by imaging studies once every 2–3 months if typical characteristics of HCC are observed in none or only one of the four radiological techniques. Follow-up should be continued if the hepatic nodules maintain in size. However, if the nodules enlarge, the corresponding handling procedures should be implemented based on the nodule size. (e) Biopsy may be considered if typical characteristics of HCC are observed in none or only one of the radiological techniques. If diagnosis is still unconfirmed after biopsy, follow-up with imaging studies should be performed once every 2–3 months. (f) If no typical characteristics of HCC are observed in any of the four radiological techniques, the patients should receive a liver biopsy. If diagnosis is still unconfirmed after biopsy, follow-up with imaging studies should be performed once every 2–3 months

examination. The tumor number and diameter should also be considered in real practice.

2. Gross description: tumor location, size, number, color, texture, relation with blood vessels and bile ducts, capsular involvement, lesions in surrounding liver tissues, satellite nodules, type of cirrhosis, distance from tumor to resection margin, and resection margin involvement should be described in detail.
3. Microscopic observation and description: according to the WHO Histological Classification of Digestive System Tumors (2010), the following contents are described in detail. Degree of differentiation: the Edmondson four-grade system divided HCC into well-differentiated, moderately differentiated, and poorly differentiated. Histological subtypes: the common histological subtypes include microtrabecular subtype, macrotrabecular subtype, pseudoglandular subtype, and compact subtype. Special cell types: such as clear cells, lipid-rich cells, spindle cells, and undifferentiated cells. Extent and degree of tumor necrosis, lymphocyte infiltration, and interstitial fibrosis. Growth pattern: pericancerous infiltration, capsular invasion or penetration, microvascular invasion, and satellite nodules. Evaluation of chronic liver diseases: HCC is often accompanied by varying degrees of chronic viral hepatitis or cirrhosis. The Scheuer scoring system or China's histological grading and staging criteria for chronic viral hepatitis are recommended.
4. Microvascular invasion (MVI): it is defined as the observation of cancer cell clusters in the vascular lumen lined by endothelial cells under the microscope, especially in the branches of the portal vein (including intracapsular blood vessels). Method of pathological grading: M0: No MVI; M1 (low-risk group): ≤5 MVI; M2 (high-risk group); >5 MVI, or MVI of distal paracancerous tissues.
5. Representative immunohistochemical markers: hepatocyte antigen (Hep Par1) is a cytoplasmic marker. Polyclonal carcinoembryonic antigen (pCEA) is a marker for bile canaliculi. CD34 is a marker for diffused liver sinusoidal microvessels, and GPC-3 is only expressed in the cytoplasm of HCC. In addition, it is also necessary to identify representative immunohistochemical markers for intrahepatic cholangiocarcinoma (ICC). Cytokeratin-19 (CK19) and mucin 1 (MUC1) are usually detected in the cytoplasm of ICC cancer cells.

5.3 Differential Diagnosis of HCC

5.3.1 Differential Diagnosis of AFP Positivity

1. Chronic liver diseases: dynamic observation of serum AFP level is required for hepatitis and cirrhosis patients. The serum levels of AFP and ALT generally have the same pattern of change (increase transiently or fluctuate repeatedly). The serum level of AFP is generally not above 400 μg/L and remains high only for a short time. HCC is suspected if the serum level of AFP changes in an opposite direction as ALT and/or AFP level remain persistently elevation.
2. Identification of pregnancy, embryonal, and gonadial tumors: these tumors are primarily identified by medical history, physical examination, abdominal and pelvic US, and CT scan.
3. Digestive system tumors: some tumors in the stomach, pancreas, and intestinal tract may also cause serum AFP elevation. Apart from a review of the medical history, physical examination, and radiological techniques, serum AFP variant detection is also helpful for identifying the origin of tumors. For example, AFP not bound to lens culinaris lectin is the predominant type of AFP generated by gastric cancer.

5.3.2 Differential Diagnosis of Space-Occupying Lesions in the Liver

1. Secondary liver cancers are mostly metastases from digestive tract tumors in patients who do not have liver diseases. The medical history of these patients may contain symptoms associated with digestive tract tumors, such as

hematochezia, abdominal distension and discomfort, anemia, and weight loss, with AFP negative. In contrast, increases may be observed in digestive tract tumor markers, such as CEA, CA19-9, and CA242. Some typical radiological characteristics include: (1) multiple space-occupying lesions are detected, while HCC is usually solitary; (2) a typical radiological feature of a metastatic tumor is the "bull's-eye sign" (tumor with a surrounding halo and low echoes or hypodensities in the center due to the lack of blood supply); (3) fewer tumor blood vessels can be displayed by contrast-enhanced CT or hepatic arteriography, with less blood supply than HCC; (4) primary lesions may be found in the gastrointestinal tract by gastrointestinal endoscopy or angiography.

2. Cholangiocarcinoma is generally found in patients without liver disease who may have increased levels of tumor markers such as CEA and CA19-9. The most useful radiological modality for cholangiocarcinoma is contrast-enhanced CT scan, with a less abundant blood supply than HCC but a larger amount of fibrous components. Cholangiocarcinoma generally has a rapid wash-in and slow wash-out feature during contrast-enhanced CT and is often accompanied by dilated distal bile duct.
3. Hepatosarcoma is commonly diagnosed in patients without liver diseases and is characterized by homogeneous solid space-occupying lesions with abundant blood supply by radiography. Hepatosarcoma may be hardly differentiable from AFP-negative HCC.
4. Benign liver tumors or nodules primarily include the following types of benign liver diseases, for which differential diagnosis should be made.
   (a) Liver cavernous hemangioma: liver cavernous hemangioma, also known as liver hemangiomas, is the most common type of benign liver tumor that gradually grows in size without a malignant tendency. The benign tumor is more common in female patients without underlying liver diseases and is more easily diagnosed when its diameter is larger than 5 cm. However, small hemangioma is likely to be confused with HCC. Both US and CT scans have a higher diagnostic rate for liver hemangioma. MRI usually offers a more accurate differentiation between liver hemangioma and other lesions. Contrast-enhanced CT scan of liver hemangioma usually features an enhancement from the periphery to the center, with a rapid wash-in and slow wash-out characteristic that differs from the rapid wash-in and rapid wash-out characteristic of HCC. The "light bulb sign" is typical upon MRI of liver hemangioma.
   (b) Hepatic adenoma: hepatic adenoma is common in female patients without underlying liver diseases who often have a history of oral contraceptive use. Hepatic adenoma is difficult to distinguish from well-differentiated HCC. 99mTc nucleotide scan is a more useful examination for differentiating hepatic adenoma as the tumor is capable of nucleotide uptake and appears strongly positive in the delayed phase. The hemorrhage rate and malignant transformation rate of hepatic adenoma are 29% and 5%, respectively. Surgery is usually recommended for hepatic adenoma.
   (c) Focal nodular hyperplasia: this condition is more common in young females, with a male-to-female ratio of about 1:8. Focal nodular hyperplasia (FNH) is occasionally accompanied by bleeding and calcification, but has no malignant tendency. FNH is generally asymptomatic. Some patients with large lesions may experience upper abdominal discomfort or pain in the liver area. FNH rupture and bleeding are very rare complications. This condition is characterized by hypodense or isodense nodule during plain CT scan, with scars in the center presenting as a stellate hypodensity. Contrast-enhanced CT scan in the arterial phase may show a hyperdense lesion

with uniform enhancement except for the scarred foci in the center. The lesion is generally isodense in the portal venous/delayed phases, but the central scar may have a delayed enhancement. Given these features, a combination of several radiological techniques may increase the diagnostic accuracy of FNH.

(d) Hepatic inflammatory pseudotumor: this condition is an inflammatory proliferative disease characterized by fibrous tissue hyperplasia and chronic inflammatory cell infiltration. The etiology of hepatic inflammatory pseudotumor still remains unclear. Infection, immune response, bleeding and necrosis of liver parenchyma, occlusive phlebitis, and secondary response caused by rupture of the intrahepatic bile ducts maybe associated with this condition. Its basic pathological change is the formation of an inflammatory hyperplastic mass. The lesion is characterized by infiltration of various inflammatory cells, including plasma cells, lymphocytes, neutrophils, and phagocytes. Normal hepatic tissues are damaged and gone, with fibrous tissue hyperplasia. However, cirrhosis is usually not observed. Hepatic inflammatory pseudotumor is a benign disease that can be treated by antibiotics and nonsteroidal antiinflammatory drugs. The treatment efficacy should be observed along with regular detection of various parameters. However, hepatic inflammatory pseudotumor is frequently misdiagnosed as liver cancer and resected.

(e) Hepatic adenomatous hyperplasia: this condition is characterized by the gradual formation of tumor-like lesions caused by hyperplasia of hepatocytes during chronic hepatitis and cirrhosis. Hepatic adenomatous hyperplasia specifically refers to pronounced regenerative nodules in cirrhotic patients. Hepatitis virus infection may be an important factor for this condition. Hepatic adenomatous hyperplasia is usually a solitary nodule larger than cirrhotic nodule. The former is typically 1–3 cm and may occasionally reach 10 cm in diameter. One feature of this disease is that the patients are often combined with pathological changes, including hepatitis, cirrhosis, portal hypertension, and splenomegaly. Hepatic adenomatous hyperplasia is considered a precancerous lesion of HCC. This condition is difficult to distinguish from small HCC before surgery, and hence active treatment should be used.

(f) Hepatic cysts: hepatic cysts are quite common and may appear as solitary or multiple cysts with a diameter of over 10 cm or as small as 2–3 mm. Most hepatic cysts can be easily differentiated from HCC. However, it is difficult to differentiate between complex hepatic cysts and HCC with cystic lesions. Hepatic cysts may be observed dynamically. Surgery can be considered if a solitary hepatic cyst grows to a certain size or when multiple hepatic cysts start to impact liver function.

(g) Hepatic abscess: this condition usually occurs in patients with a history of dysentery or suppurative disease but no history of liver disease. Patients may have had or are currently having an infection. A nonliquefied abscess may be easily confused with HCC. A liquefied abscess presents as a fluid surface, a feature that can be used to differentiate from HCC with central necrosis. In addition, hepatic arteriography generally shows no apparent staining of blood vessels in tumors.

(h) Hepatic echinococcosis: this condition is usually found in patients with many years of living history in pasturing areas and a history of exposure to dogs and sheep. One characteristic manifestation is tremor upon palpation. The Casoni test is a specific detection method for this disease, with a positive rate of 90–95%. US may show strong echoes from the floating sacs in the space-occupying cystic cavity, and

CT may reveal calcified sac walls. Aspiration may induce a severe allergic reaction, and hence biopsy is not recommended for definitive diagnosis.

Suggested Reading

1. Chinese Society of Liver Cancer, Liver Cancer Study Group, Chinese Society of Hepatology, Chinese Medical Association, Committee of Oncopathology (COP) of Chinese Anticancer Association. Guidelines for standardized diagnosis and treatment of primary liver cancer (2015 edition). Chin J Hepatobiliary Surg. 2015;21(3):145–51.
2. Zhang BC, Wang MR, Chen JG, et al. A clinical study of lung cancer discovered by screening and follow-up in high-risk populations. Chin J Clin Oncol. 1994;21(7):489–91.
3. Yu MC, Yuan JM. Environmental factors and risk for hepatocellular carcinoma. Gastroenterology. 2004;127(5 Suppl 1):72–8.
4. Cong WM. Surgical pathology of hepatobiliary tumors. Beijing: People's Medical Publishing House; 2015. p. 276–320.
5. Li D, Mallory T, Satomura S. AFP-L3: a new generation of tumor marker for hepatocellular carcinoma. Clin Chim Acta. 2001;313(1–2):15–9.
6. Chan CY, Lee SD, Wu JC, et al. The diagnostic value of the assay of des-gamma-carboxy prothrombin in the detection of small hepatocellular carcinoma. J Hepatol. 1991;13(1):21–4.
7. Xing H, Zheng YJ, Han J, et al. Protein induced by vitamin K absence or antagonist-II versus alpha-fetoprotein in the diagnosis of hepatocellular carcinoma: a systematic review with meta-analysis. Hepatobiliary Pancreatic Dis Int. 2018;17(6):487–95.
8. Yang T, Xing H, Wang G, et al. A novel online calculator based on serum biomarkers to detect hepatocellular carcinoma among patients with hepatitis B. Clin Chem. 2019;65(12):1543–53.
9. Rodriguez-Peralvarez M, Luong TV, Andreana L, et al. A systematic review of microvascular invasion in hepatocellular carcinoma: diagnostic and prognostic variability. Ann Surg Oncol. 2013;20(1):325–39.
10. Ma XL, Jiang M, Zhao Y, et al. Application of serum annexin A3 in diagnosis, outcome prediction and therapeutic response evaluation for patients with hepatocellular carcinoma. Ann Surg Oncol. 2018;25(6):1686–94.
11. Ma XL, Gao XH, Gong ZJ, et al. Apolipoprotein A1: a novel serum biomarker for predicting the prognosis of hepatocellular carcinoma after curative resection. Oncotarget. 2016;7(43):70654–68.
12. Ge T, Shen Q, Wang N, et al. Diagnostic values of alpha-fetoprotein, dickkopf-1, and osteopontin for hepatocellular carcinoma. Med Oncol. 2015;32(3):59.
13. Yu J, Ding WB, Wang MC, et al. Plasma circular RNA panel to diagnose hepatitis B virus-related hepatocellular carcinoma: a large-scale, multicenter study. Int J Cancer. 2019;146(6):1754–63.
14. Xu RH, Wei W, Krawczyk M, et al. Circulating tumour DNA methylation markers for diagnosis and prognosis of hepatocellular carcinoma. Nat Mater. 2017;16(11):1155–61.
15. Lin XJ, Chong Y, Guo ZW, et al. A serum microRNA classifier for early detection of hepatocellular carcinoma: a multicentre, retrospective, longitudinal biomarker identification study with a nested case-control study. Lancet Oncol. 2015;16(7):804–15.
16. Wei Y, Chen X, Liang C, et al. A noncoding regulatory RNAs network driven by Circ-CDYL acts specifically in the early stages hepatocellular carcinoma. Hepatology. 2020;71(1):130–47.
17. Qu C, Wang Y, Wang P, et al. Detection of early-stage hepatocellular carcinoma in asymptomatic HBsAg-seropositive individuals by liquid biopsy. Proc Natl Acad Sci USA. 2019;116(13):6308–12.
18. Yu LX, Zhang BL, Yang Y, et al. Exosomal microRNAs as potential biomarkers for cancer cell migration and prognosis in hepatocellular carcinoma patient-derived cell models. Oncol Rep. 2019;41(1):257–69.
19. Gao Q, Zhu H, Dong L, et al. Integrated proteogenomic characterization of HBV-related hepatocellular carcinoma. Cell. 2019;179(2):561–77.
20. Han J, Han ML, Xing H, et al. Tissue and serum metabolomic phenotyping for diagnosis and prognosis of hepatocellular carcinoma. Int J Cancer. 2020;46(6):1741–53.
21. Ren Z, Li A, Jiang J, et al. Gut microbiome analysis as a tool towards targeted non-invasive biomarkers for early hepatocellular carcinoma. Gut. 2019;68(6):1014–23.
22. Wong VW, Chan SL, Mo F, et al. Clinical scoring system to predict hepatocellular carcinoma in chronic hepatitis B carriers. J Clin Oncol. 2010;28(10):1660–5.
23. Wu MC, Shen F. Liver cancer. Beijing: People's Medical Publishing House; 2010. p. 58–61.
24. National Comprehensive Cancer Network (NCCN). NCCN clinical practice guidelines in oncology. Hepatobiliary cancers. Version 1. 2018 [EB/OL]. http://www.nccn.org/professionals/physician_gls/pdf/hepatobiliary.pdf. Accessed 15 Oct 2020.
25. Lin G, Gu J, Han SY, et al. Selective angiography for diagnosing primary liver cancer. Chin J Radiol. 1979;13(3):129–32.
26. Chinese Society of Clinical Oncology. Guidelines for diagnosis and treatment of primary liver. Beijing: People's Medical Publishing House; 2018. p. 4–16.

Imaging Techniques for Liver Cancer Diagnosis

6

Bibo Tan, Feng Shen, Chun Yang, Mengsu Zeng, Jianhua Wang, Changjing Zuo, and Chao Cheng

6.1 Ultrasonography

Diagnostic ultrasonography (US) involves the use of a medical ultrasound diagnostic instrument by a medical worker to scan the human body. Analog images of human organs and tissues are obtained for observation, and pathological or physiological judgments are made based on these observations. This diagnostic technique can be used to discover new lesions. B-mode US is currently the most widely used. US, X-ray, computer tomography (CT) scan, and magnetic resonance imaging (MRI) are the four major radiographic techniques. US is simple, fast, non-invasive and painless, cheap, and easily available. It is the most widely known and accepted radiographic examination. US is not only used for diagnostic purposes but is also vital in preventive health care. US plays an irreplaceable role in disease screening in the community, especially in the follow-up of patients with chronic liver disease and identification of early stage HCC.

B. Tan · F. Shen (✉)
Shanghai Eastern Hepatobiliary Surgery Hospital, Shanghai, China

C. Yang · M. Zeng · J. Wang
ZhongShan Hospital Fudan University, Shanghai, China

C. Zuo · C. Cheng
Changhai Hospital, Shanghai, China

6.1.1 History of Diagnostic US in HCC

As an important branch of medical imaging, diagnostic US is inseparable from the development of modern industrial technologies. In 1880, the Curie brothers discovered the piezoelectric effect, which laid the theoretical foundation for US technology. The piezoelectric effect and its converse were used in the early twentieth century to manufacture equipment that could emit ultrasound waves, which were soon put into industrial production. In 1942, the Austrian psychiatrist K. T. Dussik was the first to inspect the patients' heads using an A-mode ultrasound. This was the first prototype of diagnostic US in human history. With continuous improvement and progress in industrial technology, M-mode, B-mode and D-mode US technologies were successively invented and put into clinical use.

Influenced by technologies abroad, Prof. Yongchang Zhou from the Shanghai Sixth People's Hospital was among the first Chinese scholars to explore this new imaging technology in the late 1950s. His achievements have laid a solid foundation for the development of diagnostic US in China and led to an upsurge of research in this field. Studies on liver disease are one of the important directions in US application. At this stage, the characteristics of liver tumors under different US modes have been studied extensively. US is able to differentiate between cystic and solid liver tumors.

X. Chen (ed.), *Diagnosis and Treatment of Liver Cancer in China*,
https://doi.org/10.1007/978-981-97-7969-7_6

B-mode ultrasound ultimately stood out among various modes after extensive application and research and became the most suitable instrument for liver examination. Aloka produced the first color Doppler US scanner in 1982, known as the D-mode US. This mode utilizes Doppler's principle in physics to visualize blood flow and direction in the human circulation. The integration of D-mode and B-mode US gave rise to B-mode US with D-mode functions, known as the color Doppler US. By then, the prototype of B-mode had come into being. The emergence of new technologies had opened up new directions of research. In 1987, Prof. Yuhua Zhao applied color Doppler US to liver tumor examination and demonstrated for the first time that the amount of blood flow in HCC was closely related to its pathological structure. This finding was first presented in a 1988 international conference in Washington and won unanimous applause from the peers.

With rapid progress in computer technologies, diagnostic US has also enjoyed continuous modification and improvement. The accuracy and resolution of US, especially B-mode US, have taken a great leap forward due to the use of digital technologies. US has an unprecedented ability to detect hepatic space-occupying lesions. The diagnosis accuracy for small HCC has particularly increased significantly. The smallest liver tumor that can be identified by B-mode US currently available on the market is 5 mm in diameter. B-mode US is the most popular and preferred imaging examination for HCC screening worldwide. However, there are also some inherent drawbacks in US. US diagnosis results are influenced by several factors, including whether the patients are obese, whether the tumor is located near the diaphragm or sites susceptible to gas disturbance such as the stomach, and the operator's skills and experience.

6.1.2 New US-Based Technologies for HCC Diagnosis and Their Applications

The late 1980s saw the realization of three-dimensional ultrasound imaging technology. Three-dimensional US imaging was first applied in obstetrics and later gained wide acceptance. Given its unique superiority in providing 3D visualization of the human anatomy, relentless efforts have been made to use this technology in the study of liver diseases. Real-time 3D contrast-enhanced ultrasound has now been developed and put to use. This technique constructs 3D visual images in real-time based on information from contrast-enhanced US and allows for flexible multiplane imaging to obtain more tumor-related information. This technique represents one of the major directions of diagnostic US development in the future.

Contrast-enhanced US is an important milestone in the history of the diagnostic US. It is a pure-blood pool imaging technique that can show tumor microcirculation and blood perfusion, whose emergence can be dated back to the late 1960s. Contrast-enhanced US has gradually become a mature clinical diagnostic US technique after years of development. Long-term clinical studies have demonstrated that contrast-enhanced US is superior overconventional two-dimensional US. The former has a higher detection rate of liver tumors and small HCC, especially in patients with cirrhosis, fatty liver, and other complicated liver conditions. Contrast-enhanced US also has a good performance in differentiating benign and malignant liver tumors. More advanced contrast agents are currently under research and development. The diagnostic or even therapeutic purposes of contrast-enhanced US in cancer will be further optimized in the future by using microbubbles that carry various molecular probes and targeted drugs. However, much work is still warranted to achieve these goals.

US elasticity imaging is an emerging field that has gained increasing attention in recent years. This technique offers more information about the disease from a biomechanical perspective. The basic working principle of US elasticity imaging is that the human tissues can be compressed in volume by an external force, a process known as deformation; with other conditions being equal, normal tissues and diseased tissues have different deformations due to differences in their microscopic structures. The mainstream US elasticity imaging techniques include instantaneous elastography, acoustic radiation force impulse imaging, real-time tissue elastography, and real-time shear wave elastography. Given the technical features of elasticity imaging, studies have largely focused on its use in liver fibrosis. Prof. Jia Guo and her team from the Eastern Hepatobiliary Surgery Hospital used real-time tissue elastography to differentiate between benign and malignant hepatic tumors. They found that malignant tumors were harder than benign ones, which indicates that the application of this technique in liver tumors is worthy of further investigation.

6.2 Magnetic Resonance Imaging

HCC accounts for about 90% of all primary liver cancer. For early stage HCC, curative treatment can dramatically prolong survival and reduce tumor recurrence. However, patients with middle and late-stage HCC generally miss the best chance for surgery or have a higher risk of postoperative recurrence. Therefore, reasonable use of radiological examination is essential for early discovery, early diagnosis, and early treatment of HCC, thereby improving treatment efficacy.

At present, the commonly used noninvasive radiological examinations for HCC include US, CT, and MRI. Each radiographic examination has its advantages and drawbacks. Therefore, emphasis should be placed on the complementary use of these examinations to provide a comprehensive evaluation of tumors. US and serum alpha-fetoprotein (AFP) are currently used to screen high-risk populations (individuals with hepatitis B, hepatitis C, carriers of HBV and HCV, cirrhosis, a family history of HCC, alcohol abuse, and metabolic syndrome). Dynamic contrast-enhanced CT scans and MRI can be performed in case of a need for diagnostic confirmation. MRI does not use ionizing radiation, has high soft tissue resolution, and is capable of multi-parameter imaging. Meta-analyses and clinical trials in the past 5 years have demonstrated that dynamic contrast-enhanced MRI is the preferred imaging technique with a 77–90% overall sensitivity and 84–97% specificity for HCC.

In 1985, Nanfang Hospital affiliated to the First Military Medical University (currently Nanfang Hospital affiliated to South Medical University) introduced China's first whole-body MRI scanner and put it to clinical use. Over the past 30 years, Chinese radiologists have accumulated extensive clinical experience in MRI-based HCC diagnosis and published numerous articles in various journals. Prof. Tianzhen Shen published the article *MRI diagnosis of primary HCC* in 1990 in the *Chinese Journal of Radiology*. Later, many Chinese abdominal radiologists have successively published articles and monographs on this topic. One outstanding achievement was made by the radiology team led by Prof. Kangrong Zhou from the Zhongshan Hospital of Fudan University. This team was engaged in the systematic study of radiographic diagnosis of HCC and published a series of articles and monographs, proposing the diagnostic methods and criteria for small HCC based on MRI. The team was rewarded the second prize of the 2005 National Award for Science and Technology Progress because of their findings, which laid a solid foundation for the clinical application of MRI in HCC diagnosis, efficacy evaluation, and prognostic prediction.

At present, the primary MRI sign for HCC diagnosis is the "rapid wash-in and rapid wash-out" enhancement pattern, which is characterized by significantly inhomogeneous tumor enhancement or occasional homogeneous enhancement (especially in small HCCnodule ≤3.0 cm) in the arterial phase (typically the late arterial phase), and significantly attenuated or decreased tumor enhancement in the portal venous and/or delayed phase (parenchyma balance phase). Secondary signs include capsule-like structure, slight T2WI hyperintensity, and restricted diffusion. The radiographic feature of "rapid wash-in and rapid wash-out" has a 66–82% diagnostic sensitivity and over 90% specificity for nodules above 1.0 cm in cirrhotic patients. Although the diagnostic efficacy has now been considerably improved, detection of micro-HCC nodules (≤1.0 cm), especially the diagnosis of nodules without the typical rapid wash-in and rapid wash-out feature, remains a significant challenge in the MRI-based diagnosis of HCC. The applications of functional and quantitative MRI, especially the gradual popularization of hepatobiliary-specific MRI contrast medium, and the standardized evaluation of liver nodules using the concepts and rules of the liver imaging reporting and data system (LI-RADS), have dramatically improved the diagnostic efficacy of MRI in liver tumor evaluation.

6.2.1 Functional and Quantitative MRI

6.2.1.1 Diffusion-Weighted Imaging (DWI)

DWI involves application of diffusion-sensitive gradient fields in opposite directions in the image sequence to quantify the diffusion movement of water molecules. As cell density increases or cellular edema occurs, diffusion of water molecules in the extracellular space is restricted, resulting in hyperintense signals. DWI has now become a conventional clinical examination for liver diseases and yields the quantitative parameter apparent diffusion coefficient (ADC). This parameter has a certain application value in differential diagnosis of benign and malignant lesions, HCC grading, and prediction of microvascular invasion in HCC. DWI has a higher sensitivity than conventional T2-weighted imaging, especially for diagnosing small HCC. However, the specificity of DWI is only moderate. Hence, dynamic contrast-enhanced MRI is usually required for comprehensive judgment. In addition, DWI also plays an essential role in efficacy assessment after nonsurgical treatments for HCC (transarterial chemoembolization, radiofrequency ablation, targeted drug therapy, radiotherapy). Chinese scholars have conducted extensive research on DWI, and the findings have been gradually translated into clinical practice.

6.2.1.2 Susceptibility-Weighted Imaging (SWI)

SWI is a high-resolution three-dimensional gradient echo sequence with a long echo time. A flow compensation is applied across three gradients, namely, the slice-selection, phase-encoding, and read-out gradients, to simultaneously obtain the amplitude and phase spectra with exactly the same anatomical positions. The advantage of SWI lies in the visualization of magnet-sensitive materials, such as nonheme iron, hemorrhage, and vein structure. Cirrhosis is often accompanied by endogenous iron deposition, which can be found in 22–67% of all patients with nonbiliary cirrhosis. Iron usually deposits in cirrhotic nodules in a selective manner, collectively known as siderite nodules (SNs). Iron deposition can be found in both regenerative nodule (RN) and dysplastic nodule (DN). Nodules with iron deposition are mostly benign. In contrast, the levels of tissue iron and stainable iron are usually significantly decreased in cancerous nodules. Internationally, the team led by Prof. Mengsu Zeng was among the first to apply SWI to study the changes in iron deposition pattern as cirrhotic nodules transform into DNs, early HCCs and small HCCs (sHCCs). The researchers reported that cirrhotic nodules with nodules positive for iron deposition show hypodensities in SWI. On the other hand, high-grade DNs, early HCC, and sHCCs appear as focal iron-deficient areas on a background of iron deposition due to iron washout (Fig. 6.1). The endogenous iron deposition information provided by SWI is independent of the blood supply characteristics of nodules. Thus, SWI can work synergistically with dynamic contrast-enhanced MRI using gadolinium-based contrast agents. SWI has a particularly high diagnostic value in the follow-up of high-risk populations.

6.2.1.3 Perfusion-Weighted Imaging (PWI)

PWI uses MRI sequences with a high temporal resolution to continuously and dynamically collect liver images before and after contrast agent injection. Semiquantitative and quantitative tissue microperfusion data, including arterial fraction (ART), transfer constant (Ktrans), rate constant (Kep), and extracellular volume fraction (Ve), are acquired using the two-compartment pharmacokinetic model of drug elimination in the postprocessing software (Fig. 6.2). PWI

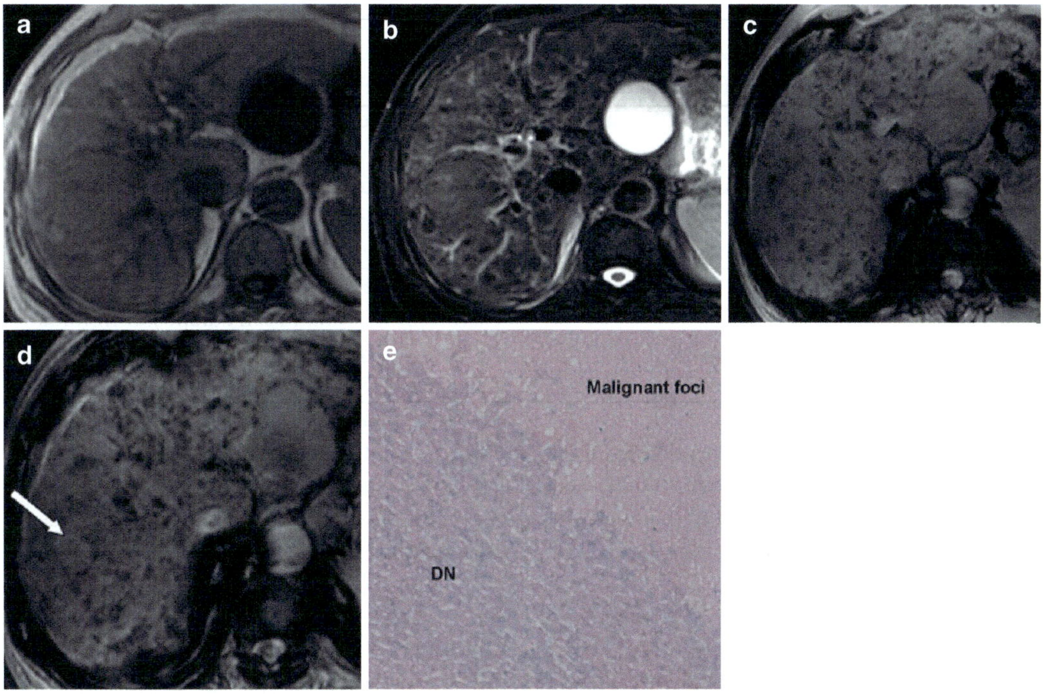

Fig. 6.1 Application value of SWI in sHCC diagnosis. (**a**–**c**) Plain T1WI images, fat-suppression T2WI, and SWI images at initial diagnosis. The lesion is shown as isodensity in T1WI and T2WI. SWI shows iron deposition in nodule in the background liver and also within the nodule, which is similar to that in the background liver; (**d**) SWI image 14 months later shows a hyperdense nodule within the nodule (indicated by the arrowhead); (**e**) Prussian blue staining (×50) indicating no iron deposition in the cancerous lesion but grade 3 iron deposition in the background nodule

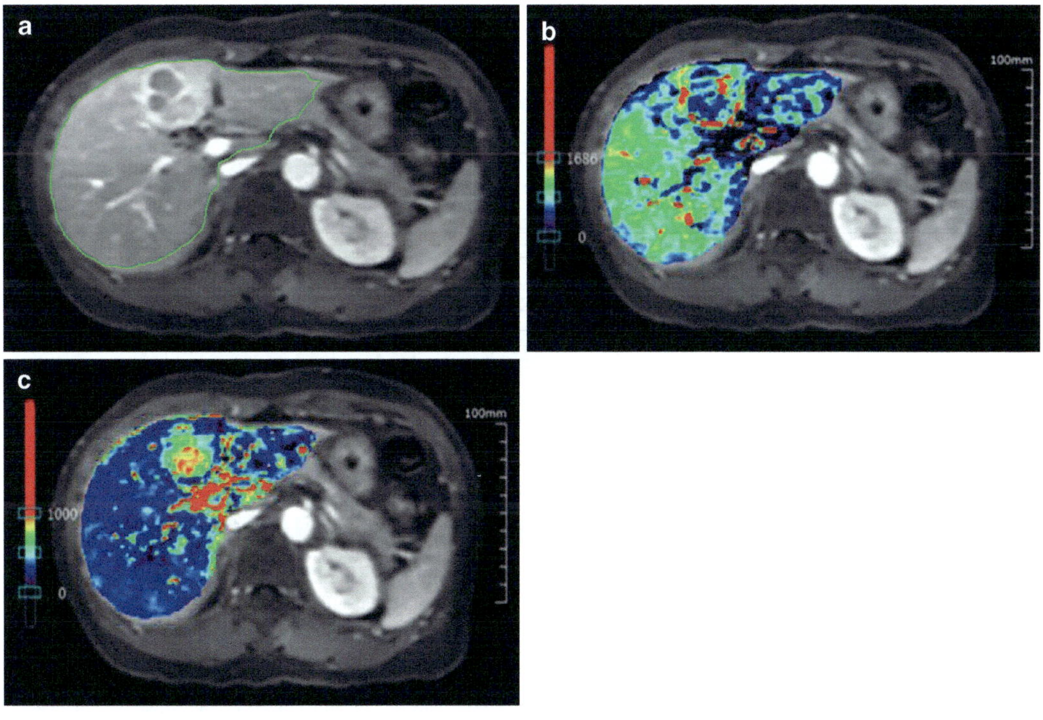

Fig. 6.2 Perfusion-weighted imaging of the liver. (**a**) HCC in the left lobe; (**b**) blood flow image of the portal vein; (**c**) perfusion fraction map of the hepatic artery

reflects angiogenesis in HCC by assessing microvessel density quantitatively, thus offering more accurate and objective HCC pathological grading, efficacy evaluation, and prognostic prediction. With continuous MRI hardware advancement, sequence optimization, and postprocessing software updates, the practicality and feasibility of PWI are expected to be greatly improved.

6.2.2 Hepatobiliary-Specific Contrast Agents

Organic anion transporting polypeptide-8 (OATP-8) on the surface of liver cancer cells is downregulated before angiogenesis in the liver tumor. As a result, the ability of OATP-8 to transport hepatobiliary-specific contrast medium to the liver cells decreases, thus making the early detection of HCC possible. Gadoxetate disodium (Gd-EOB-DTPA) is a hepatobiliary-specific MRI contrast medium prepared by adding a fat-soluble ethoxybenzyl (EOB) onto the Gd-DTPA molecule. About 50% of the injected Gd-EOB-DTPA binds to OATP-8 and enters hepatocytes where it is metabolized and excreted via the biliary system. Gd-EOB-DTPA can provide similar multi-phase dynamic enhancement as the conventional extracellular contrast agent Gd-DTPA by shortening the T1 relaxation time of the tissue. Therefore, Gd-EOB-DTPA allows the observation of the multi-phase dynamic enhancement pattern of liver lesions. In addition, while the liver parenchyma is enhanced maximally at 10–20 min after Gd-EOB-DTPA injection in individuals with normal liver function, the contrast agent is not absorbed by HCC and appears as a hypodensity. Therefore, this contrast medium is favorable for the detection of small HCC nodule (<2 cm) and visualization of the biliary system. This corresponding phase is known as the hepatobiliary phase. A multicenter clinical study conducted by Prof. Mengsu Zeng and his team in China has confirmed the superiority of hepatobiliary-specific MRI contrast medium in the detection and diagnosis of sHCC and micro-HCC. Gd-EOB-DTPA has been widely used worldwide. The application of Gd-EOB-DTPA has expanded from the diagnosis of sHCC/micro-HCC and differential diagnosis of intrahepatic focal lesions to the diagnosis and assessment of cirrhosis, liver function, and biliary disorders. Gd-EOB-DTPA also has excellent clinical and scientific values for assessing and predicting the biological behaviors of HCC, such as the degree of differentiation and microvascular invasion (Fig. 6.3).

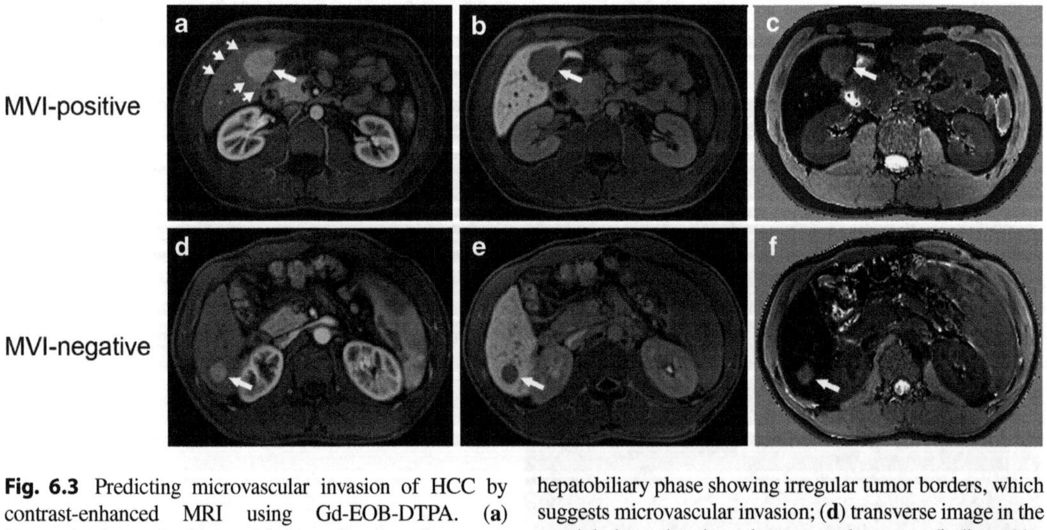

Fig. 6.3 Predicting microvascular invasion of HCC by contrast-enhanced MRI using Gd-EOB-DTPA. (**a**) Transverse image in the arterial phase showing a hypervascular tumor (indicated by the long arrowhead) and peritumoral enhancement (indicated by the short arrowhead); (**b**) T1WI in the hepatobiliary phase; (**c**) T1 mapping in the hepatobiliary phase showing irregular tumor borders, which suggests microvascular invasion; (**d**) transverse image in the arterial phase showing a hypervascular tumor (indicated by the long arrowhead); (**e**) T1WI in the hepatobiliary phase; (**f**) T1 mapping in the hepatobiliary phase showing regular tumor borders, which suggests no microvascular invasion

6.2.3 LI-RADS Classification

The American College of Radiology (ADR) proposed the LI-RADS classification for the first time in 2011. Later, revisions of this classification were released in 2013, 2014, 2017, and 2018, respectively. The LI-RADS classification introduces secondary auxiliary diagnostic signs in addition to primary radiographic features, such as rapid wash-in/rapid wash-out and tumor size, to assess the probability of benign or malignant liver tumor in high-risk populations. This classification system is intended to provide the framework and strategy for standard diagnosis and differential diagnosis for resident physicians as well as for education and training purposes. More importantly, the LI-RADS classification offers a standard and uniform set of terminology and assessment methods for the academic community, which facilitates academic exchange and manuscript publication. In 2018, the American Association for the Study of Liver Diseases (AASLD) integrated the LI-RADS classification into its AASLD Clinical Practice Guideline for HCC (2018 Edition). This act highlights the importance and value of LI-RADS and radiologists in HCC diagnosis. The release of the LI-RADS classification has made the reporting of MRI diagnosis of liver tumor lesions more standardized. Chinese radiologists have conducted numerous studies on the LI-RADS classification since its release and published many articles in journals at home and abroad, including interpretation of the LI-RADS guideline. These scholars have highlighted the strengths and limitations of this guideline based on the features of HCC in Chinese population in order to provide more objective and scientific assessment of its application value in HCC diagnosis and improve MRI-based diagnosis of HCC in China.

A large body of work has been done on liver MRI imaging under the joint efforts of Chinese radiologists in recent years. These studies include clinical applications, such as on MRI-based diagnosis of sHCC/micro-HCC, and applications of new technologies such as radiomics and AI in liver MRI.

6.2.4 Studies on the Clinical Application of MRI in the Diagnosis of Small and Micro-HCC

HCC has a poor prognosis, with the 5-year survival rate of progressive HCC <20%. In contrast, the overall 5-year survival rate of small HCC is up to 50–60%. Therefore, early identification of precancerous lesions and early stage HCC nodules in cirrhotic patients followed by active interventional therapy are vital for improving prognosis. Gd-EOB-DTPA-enhanced MRI can improve the detection rate and the accuracy of diagnosis and differential diagnosis of HCC ≤1.0 cm. Meta-analyses and several studies have indicated that Gd-EOB-DTPA-enhanced MRI has superior accuracy than multi-slice multiphase spiral dynamic contrast-enhanced CT, plain MRI scan, and dynamic contrast-enhanced scan using conventional extracellular contrast medium in the diagnosis of small HCC (≤2.0 cm). The combined use of hypodensity in the hepatobiliary phase, enhancement in the arterial phase, and restricted diffusion signs not only significantly improves the diagnostic sensitivity for small HCC but also helps with the identification of precancerous lesions, including high-grade dysplastic nodules.

6.2.5 Application Value of Radiomics and Artificial Intelligence (AI) in HCC Diagnosis

Lambin et al. proposed the concept of radiomics in 2012. Radiomics uses computer assistance to extract a large number of high-throughput quantifiable features from medical images and make predictions on clinical concerns and issues (e.g., diagnosis, efficacy assessment, and prognosis) through AI algorithm training and model construction. Compared with conventional radiology, radiomics can extract plentiful features hardly visible to the human eyes with the use of a computer. The application of radiomics in HCC, including microvascular invasion prediction, tumor classification, immune response, and postoperative recurrence assessment, is currently being investigated.

Despite the constant progress in diagnostic and therapeutic techniques, HCC remains the fourth leading cause of cancer-related deaths and ranks sixth in the cancer incidence in the world. According to the WHO estimation, over one million people will die of HCC in 2030. Therefore, a large body of research data will be needed to further optimize diagnostic performance, improve prognosis and quality of life, and reduce the disease burden of HCC. Maximization of the value of radiology in multidisciplinary team (MDT) diagnosis, exploration of simple and highly effective preoperative liver function assessment methods, and application of new MRI techniques and contrast agents will be the focus of future investigations.

6.2.6 Application of Radiology in MDT Diagnosis of HCC

HCC is usually highly malignant, with limited efficacy by a single, conventional diagnostic and therapeutic measure. Studies from western countries have demonstrated that the MDT approach for diagnosis and treatment can significantly improve treatment efficacy for HCC and the patients' quality of life while reducing medical costs. Precise preoperative staging of HCC is the cornerstone for selecting an appropriate treatment modality. Given the uniqueness of HCC, preoperative biopsy for pathological examination is not recommended for patients who may undergo surgical resection. In addition, since the identification of vascular invasion and lymph node metastases relies on radiological judgment (typically MRI), accurate preoperative staging is largely dependent on the precise interpretation of radiologists in the MDT. During an MDT meeting, radiologists are mainly responsible for: (1) the diagnosis and differential diagnosis of HCC and other benign and malignant liver tumors; (2) locating the hepatic segments invaded by the tumor; (3) determining whether there are vascular and lymph node involvements; (4) determining whether there are distant metastases; (5) clinical staging of HCC; and (6) evaluating whether the tumor is resectable. For non-resectable patients, the assessments are more focused on efficacy as well as presence of new lesions and metastases.

6.2.7 Liver Function Assessment

An accurate evaluation of liver functional reserve is critical. At present, the commonly used liver function assessment methods include several liver function grading systems and serological testing. However, these methods are only capable of assessing overall liver function but do not provide local liver function evaluation or prediction. Recent studies have shown that Gd-EOB-DTPA can also be used to assess liver functions apart from the differential diagnosis of liver lesions. The uptake of Gd-EOB-DTPA in the liver parenchyma can be quantified by measuring the changes in signal intensity (SI) in the liver parenchyma or T1 relaxation time of liver tissues after Gd-EOB-DTPA-enhanced MRI, which indirectly reflect the liver function reserve. The T1 value measured by T1 mapping reflects the change in relaxation time of liver tissues, and this measurement is independent of the influence of various parameters. Thus, T1 can more accurately and objectively reflect the changes in Gd-EOB-DTPA uptake in the liver. Haimerl et al. pointed out that T1-based parameter offers a more accurate quantitative evaluation of liver functions than SI-related parameters. The study by Zhou et al. reported heterogeneity in liver damage caused by chronic liver diseases, and the impaired degree of liver function varies among different hepatic segments. Comprehensive analysis of the liver function and volume of each hepatic lobe/segment is of avail to the precise development of therapeutic regimen and efficacy monitoring.

6.2.8 Clinical Applications of Highly Concentrated Macrocyclic Contrast Medium

The increases in nephrogenic systemic fibrosis and gadolinium deposition in recent years have raised concerns in the safety of gadolinium-based contrast agents among radiologists. Existing studies have shown that linear gadolinium-based contrast mediums are more likely to deposit in the brain than macrocyclic ones. However, the clinical and biological significance of gadolinium deposition in the brain remains unclear. Gadobutrol is the only macrocyclic gadolinium-based contrast agent with a concentration of up to 1.0 mol/L. Gadobutrol has a higher relaxation rate and higher concentration compared with other gadolinium-based contrast agents, and its ability to significantly shorten the T1 relaxation time can dramatically improve tissue enhancement. Therefore, gadobutrol can detect lesions more accurately and offer a clearer visualization of lesion details. Gadobutrol is particularly advantageous in central nervous system imaging, perfusion imaging, and contrast-enhanced MR angiography (CE-MRA). However, its applications in liver tumors remain to be further investigated.

6.3 Hepatic Arteriography

The development of interventional radiology has fueled the clinical application of digital subtraction angiography (DSA). At present, DSA equipment has become a necessity for interventional diagnosis and treatment. Hepatic arteriography can assist in the diagnosis and treatment of HCC. This technique can determine the number and size of liver lesions as well as visualize arterial blood supply to the tumor and the presence of venous fistula or vein tumor thrombosis, thereby facilitating the decision on surgical resection or appropriate interventional treatment.

6.3.1 Procedures of Hepatic Arteriography

6.3.1.1 DSA Device

The high-power (≥1000 mA) biplane digital subtraction angiography (DSA) equipment is usually recommended.

6.3.1.2 Angiography Equipment

Apart from the surgery pack, puncture needle, and guidewire used for conventional vascular intervention, catheters and microcatheters for conventional hepatic arteriography should also be prepared.

6.3.1.3 Angiography Procedures

Selective hepatic arteriography is more commonly performed, with the end of the catheter placed in the abdominal artery or common hepatic artery. The total volume and flow rate of the contrast medium should be determined based on the thickness of the hepatic artery. The total volume of contrast agent injected for selective hepatic arteriography is usually 20–25 mL, with a flow rate of 4–5 mL/s. The image acquisition time is 15–25 s. The filming procedure is as follows: After a delay of 1 s, images are collected continuously for 25 s at a speed of 4–6 frames per second in the arterial, parenchymal, and venous phases. Next, a microcatheter is inserted into the right hepatic artery or the left hepatic artery for arteriography. The total volume is 6–12 mL each time with a flow rate of 2 mL/s. Collateral blood supply to the tumor lesions needs to be identified, such as exploration of the superior mesenteric artery, left gastric artery, and inferior phrenic artery. Blood supply to the tumors should be embolized as much as possible. If hepatic arteriography finds any sparsity or absence of blood vessels within a specific region of the liver, the hepatic artery or collateral blood vessels originating from the ectopic site will need to be located.

6.3.2 Main Angiographic Manifestations of HCC

HCC is usually rich in blood supply upon hepatic arteriography.

1. The liver-supplying arteries and their branches are thickened and distorted.
2. The tumor vessels and the tumor are positively stained. These are the most characteristic manifestations of HCC, with a visualization rate of 92.5% and 98.8%, respectively. The tumor blood vessels are generally neovessels that are disorganized and vary in lumen thickness with abnormal dilation and distortion in the tumor regions. Tumor lake (also known as the vascular lake) may appear in the arterial phase, which is a "lake- or pool-like" contrast medium accumulation. This sign disappears slowly and may linger even after the contrast

agent has been eliminated from the artery. Although the mechanism of the formation of tumor lake is not fully understood yet, some researchers believe that it was caused by the retention of the contrast medium in the necrotic region or by vascular degeneration. An experiment by Prof. GuiLinin 1985 showed that "tumor lake" was actually formed by dilated abnormal blood vessels lined with a monolayer of endothelial cells. Tumor staining occurs in the capillary phase in three patterns, namely, nodular, nonuniform, and uniform. These staining patterns are associated with contrast agent accumulation in the tumor interstitial space and retention in the tumor blood vessels. A large tumor may present with a higher density in the periphery and lower density or nonuniformity in the center when it has necrosis in the center. If a large tumor has two supplying arteries with little communication, the tumor may be shown as a hemisphere due to the partial lack of tumor blood vessels and staining (Figs. 6.4, 6.5 and 6.6).

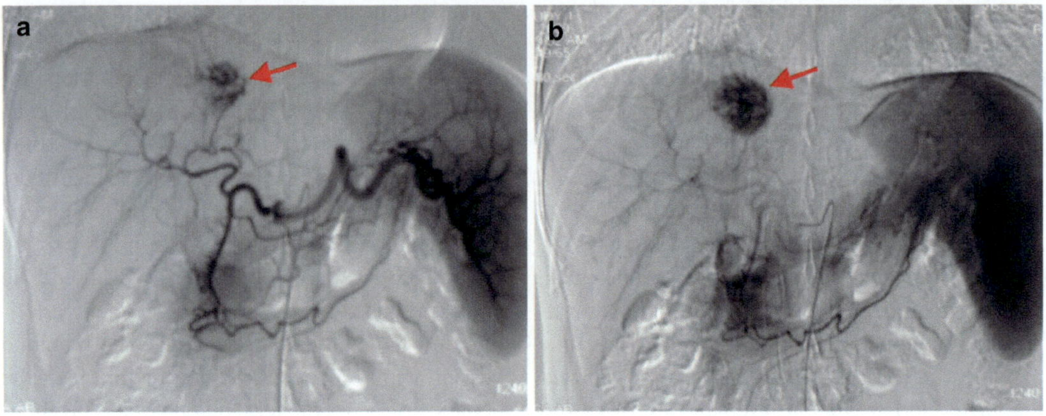

Fig. 6.4 HCC (I). (**a**) The medial branch of the left hepatic artery is mildly thickened in the arterial phase, and the tumor is rich in distorted and irregular blood vessels; (**b**) The tumor is densely stained in the parenchymal phase, with a diameter of about 30 mm. The tumor contour is traced

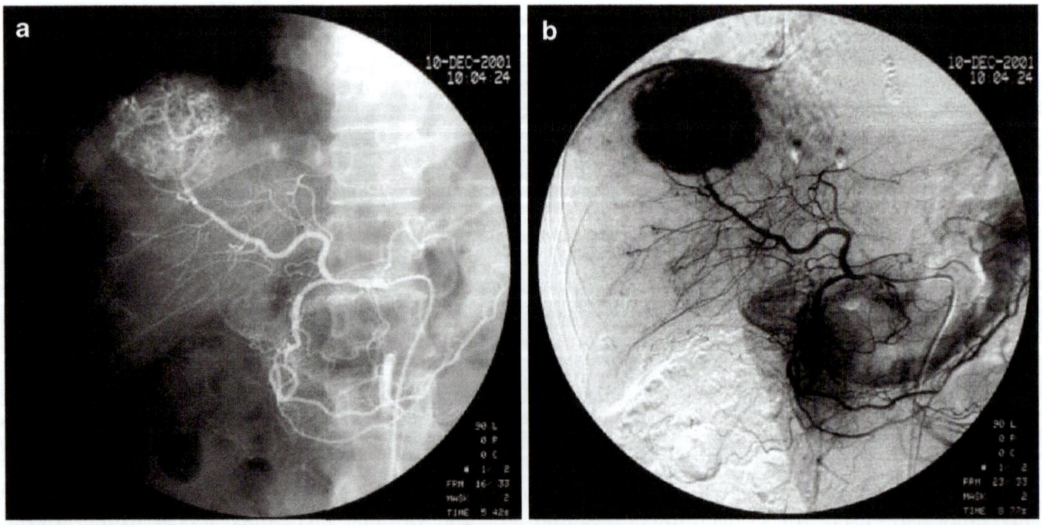

Fig. 6.5 HCC (II). (**a**) The right hepatic artery is thickened in the arterial phase, and the tumor is rich in distorted and irregular blood vessels. Small branches of the portal vein with APS are visible; (**b**) the tumor is densely stained in the parenchymal phase (6 cm in diameter)

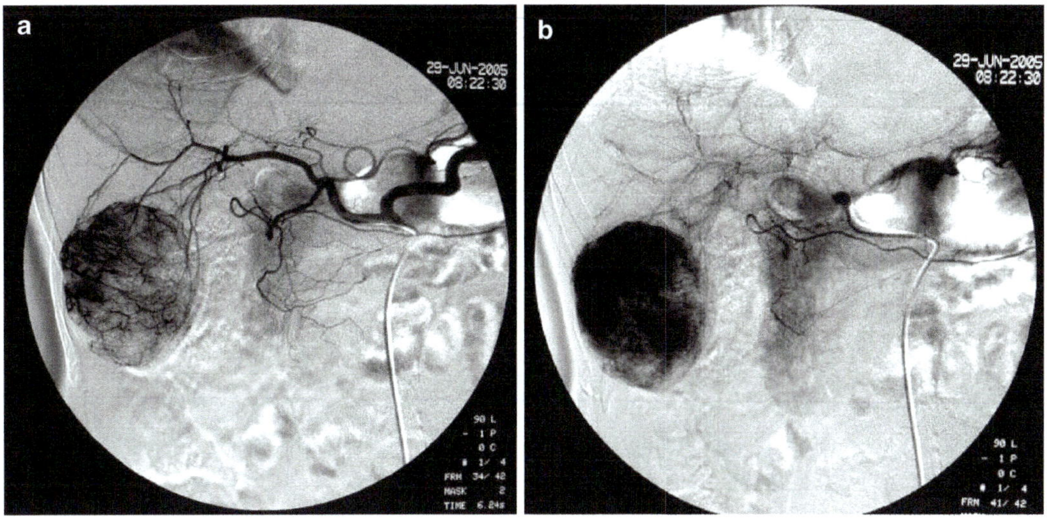

Fig. 6.6 HCC (III). (**a**) A large liver lesion (7.5 cm in diameter) is visible in the right lobe in the arterial phase, and the tumor is rich in blood vessels; (**b**) The tumor is densely stained in the parenchymal phase

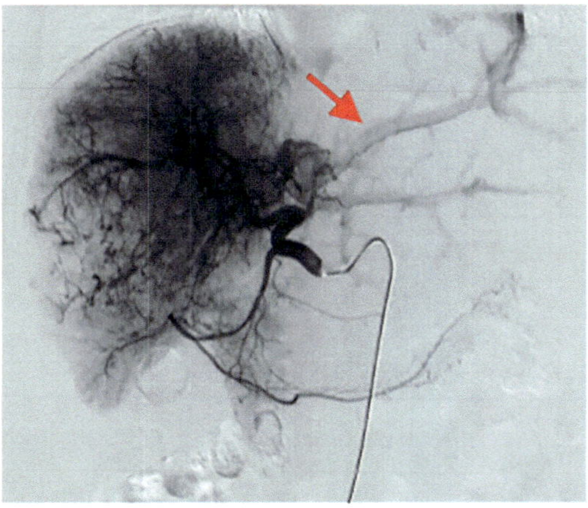

Fig. 6.7 A large liver lesion is visible in the right lobe in the arterial phase. The tumor is rich in blood vessels with APS. The left branch of the portal vein can also be visualized

3. Arterial-portal venous shunt (APS), also known as an arteriovenous fistula, is the establishment of blood flow between the hepatic artery and the portal vein. Portal vein branches and even the main trunk of the portal vein can be visualized in the arterial phase. As the hepatic artery and the portal vein are visualized simultaneously, the double-track sign can be observed. If there is substantial blood flow between the hepatic artery and portal vein, the hepatic artery and the portal vein may appear to overlap and manifest as blurred vascular shadows. The detection rate of arteriovenous shunt could be as high as 63.2%, and 52% of which is APS. Artery-hepatic vein shunt is rare (<3%) and presents as early visualization of the hepatic vein. The pathological basis of APS is intravenous tumor thrombosis (Fig. 6.7).
4. Straightening, displacement, and distortion of arteries caused by compression from large tumors.
5. Tumor encasement of arteries. The tumor encases and infiltrates the arteries, causing stiffness, stenosis, and irregularity of the arterial wall. This condition is more commonly seen in massive HCC (Fig. 6.8).
6. Tumor thrombus of the portal vein and hepatic veins. Tumor thrombus in the main trunk and the left and right branches of the portal vein present as a filling defect in the portal vein. In case of significant obstruction of the portal vein, the filling defect in the portal vein becomes more pronounced as the amount of contrast agent in the portal vein increases in the middle and late arterial phase. Tumor thrombus are supplied by arteries. Therefore, a filling defect can be seen in the dilated portal vein where the tumor thrombus is located in the middle arterial phase. In

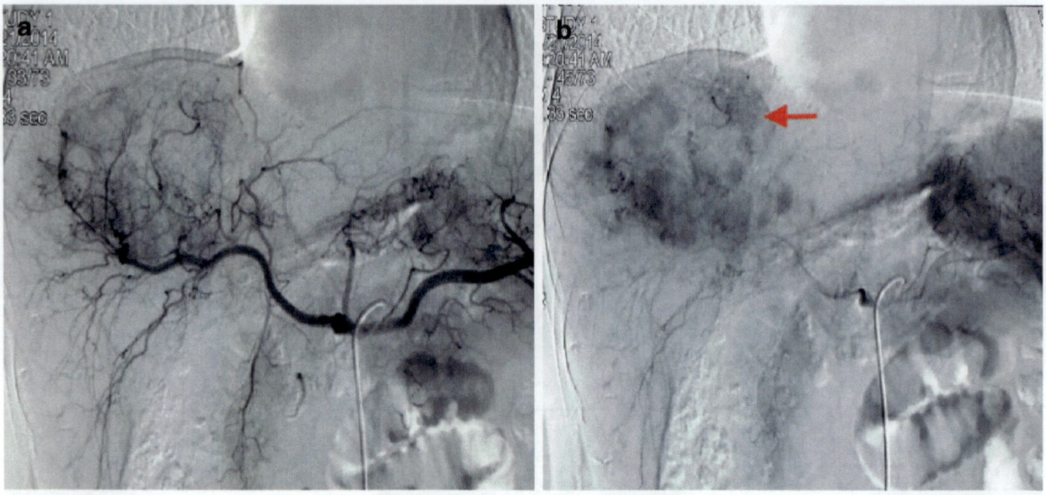

Fig. 6.8 (**a**) Large HCC in the right lobe near the diaphragmatic dome in the arterial phase presents as tumor encasement (indicated by the arrowhead), with rich blood supply; (**b**) tumor lesion is dense but non-uniformly stained (8.4 cm in diameter) in the parenchymal phase

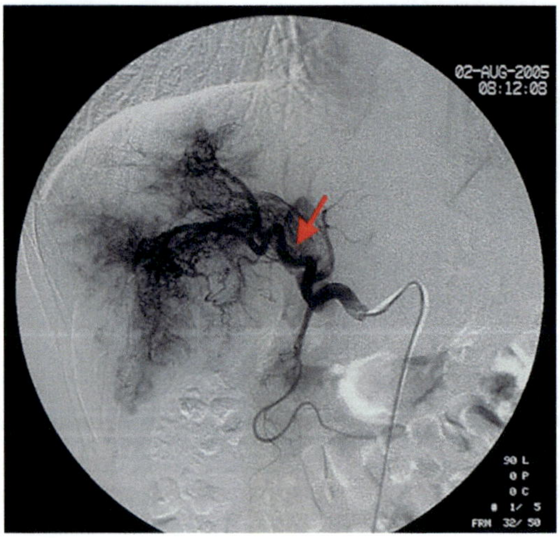

Fig. 6.9 APS is observed in the arterial phase. There are tumor thrombi in the main trunk and right branch of the portal vein, presenting as a stripe sign

addition, several parallel blood vessels traveling in the direction of the vein are visible within the tumor thrombus, which is a typical manifestation of the arteries supplying the tumor thrombus, known as the “stripe sign” (also known as the “linear sign”). Portal vein tumor thrombosis presents as a stripe sign in the hepatic vein, which may extend to the inferior vena cava, or sometimes even to the right atrium (Figs. 6.9, 6.10 and 6.11).

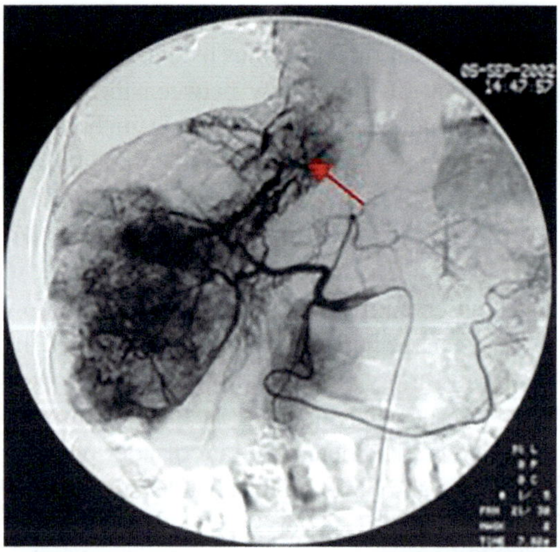

Fig. 6.10 A massive liver tumor in the right lobe of the liver is visible in the arterial phase. The tumor has a rich blood supply, and tumor lake is visible. Anartery-hepatic vein shunt is also present. There is a tumor thrombus in the right hepatic vein, presenting as a track sign. The tumor thrombus extends downwards to the inferior vena cava (indicated by the arrowhead)

Among the above findings in hepatic arteriography, tumor blood vessels and tumor staining are the most common, accounting for 92.5% and 98.8%, respectively. Arteriovenous shunt, tumor encasement of the artery, and portal vein tumor thrombosis are less common. Although these

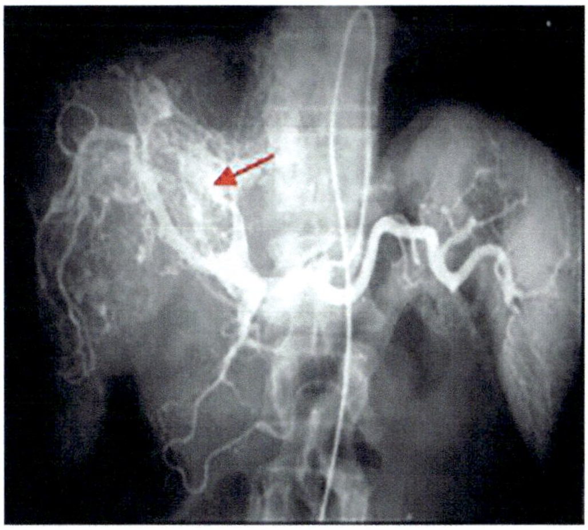

Fig. 6.11 A large liver tumor in the right lobe of the liver is visible in the arterial phase. APS is conspicuous, with a large tumor thrombus in the main trunk of the portal vein, which presents as a cup-like filling defect (indicated by the arrowhead)

three manifestations account for 33.3%, 53.6%, and 23.8% of all findings, respectively, they are the characteristic changes in malignant liver tumors.

6.3.3 Manifestations of Intrahepatic Cholangiocarcinoma (ICC) in Hepatic Arteriography

ICC is relatively rare and originates from the intrahepatic bile duct epithelial cells in secondary branches of the bile duct, only accounting for 5–10% of primary liver cancer. ICC is grossly classified as nodular (60–80%), periductal infiltration (15–35%), nodular infiltration, and intraductal growth (8–29%). Histopathologically, ICC is mostly adenocarcinoma with varying degrees of differentiation.

ICC usually manifests as a lack of blood supply in hepatic arteriography. The tumor blood vessels appear in the middle and late arterial phases, generally as increased number of tiny, disordered, newly formed vessels. The tumor is lightly and nonuniformly stained with denser staining in the periphery. The center of the tumor is vacuolated, sometimes with mild bile duct dilatation near the tumor. In some cases, ICC only presents as a tumor that encases artery. The invaded hepatic artery has rigid, stenotic, and irregular walls (Fig. 6.12).

Mixed liver cancer: HCC-ICC mixed liver cancer is a rare condition.

6.3.4 Infusion Hepatic Arteriography (IHA)

One difference between infusion and conventional hepatic arteriography is the use of a large volume, typically 20–30 mL, of iodinated contrast agent at a flow rate of 2–3 mL/s. This imaging technique is able to detect small hypervascular tumors (<0.5 cm in diameter) and small hypovascular tumors (<2 cm in diameter) that are likely missed by conventional hepatic arteriography. The working mechanism of this technique is that a larger amount of the contrast medium will accumulate in the tumor primarily supplied by the hepatic artery. In contrast, 75% of the blood supply to the normal liver tissue comes from the portal vein containing no contrast medium, while only a small amount of the contrast medium (25%) is carried into the tissue by the hepatic artery. Under a slow-rate injection, this small portion of the contrast medium will be quickly diluted by the portal vein blood, which contrasts with the densely stained tumor.

Differential diagnosis: primary liver cancer should be differentiated from metastatic liver cancer, hepatic adenoma, hepatic cavernous hemangioma, and focal nodular hyperplasia.

1. It is sometimes difficult to differentiate metastatic liver cancer from primary liver cancer, especially hypervascular metastatic tumors. The two conditions share similar radiological changes and patterns of iodine oil deposition. Nevertheless, primary lesions can be found in most cases by reviewing the patient's medical history and performing thorough examinations. The angiographic manifestations of hepatic metastases vary with the type of primary cancer. Metastatic liver cancers are divided into the following three categories based on blood supply.

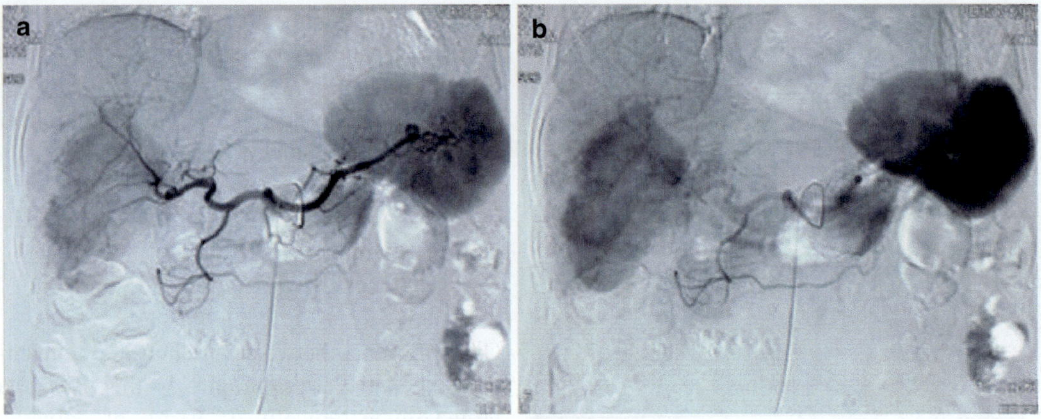

Fig. 6.12 Intrahepatic cholangiocarcinoma. (**a**) The right hepatic artery is invaded by the tumor in the arterial phase and becomes rigid and thin. The tumor lacks blood supply; (**b**) the tumor is nonuniformly stained in the parenchyma phase, with much denser staining in the periphery than in the center

(a) Hypervascular metastatic cancer: the hepatic artery is significantly thickened, with abundant tumor blood vessels. Tumor lake and APS are visible, and the tumor is clearly stained. The radiological manifestations are similar to those of HCC. The primary lesions leading to the hypervascular metastatic cancer are mostly renal cancer, chorionic epithelioma, pancreatic islet cell tumor, thyroid cancer, intestinal carcinoid, and a small portion of gastric and colonic cancers.

(b) Moderately vascular metastatic cancer: the hepatic artery is thickened. The tumor blood vessels are tiny and tortuous, presenting with a network-like distribution. The tumor is lightly stained with a ring-like pattern. Primary lesions leading to moderately vascular metastatic cancer are mostly colon cancer, rectal cancer, breast cancer, adrenal cancer, seminoma, and melanoma, as well as some gastric, esophageal, and pancreatic cancers (Fig. 6.13).

(c) Hypovascular metastatic cancer: the tumor has sparse blood vessels and no clear staining. Filling defect shadows of varying numbers and sizes are visible in the parenchymal phase. Such metastatic cancers result from some primary gastric, pancreatic, esophageal, and lung cancers. All solid tumors have blood vessels, while avascular lesions are only present in simple hepatic cysts that have avascular regions.

2. Hepatic arteriography of hepatic adenoma usually shows thin, disordered tumor blood vessels, some of which may be stained. However, there are no characteristic changes associated with hepatic malignancy, such as arteriovenous fistula.
3. Hepatic hemangioma is composed of dilated hepatic sinusoids. Lesion is densely stained in a small cotton ball- or popcorn-like pattern by contrast medium that enters through the hepatic sinusoids. Typical staining has a semi-arc or horseshoe-like pattern. The imaging (staining) of blood sinuses is characterized by the rapid "wash-in" and slow "wash-out" feature, which involves early visualization in the arterial phase that lasts for 20 s or longer before disappearing. This feature is unique to hepatic hemangioma, and the condition is not associated with an elevation of hepatic malignancy markers such as AFP.
4. Focal nodular hyperplasia (FNH) is a benign mass composed of hyperplastic hepatic parenchyma. The fibrous scar in the mass contains blood vessels and radiating septa that constitute a stellate or wheel-shaped pattern. Hepatic arteriography of FNH usually reveals a rich blood supply. The branches of the supply artery

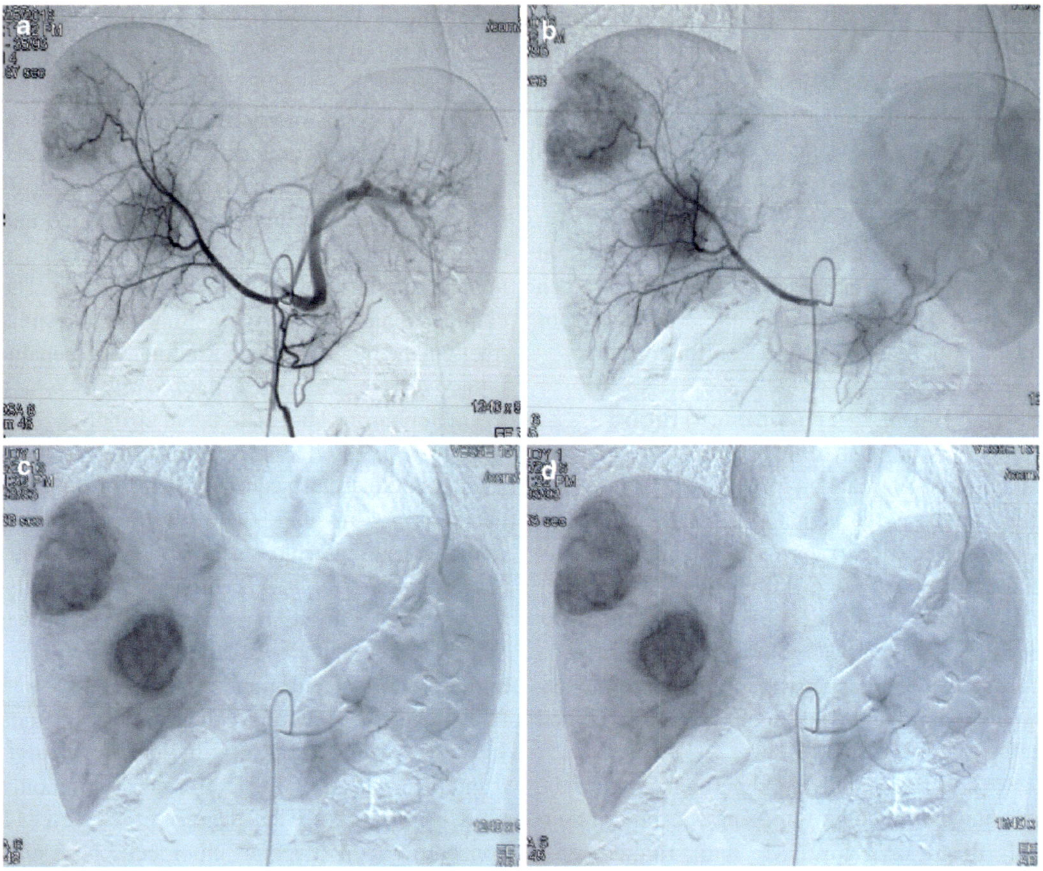

Fig. 6.13 Liver metastases after surgery for colon cancer. (**a** and **b**) Two metastatic lesions are visible in the right lobe of the liver in the arterial phase, with a mild to moderate increase in tumor blood vessels; (**c** and **d**) The tumor is more densely stained in the periphery than in the center in the parenchyma phase

are thickened and apparently tortuous. The tumor is clearly stained, and the intratumoral septa form a grid-like pattern. No characteristic changes associated with hepatic malignancy, such as elevated AFP, are observed.

6.4 Radionuclide Imaging

6.4.1 Radionuclide Hepatobiliary Imaging

The liver tissue is composed of hepatocytes that constitute the parenchyma and Kupffer cells and has a dual blood supply and hepatic sinusoids. Radionuclide imaging can visualize the liver based on the differential uptake and phagocytosis of radionuclides by hepatocytes and Kupffer cells. The technique can also observe blood flow and radionuclide distribution in the liver through blood perfusion. With the rapid development in US, CT and MRI techniques and improvements in their resolution in recent years, the clinical use of radionuclides in hepatobiliary imaging has declined. Nonetheless, this technique retains unique value in specific clinical scenarios.

6.4.1.1 Liver Colloid Imaging

Radioactive colloids with an appropriate particle size (1–5000 nm in diameter) are phagocytized by Kupffer cells in the liver after being injected intravenously into the blood circulation. These colloids remain in the liver for an extended period, and images of the liver can therefore be captured by nuclear medicine imaging equipment. Intrahepatic lesions (liver cancer, hepatic cyst, liver abscess, and Hepatic hemangioma) cannot retain colloidal imaging agents due to a lack of Kupffer cells, thus shown as regions with defects or reduction in radioactivity. Since the mononuclear phagocyte system is also present in the spleen and bone marrow radionuclide colloid imaging of the liver is also known as liver/spleen imaging. The most commonly used agent for liver colloid imaging is ^{99m}Tc sulfur colloid.

6.4.1.2 Hepatic Perfusion and Blood Pool Imaging

In a normal liver, about 75% of the blood is supplied by the portal vein and 25% by the hepatic artery, respectively. In case of blood supply changes in the liver or the presence of intrahepatic lesions, radionuclide imaging can assess hepatic perfusion and blood flow distribution during the equilibrium phase. The most commonly used radionuclide agent is ^{99m}Tc-red blood cells (^{99m}Tc-RBC).

^{99m}Tc-RBC hepatic blood pool imaging can be combined with colloid imaging for the differential diagnosis of HCC and Hemangioma (Table 6.1).

Palliative treatments, including transarterial chemoembolization (TACE) and transarterial radioembolization (TARE), are currently important treatment modalities for unresectable HCC (including some unresectable metastatic liver cancer). ^{99m}Tc-MAA hepatic angiography (perfusion imaging) (macroaggregated albumin, with a particle size of 10–90 μm) can be used to observe blood supply, collateral circulation, and arteriovenous fistula in tumors and mitigating the complications associated with selective internal radiation therapy.

Table 6.1 Radiographic Characteristics of HCC and Hemangioma on ^{99m}Tc-RBC blood pool imaging and colloid imaging

Items	HCC	Hemangioma
Perfusion imaging	Increased perfusion	Normal or mild perfusion
Blood pool imaging	Normal Filled	Excessively filled
Liver colloid imaging	Focal filling defect	Focal filling defect

6.4.1.3 Hepatobiliary Imaging

Hepatocytes (polygonal cells) selectively uptake radioactive hepatobiliary radiopharmaceuticals from the blood circulation and metabolize and excrete the radiopharmaceutical the bile in a manner similar to the secretion of bilirubin. The contrast agent is then excreted into the intestinal tract via the biliary system. Radionuclide hepatobiliary imaging can assess the process by which the radiopharmaceuticals is taken up and secreted by the liver as well as excreted into the intestine. This technique can acquire a series of dynamic hepatobiliary imaging features for the evaluation of the morphology and function of the hepatobiliary system. Radiopharmaceuticals for hepatobiliary imaging are mainly divided into two categories, namely, ^{99m}Tc-labeled dimethyl-acetanilide-iminodiacetic acids (^{99m}Tc-IDAs) and ^{99m}Tc-labeled pyridoxylideneamino acids (^{99m}Tc-PAAs). ^{99m}Tc-Sn-N-pyridoxy-5-methyltryptophan (^{99m}Tc-PMT) is the most commonly used ^{99m}Tc-PAA. The degree of ^{99m}Tc-PMT concentration in hepatic tumor cells is related to the pathological type and level of differentiation of liver cancers. The imaging process lasts until the late intestinal excretion phase, which is also known as delayed imaging of liver cancer.

6.4.1.4 Hepatic Receptor Imaging (^{99m}Tc-GSA)

Patients with HCC often have concomitant hepatitis and cirrhosis, leading to liver function impairment. Preoperative assessment of liver functional reserve is a basis for determining the extent of surgical resection and selecting an appropriate treatment. Asialoglycoprotein receptors (ASGPRs) are specifically located on the surface of human hepatocytes, and the number of ASGPRs on hepatocytes is closely related to liver function. ^{99m}Tc-galactosyl-human serum albumin (^{99m}Tc-GSA) can be rapidly taken up by hepatocytes and then slowly excreted via the bile and urinary tract. ^{99m}Tc-GSA imaging can be used in combination with single-photon emission computed tomography (SPECT) to extract parameters for liver function assessment, including functional liver volume (FLV), liver uptake ratio (LUR), and liver uptake density (LUD). This imaging modality is not affected by bilirubin levels or hepatic blood flow, thus having a high evaluation accuracy for liver reserve function. Studies have found that ^{99m}Tc-GSA SPECT/CT is used preoperatively for image fusion to simulate surgical resection in HCC patients. In the meantime, the expression level of ASGPR in the residual liver is determined after surgery, which is combined with a postoperative liver function tests. A good correlation is reported between the preoperative and postoperative assessments. Thus, ^{99m}Tc-GSA SPECT/CT imaging proves to be useful for surgical decision-making.

6.4.2 Applications of Positron Emission Tomography (PET), PET/CT, and PET/MR in Liver Cancer Diagnosis

6.4.2.1 Technical Features and Clinical Application and Development of PET, PET/CT, and PET/MR

PET imaging is a functional (metabolic) imaging technique for organs or tissues, using compounds labeled with a positron-emitting radionuclides as the imaging agent. The labeled compounds are mostly analogs of physiologically relevant substances, such as glucose, water, amino acids, and neurotransmitters. PET/CT imaging is a advanced molecular imaging technique that integrates high-sensitivity PET functional imaging with high-spatial-resolution CT imaging. PET/MR is an integration of PET functional imaging and MRI with a high soft-tissue resolution. MRI can provide high-resolution anatomical images and also functional imaging results. These integrated imaging techniques provide imaging on lesion metabolism and receptor function and expression while providing information on precise anatomical structure. At present, the most widely used PET-radiotracer is the glucose analog ^{18}F-fluorodeoxyglucose (^{18}F-FDG).

PET and PET/CT have undergone rapid development in recent years. The first commercial PET scanner was put into clinical use in 1974, and the first commercial PET/CT scanner into clinical use in 2001. The first PET scanner became available in China in 1995 and was soon put into clinical practice. The first PET/CT scanner became available in 2002. In the past 5–10 years, PET/CT has been extensively popularized in China. Impressive progress has also been made in the development and application of domestically made PET/CT equipment.

PET/MR is one of the cutting-edge technologies in functional and molecular imaging. This technology currently features an integration of PET with whole-body 3.0 T MR and real-time synchronous data acquisition. PET/MR not only reduces the radiation dose dramatically but also provides more information for tumor diagnosis. PET/MR was first introduced in China in 2012, and much experience on its use has been gained through team collaboration and clinical applications.

6.4.2.2 Applications of PET/CT and PET/MR in HCC Diagnosis

^{18}F-FDG PET/CT has limited clinical applications and must be used selectively in HCC patients. Moderately differentiated and poorly differentiated HCCs are mostly shown as hypermetabolic lesions by the ^{18}F-FDG PET/CT. This imaging modality has a high value for the diagnosis, staging, efficacy evaluation, and posttreatment recurrence monitoring of hypermetabolic HCC. However, ^{18}F-FDG PET may reveal an absence of significant metabolic abnormalities in highly differentiated HCCs, resulting in missed diagnoses. This technique also has a low diagnostic sensitivity for small HCC. Neither the National Comprehensive Cancer Network (NCCN) guidelines for the diagnosis and treatment of HCC nor the guidelines proposed by the Chinese Society of Nuclear Medicine recommend ^{18}F-FDG PET/CT for early diagnosis of HCC. Whole-body ^{18}F-FDG PET/CT has a high value in determining the causes of significant elevation in serum tumor markers after HCC treatment that are otherwise indeterminable by conventional radiology and in assessing the suitability for liver transplantation.

Guidelines for Diagnosis and Treatment of Primary Liver Cancer in China (2019 Edition) have described the following advantages of whole-body ^{18}F-FDG PET/CT: (1) staging of HCC and comprehensive assessment of any lymph node metastases or distant organ metastases; (2) re-staging of HCC. As functional PET/CT imaging is independent of the influences from the anatomical structure, this imaging modality can clearly show recurrent and metastatic lesions in altered or complex anatomical structures; (3) evaluating therapeutic efficacy. More sensitive and accurate evaluation of the efficacy of antitumor targeted drugs; (4) guiding target volume delineation in radiotherapy and locating the puncture site for biopsy; (5) assessing the malignancy and prognosis of tumors.^{18}F-FDG PET/MRI can acquire the anatomical and functional information of the lesions simultaneously, thereby improving the diagnostic sensitivity for HCC.

The invention of new imaging agents is an key area of PET/CT development. ^{11}C-acetate, a precursor for the synthesis of amino acids and sterol, is involved in intracellular fatty acid metabolism and free from the influence of glucose dephosphorylation. Given high lipid metabolism in tumor cells, ^{11}C-acetate can be concentrated in tumor tissues. Therefore, C-acetate PET/CT has a higher value for the imaging of highly differentiated, low-malignancy HCC than ^{18}F-FDG. Most malignant tumor cells are highly proliferative and hypermetabolic. A high choline content is considered an effective tracer for lipids. ^{11}C-choline has a high affinity for HCC and is mainly used for the imaging of highly and moderately differentiated tumors. ^{11}C-choline can make up for the shortcomings of ^{18}F-FDG imaging in HCC diagnosis. Furthermore, HCC uptake of ^{68}Ga-prostate-specific membrane antigen (PSMA) and ^{68}Ga-somatostatin analog (SSA) during PET/CT imaging have been previously reported. However, given the small number of studied cases, the application of these imaging modalities in HCC diagnosis remains to be further investigated.

6.4.2.3 Applications of PET and PET/CT in the Diagnosis of ICC

Adenocarcinoma is the predominant histologic type of ICC, and the lesion is usually found with an increased uptake on ^{18}F-FDG PET/CT imaging. This technique has greater value and advantages in liver lesion visualization and TNM staging and provides critical information for clinical decision-making. Studies have shown that detecting metastatic lesions can alter treatment strategies for some patients. Some studies have found that 18F-FDG PET/MR can improve the accuracy of the local and systemic staging of ICC compared with conventional radiology, such as CT and MRI, thereby aiding in treatment decision-making in some patients.

6.4.2.4 Applications of PET and PET/CT in the Diagnosis of Metastatic Liver Cancer

The radiographic manifestations and blood supply enhancement pattern of metastatic cancers are complex due to the blood supply characteristics and diverse origins of metastatic tumors in the liver. If a diagnosis cannot be made with CT or MRI, ^{18}F-FDG PET/CT can be considered for whole-body scan and evaluation. PET/CT has unique values in identifying primary lesions and extrahepatic metastases, especially those in hidden positions. This imaging modality is highly valuable for patients with a significant elevation in serum tumor markers but with negative findings on conventional radiology. However, PET/CT has a limited sensitivity for metastatic hepatic tumors <1 cm and should be combined with other imaging techniques.

Suggested Reading

1. Middleton ML. Scintigraphic evaluation of hepatic mass lesions: emphasis on hemangioma detection. Semin Nucl Med. 1996;26(1):4–15.
2. Ho S, Lau WY, Leung WT, et al. Arteriovenous shunts in patients with hepatic tumors. J Nucl Med. 1997;38(8):1201–5.
3. Oyamada H, Yamazaki S, Makuuchi M, et al. Clinical significance of 99mTc-Npyridoxyl-5-methyltryptophan (99mTcPMT) in the diag-

nosis of intrahepatic masses. Radioisotopes. 1989;38(5):244–51.
4. Iimuro Y, Kashiwagi T, Yamanaka J, et al. Preoperative estimation of asialoglycoprotein receptor expression in the remnant liver from CT/99mTc-GSA SPECT fusion images correlates well with postoperative liver function parameters. J Hepatobiliary Pancreat Sci. 2010;17(5):673–81.
5. Kaibori M, Ha-Kawa SK, Maehara M, et al. Usefulness of Tc-99m-GSA scintigraphy for liver surgery. Ann Nucl Med. 2011;25(9):593–602.
6. Ferrone C, Goyal L, Qadan M, et al. Management implications of fluorodeoxyglucose positron emission tomography/magnetic resonance in untreated intrahepatic cholangiocarcinoma. Eur J Nucl Med Mol Imaging. 2020;48(8):1871–84.
7. Kuyumcu S, Has-Simsek D, Iliaz R, et al. Evidence of prostate-specific membrane antigen expression in hepatocellular carcinoma using 68Ga-PSMA PET/CT. Clin Nucl Med. 2019;44(9):702–6.
8. Ulaner GA, Bodei L. Hepatocellular carcinoma mimicking neuroendocrine tumor metastasis on 68Ga-DOTATATE PET/CT. Clin Nucl Med. 2019;44(4):330–1.
9. Yoh T, Seo S, Morino K, et al. Reappraisal of prognostic impact of tumor SUVmax by 18F-FDG-PET/CT in intrahepatic cholangiocarcinoma. World J Surg. 2019;43(5):1323–31.
10. Shen W, Tan B, Guo J. Progress in the application of 3D-CEUS of the liver. Chin J Med Imaging Technol. 2014;30(1):157–60.
11. Claudon M, Dietrich CF, Choi BI, et al. Guidelines and good clinical practice recommendations for contrast enhanced ultrasound (CEUS) in the liver-update 2012: a WFUMB-EFSUMB initiative in cooperation with representatives of AFSUMB, AIUM, ASUM, FLAUS and ICUS. Ultraschall Med. 2013;34(1):11–29.
12. Ji JF, Zhou W, Guo J. Application value of strain ratio in the diagnosis of liver tumors by ultrasonic elastography. World Chin J Digestol. 2010;18(30):3254–8.
13. Ji JF, Zhou W, Guo J, et al. Value of ultrasonic elastography in differentiating benign and malignant liver tumors. Chin J Ultrasound Med. 2011;27(3):243–5.
14. Torre LA, Bray F, Siegel RL, et al. Global cancer statistics, 2012. CA Cancer J Clin. 2015;65(2):87–108.
15. Zhou M, Wang H, Zeng X, et al. Mortality, morbidity, and risk factors in China and its provinces, 1990-2017: a systematic analysis for the Global Burden of Disease Study 2017. Lancet. 2019;394(10204):1145–58.
16. Wang YM, Qian GJ, Xu Z, et al. Efficacy of microwave ablation in the treatment of hepatocellular carcinoma within the Milan criteria: a report of 696 cases. Chin J Hepatol. 2017;25(5):344–8.
17. Bureau of Medical Administration, National Health and Family Planning Commission of the PRC. Guidelines for diagnosis and treatment of primary liver cancer (2017 edition). Chin J Dig Surg. 2017;16(7):635–47.
18. Jiang HY, Chen J, Xia C, et al. Noninvasive imaging of hepatocellular carcinoma: from diagnosis to prognosis. World J Gastroenterol. 2018;24(22):2348–62.
19. Gao H, Gao PY. Development of medical MRI technology and its clinical application in China. Chin J Radiol. 2013;47(1):58–61.
20. Dai JZ, Shen TZ, Chen XR. MRI of primary hepatocellular carcinoma. Foreign Med Sci Clin Radiol Fascicle. 1990;13(2):65–8.
21. Chen B, Murakami T, Shih T, et al. Novel imaging diagnosis for hepatocellular carcinoma: consensus from the 5th Asia-Pacific Primary Liver Cancer Expert Meeting (APPLE 2014). Liver Cancer. 2015;4(4):215–27.
22. Merkle EM, Zech CJ, Bartolozzi C, et al. Consensus report from the 7th International forum for liver magnetic resonance imaging. Eur Radiol. 2016;26(3):674–82.
23. Roberts LR, Sirlin CB, Zaiem F, et al. Imaging for the diagnosis of hepatocellular carcinoma: a systematic review and meta-analysis. Hepatology. 2018;67(1):401–21.
24. Chernyak V, Fowler KJ, Kamaya A, et al. Liver imaging reporting and data system (LI-RADS) version 2018: imaging of hepatocellular carcinoma in at-risk patients. Radiology. 2018;289(3):816–30.
25. Van Beers BE, Daire JL, Garteiser P. New imaging techniques for liver diseases. J Hepatol. 2015;62(3):690–700.
26. Yang C, Wang H, Tang Y, et al. ADC similarity predicts microvascular invasion of bifocal hepatocellular carcinoma. Abdom Radiol. 2018;43(9):2295–302.
27. Yang C, Wang H, Sheng R, et al. Microvascular invasion in hepatocellular carcinoma: is it predictable with a new, preoperative application of diffusion weighted imaging? Clin Imaging. 2017;41:101–5.
28. Parikh T, Drew SJ, Lee VS, et al. Focal liver lesion detection and characterization with diffusion-weighted MR imaging: comparison with standard breath-hold T2-weighted imaging. Radiology. 2008;246(3):812–22.
29. Qu JR, Li HL, Shao N, et al. Additional diffusion-weighted imaging in the detection of new, very small hepatocellular carcinoma lesions after interventional therapy compared with conventional 3 T MRI alone. Clin Radiol. 2012;67(7):669–74.
30. Wu LF, Rao SX, Xu PJ, et al. Pre-TACE kurtosis of ADC total derived from histogram analysis for diffusion-weighted imaging is the best independent predictor of prognosis in hepatocellular carcinoma. Eur Radiol. 2019;29(1):213–23.
31. Zeng MS, Li RK. Clinical application of susceptibility-weighted imaging for studying the multi-step hepatocarcinogenic process of cirrhotic liver nodules. J Clin Hepatol. 2013;29(1):38–41.
32. Ludwig J, Hashimoto E, Porayko MK, et al. Hemosiderosis in cirrhosis: a study of 447 native livers. Gastroenterology. 1997;112(3):882–8.
33. Terada T, Nakanuma Y. Iron-negative foci in siderotic macroregenerative nodules in human cirrhotic liver.

A marker of incipient neoplastic lesions. Arch Pathol Lab Med. 1989;113(8):916–20.
34. Honda H, Kaneko K, Kanazawa Y, et al. MR imaging of hepatocellular carcinomas: effect of Cu and Fe contents on signal intensity. Abdom Imaging. 1997;22(1):60–6.
35. Li RK, Zeng MS, Rao SX, et al. Using a 2D multibreath-hold susceptibility-weighted imaging to visualize intratumoral hemorrhage of hepatocellular carcinoma at 3T MRI: correlation with pathology. J Magn Reson Imaging. 2012;36(4):900–6.
36. Li RK, Zeng MS, Qiang JW, et al. Diagnostic value of susceptibility-weighted imaging in small liver cancers with a cirrhotic background. Chin J Radiol. 2015;49(7):520–4.
37. Li RK, Zeng MS, Qiang JW, et al. Susceptibility-weighted imaging of multistep hepatocarcinogenesis in cirrhotic livers: correlation with pathology. Chin J Radiol. 2013;47(11):1014–8.
38. Song Q, Ma J, Rao SX, et al. Evaluation of microcirculation function status of HCC using 3D-DCE-MRI perfusion of Tofts model. Radiol Pract. 2013;28(6):662–5.
39. Chen J, Qian T, Zhang H, et al. Combining dynamic contrast enhanced magnetic resonance imaging and microvessel density to assess the angiogenesis after PEI in a rabbit VX2 liver tumor model. Magn Reson Imaging. 2016;34(2):177–82.
40. Kierans AS, Kang SK, Rosenkrantz AB. The diagnostic performance of dynamic contrast-enhanced MR imaging for detection of small hepatocellular carcinoma measuring up to 2cm: a meta-analysis. Radiology. 2016;278(1):82–94.
41. Abdominal Group of the Chinese Society of Radiology. Expert consensus on clinical application of hepatobiliary-specific MRI contrast agent Gd-EOB-DTPA. Chin J Radiol. 2016;50(9):641–6.
42. Ding Y, Rao SX, Meng T, et al. Usefulness of T1 mapping on Gd-EOB-DTPA-enhanced MR imaging in assessment of non-alcoholic fatty liver disease. Eur Radiol. 2014;24(4):959–66.
43. Ding Y, Rao SX, Chen C, et al. Potential of Gd-EOB-DTPA-enhanced MR imaging for evaluation of bile duct ligation-induced liver injury in rabbits. Hepatol Int. 2015;9(2):303–9.
44. Ding Y, Rao SX, Zhu T, et al. Liver fibrosis staging using T1 mapping ongadoxetic acid-enhanced MRI compared with DW imaging. Clin Radiol. 2015;70(10):1096–103.
45. Ding Y, Rao SX, Chen C, et al. Assessing liver function in patients with HBV-related HCC: a comparison of T1 mapping on Gd-EOB-DTPA-enhanced MR imaging with DWI. Eur Radiol. 2015;25(5):1392–8.
46. Wu L, Cai HS, Peng XY, et al. Correlation between gadoxetate disodium-enhanced magnetic resonance cholangiography and liver function. Chin J Radiol. 2013;47(8):726–30.
47. Xie S, Ji Q, Hou JC, et al. Influence of liver function on liver enhancement in the hepatobiliary phase during gadoxetate disodium-enhanced MRI. Chin J Radiol. 2014;48(8):655–8.
48. Ding Y, Zeng MS, Rao SX, et al. Assessment on T1 mapping values using gadoxetic acid-enhanced MRI examination in comparison with organic anion transporters and multi-drug resistance proteins values on the hepatocytes on colorectal liver metastases. Chin J Radiol. 2015;49(3):195–8.
49. Liang ML, Zhang L, Zhang JQ, et al. Evaluation of liver function reserve with gadoxetate disodium-enhanced MR. Chin J Radiol. 2013;47(6):522–5.
50. Wang W, Yang C, Zhu K, et al. Recurrence after curative resection of HBV-related hepatocellular carcinoma: diagnostic algorithms on gadoxetic acid-enhanced MRI. Liver Transpl. 2020;26(6):751–63.
51. Zou XL, Hai YC, Shen YQ, et al. Updates of liver imaging report and data system (LI-RADS): an interpretation of the 2018 edition. Radiogr Pract. 2018;33(11):1114–7.
52. Yin DL, Liu LX. Application value of liver imaging reporting and data system in HCC diagnosis. Chin J Dig Surg. 2017;16(2):130–3.
53. Mehmet Emin M, Zhang Q, Wang JX, et al. Comparative analysis of CT and MRI features of hepatocellular carcinoma by using liver imaging reporting and data system (LI-RADS). ModMedImage. 2019;28(1):8–11.
54. Du J, Yang DW, Zhang N, et al. Consistency of MRI sign interpretation of HCC based on the liver imaging reporting and data system. Chin J Med Imaging. 2019;27(7):481–6.
55. Ding Y, Rao SX, Wang WT, et al. Comparison of gadoxetic acid versus gadopentetate dimeglumine for the detection of hepatocellular carcinoma at 1.5 T using the liver imaging reporting and data system (LI-RADS v. 2017). Cancer Imaging. 2018;18(1):48.
56. Hytiroglou P, Park YN, Krinsky G, et al. Hepatic precancerous lesions and small hepatocellular carcinoma. Gastroenterol Clin N Am. 2007;36(4):867–87.
57. Zeng MS, Ye HY, Guo L, et al. Gd-EOB-DTPA-enhanced magnetic resonance imaging for focal liver lesions in Chinese patients: a multicenter, open-label, phase III study. Hepatobiliary Pancreatic Dis Int. 2013;12(6):607–16.
58. Lee YJ, Lee JM, Lee JS, et al. Hepatocellular carcinoma: diagnostic performance of multidetector CT and MR imaging-a systematic review and meta-analysis. Radiology. 2015;275(1):97–109.
59. Renzulli M, Biselli M, Brocchi S, et al. New hallmark of hepatocellular carcinoma, early hepatocellular carcinoma and high-grade dysplastic nodules on Gd-EOB-DTPA MRI in patients with cirrhosis: a new diagnostic algorithm. Gut. 2018;67(9):1674–82.
60. Lambin P, Rios-Velazquez E, Leijenaar R, et al. Radiomics: extracting more information from medical images using advanced feature analysis. Eur J Cancer. 2012;48(4):441–6.
61. Yang L, Gu D, Wei J, et al. A radiomics nomogram for preoperative prediction of microvascular inva-

sion in hepatocellular carcinoma. Liver Cancer. 2019;8(5):373–86.
62. Zhang Z, Jiang H, Chen J, et al. Hepatocellular carcinoma: radiomics nomogram on gadoxetic acid-enhanced MR imaging for early postoperative recurrence prediction. Cancer Imaging. 2019;19(1):22.
63. Chen S, Feng S, Wei J, et al. Pretreatment prediction of immunoscore in hepatocellular cancer: a radiomics-based clinical model based on Gd-EOB-DTPA-enhanced MRI imaging. Eur Radiol. 2019;29(8):4177–87.
64. Oyama A, Hiraoka Y, Obayashi I, et al. Hepatic tumor classification using texture and topology analysis of non-contrast-enhanced three-dimensional T1-weighted MR images with a radiomics approach. Sci Rep. 2019;9(1):8764.
65. Wang HQ, Yang C, Zeng MS, et al. Magnetic resonance texture analysis for the identification of cytokeratin 19-positive hepatocellular carcinoma. Eur J Radiol. 2019;117:164–70.
66. Wang ZG, Zhou WP. Some thoughts on the integrated treatment strategies and multidisciplinary treatment model for different stages of liver cancer. Chin J Hepatobiliary Surg. 2018;26(6):401–4.
67. Professional Committee of Gastrointestinal Tumors of Chinese Research Hospital Association, Professional Committee of Multidisciplinary Integrated Treatment of Chinese College of Surgeons. Expert consensus on multidisciplinary collaborative team care service model for liver and biliary tract cancers. Chin Arch Gen Surg, Electron Ed. 2017;11(1):1–3.
68. Haimerl M, Verloh N, Zeman F, et al. Gd-EOB-DTPA-enhanced MRI for evaluation of liver function: comparison between signal-intensity-based indices and T1 relaxometry. Sci Rep. 2017;7:43347.
69. Zhou ZP, Long L, Qiu WJ, et al. Evaluating segmental liver function using T1 mapping on Gd-EOB-DTPA-enhanced MRI with a 3.0 Tesla. BMC Med Imaging. 2017;17(1):20.
70. Kanda T, Osawa M, Oba H, et al. High signal intensity in dentate nucleus on unenhanced T1-weighted MR images: association with linear versus macrocyclic gadolinium chelate administration. Radiology. 2015;275(3):803–9.
71. Mcdonald RJ, Mcdonald JS, Kallmes DF, et al. Gadolinium deposition in human brain tissues after contrast-enhanced MR imaging in adult patients without intracranial abnormalities. Radiology. 2017;285(2):546–54.
72. Pollard J, Fleischli DJ, Nebesar RA. Angiography of hepatic neoplasms. Semin Roentgenol. 1983;18(2):114–22.
73. Kido C, Sasaki T, Kaneko M. Angiography of primary liver cancer. Am J Roentgenol Radium Therapy, Nucl Med. 1971;113(1):70–81.
74. Jewel KL. Primary carcinoma of the liver: clinical and radiologic manifestations. Am J Roentgenol Radium Therapy, Nucl Med. 1971;113(1):84–91.
75. Lin G. Microvascular structure and blood supply of liver tumors. Chin J Radiol. 1985;19(5):257.
76. Chen XR, Lin G, Duan CX, et al. Selective angiography. Shanghai: Shanghai Science and Technology Press; 1990.
77. Liu Q, Lv TZ. Imaging findings of liver cancer invading the portal vein and the clinical significance. Chin J Radiol. 1991;25(3):152–5.
78. Wang JH, Wang XL, Yan ZP. Abdominal interventional radiology. Shanghai: Shanghai Medical University Press; 1998.
79. Ouyang Y. Digital subtraction angiography diagnostics. Beijing: People's Medical Publishing House; 2000.
80. Li YH. Illustrations of practical interventional diagnostic and therapeutic technologies. Beijing: Science Press; 2002.
81. Duan CX, Wang PJ, Li JD. Hepatobiliary and pancreatic imaging. Shanghai: Shanghai Science and Technology Literature Publishing House; 2004.

7 Advances in the Clinical Staging of Liver Cancer

Zhangjun Cheng and Feng Shen

A clinical staging system for hepatocellular carcinoma (HCC) is usually developed based on the primary liver tumor, the extent of tumor involvement, and the impact of the tumor on prognosis. The staging system can be used for prognostic stratification and describing the severity of malignancy in individuals. Accurate clinical staging of HCC is not only helpful for the formulation of a reasonable treatment procedure and prognostic assessment by clinicians but also for the design of a clinical study, such as subject selection and grouping. There have been various clinical staging systems of HCC. Nearly all of these systems were developed based on HCC cohorts and clinical practice in a specific country or region. By 2018, approximately 20 staging systems of HCC had been proposed worldwide. The multiplicity of the staging systems highlights the fact that a single widely accepted staging system is still lacking and that HCC staging is extremely complicated.

Z. Cheng
Zhongda Hospital Southeast University, Nanjing, China

F. Shen (✉)
Shanghai Eastern Hepatobiliary Surgery Hospital, Shanghai, China

7.1 History of Clinical Staging of HCC

The Okuda staging system proposed by a Japanese group in 1985 is the world's first published clinical staging system for HCC. The American Joint Committee on Cancer (AJCC) and the Union for International Cancer Control (UICC) proposed a separate clinical staging system for HCC in the fifth edition of the TNM staging system in 1997. This TNM system was developed based on the anatomical scope of HCC, namely, the primary tumor (T), node (N), and metastasis (M), and was updated every 6–8 years. The eighth edition is the latest edition released in 2018. The Cancer of the Liver Italian Program (CLIP) published the CLIP staging system in 1998. The Barcelona Clinic Liver Cancer (BCLC) staging system was first proposed in 1999. By 2018, nearly 20 staging systems for HCC had been published worldwide. Apart from the aforementioned staging systems, other classifications include the GRETCH staging system in France, CUPI and HKLC staging systems in Hong Kong, JIS staging system in Japan, MESIAH staging system in the United States, and ITA. LI. CA staging system in Italy. The first recommendation for primary liver cancer staging in China was proposed during the National Collaborative Conference on Liver Cancer Prevention and Treatment Research in 1977. Later, experts in the Committee of Liver Cancer Society of Chinese Anti-Cancer Association

X. Chen (ed.), *Diagnosis and Treatment of Liver Cancer in China*,
https://doi.org/10.1007/978-981-97-7969-7_7

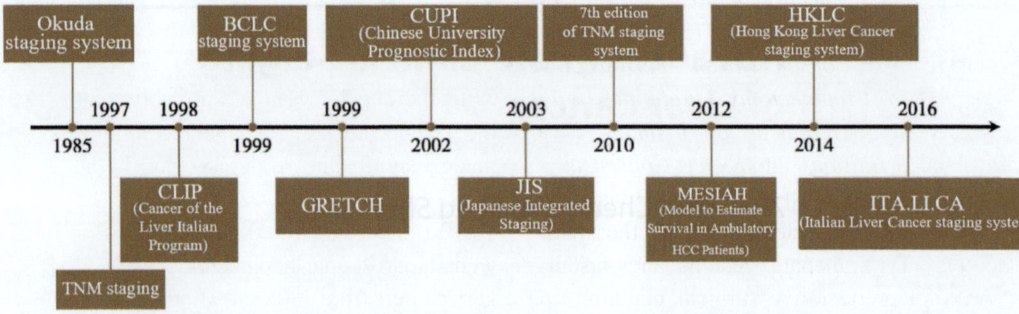

TNM: Tumor, Node, Metastasis; BCLC: Barcelona Clinic Liver Cancer; CRETCH: Groupe d'Etude et de Traitement du Carcinome Hépatocellulaire; CLIP: Cancer of the Liver Italian Program; JIS: Japanese Integrated Staging Score; CUPI: Chinese University Prognostic Index; MESIAH: Model to Estimate Survival in Ambulatory HCC Patients; HKLC: Hong Kong Liver Cancer; ITA.LL.CA: Italian Liver Cancer.

Fig. 7.1 The developmental history of the main clinical staging systems for HCC in the world

developed a new edition of China's clinical staging criteria for primary liver cancer based on the old version published in 1977 and the AJCC/UICC TNM staging system, with incorporation of the modified Child-Pugh score. The new edition was published in September 2001. In 2011, the Ministry of Health (currently the National Health Commission) asked a group of multidisciplinary liver cancer experts to develop the Guidelines for Diagnosis and Treatment of Primary Liver Cancer. The Guidelines were updated in 2017 and 2019, respectively. The Guidelines took into consideration China's national conditions and clinical practice and developed a liver cancer staging system and treatment roadmap. At present, the 2019 Edition has already been put into routine clinical practice (Fig. 7.1).

7.2 Main Parameters Included in the Clinical Staging of HCC

The clinical staging of malignancies is primarily a prognostic stratification based on the difference in patient survival in order to reflect the stage of the disease. However, there are various factors that can impact the prognosis of HCC patients. In addition to factors related to the tumor itself, such as the tumor burden and metastasis (e.g., T, N, and M), liver function, performance status, and complications all have an impact on the selection of HCC treatment, which in turn affects patient prognosis. Furthermore, geography, environment, lifestyle, and race all influence patient prognosis. The clinical staging of HCC is made even more complicated due to the presence of numerous prognostic risk factors. The HCC staging systems currently in use are generally developed based on the aforementioned independent prognostic risk factors. Since different staging systems are based on the observations of independent cohorts, factors that impact prognosis also vary. Therefore, there may be large differences in the variables included in the staging system (Table 7.1).

Table 7.1 Variables included in different major staging systems

	Tumor-related variables							Patient-related variables		Liver function-related variables						Other
Staging	Diameter	Quantity	Macrovascular invasion	Microvascular invasion	Distant metastasis	Lymph node metastasis	AFP	PS score	Age	Modified Child-Pugh score	TBIL	ALB	PT/INR	Ascites	ALP	Creatinine
Okuda	√										√	√		√		
CLIP	√		√				√			√						
BCLC	√	√	√		√			√		√						
HKLC	√	√	√					√		√						
MESIAH	√	√	√		√				√		√	√	√			√
Alberta algorithm	√	√	√		√			√		√						
GRETCH							√				√				√	
CUPI	√				√	√	√				√			√	√	
ITA. LI. CA	√	√	√		√		√	√		√						
JIS	√	√	√		√			√		√						
AJCC TNM	√	√	√		√	√										
Chinese staging system	√	√	√		√			√		√						

Note: *AFP* Alpha-fetoprotein, *PS* performance status, *TBIL* total bilirubin, *ALB* albumin, *PT* prothrombin time, *INR* international normalized ratio, *ALP* alkaline phosphatase

7.3 Characteristics of Different Major Staging Systems

7.3.1 Okuda Staging System

The Okuda staging system published in 1985 included four variables, namely, tumor size, ascites, albumin, and bilirubin, which divided HCCs into three stages. It was the world's first HCC staging system that included liver function and served as an important reference for the development of subsequent HCC staging systems. However, this system was developed at a much earlier time when diagnostic and therapeutic measures were very limited. Tumor size was the only tumor-related factor included, and stratification was performed based only on whether the lesion occupied more than half the liver. Without considering many critical prognostic factors, such as tumor number, vascular invasion, portal vein tumor thrombosis, and extrahepatic metastases, the Okuda system, thus, provided prognostic prediction only suitable for patients with advanced HCC. The accuracy of staging was poor in early HCC patients who are suitable for surgery or other treatments. Moreover, too much weight was assigned to liver function in this system. Excessive emphasis on the impact of liver function on prognosis makes the staging system unable to accurately reflect the tumor burden.

7.3.2 AJCC/UICC TNM Staging

The first edition of the AJCC/UICC TNM staging system was proposed in 1977. The fifth edition, published in 1997, included the first staging system for HCC. After a series of updates, the seventh edition was released in 2010. The eighth edition released in 2018 is currently in clinical use. The TNM system focuses on pathological staging, which involves comprehensive evaluation of the primary tumor (T), lymph node involvement (N), and metastasis (M). The eighth edition of the TNM system placed a greater emphasis on the influence of tumor size, tumor number, vascular invasion, and invasion of adjacent organs on prognosis and refined the T classification. AJCC recommends collecting variables that may influence patient prognosis, such as AFP, histological grade, hepatic fibrosis score, prothrombin time, and serum bilirubin. However, these variables are not included in the staging system. Under the TNM system, postoperative histopathology is usually required to determine N status. Therefore, this system is mainly applicable to the prognostic prediction of HCC patients who undergo surgical treatment such as liver resection and liver transplantation. The TNM system is less extensively used in clinical practice compared with the BCLC staging system because the former only includes tumor burden but does not consider the influence of liver function and tumor markers on prognosis, which affects the accuracy of prognostic prediction. In addition, lymph node metastasis may be hard to assess before surgery. Hence, this system is usually not routinely used to provide disease staging and guide treatment decision-making before surgery.

7.3.3 CLIP Staging

To address the defects of the TNM staging system, the CLIP group proposed the CLIP score in 1998, which provides a more precise quantification of the prognostic effect of different variables. The modified Child-Pugh score is incorporated into this system. The extent of tumor involvement is refined in the CLIP staging system based on the Okuda staging system by including tumor number and extent as well as portal vein tumor thrombosis. In addition, the CLIP staging system also integrates serum AFP, which highlights the importance of tumor biological characteristics in prognostic prediction. Since the CLIP system integrates more prognostic risk factors than the Okuda system, the former can perform a better prognostic stratification with better accuracy. The CLIP system can assist surgeons with clinical decision-making. Patients with a favorable prognosis are selected for curative-intent surgical resection, while those predicted to have a poor prognosis are recommended for other treatments or included in clinical trials to prolong their survival. However, since over 50% of the source patients for the CLIP system underwent transarterial chemoembolization (TACE) or local ablation and only 2.8% of them received surgery, the accuracy of this system in predicting the prognosis of surgically treated patients is still debated. Furthermore, the CLIP system only offers a rough classification of the extent of the tumor, and stratification of early and very early HCC remains difficult. Moreover, given that giant tumor is still a broad concept and cannot be objectively quantified, the accuracy and reliability of the CLIP system still warrant further improvement.

7.3.4 BCLC Staging

The BCLC staging system was proposed by the Barcelona Clinic Liver Cancer (BCLC) Group in 1999 based on the data of patients who received surgical resection or no treatment (Table 7.2). This system was intended for prognostic prediction and treatment decision-making for surgical resection, liver transplantation, and ablation therapy. It offers a more refined classification of tumor burden and includes tumor size, tumor number, vascular invasion, and extrahepatic metastasis. It is the first staging system that integrates general performance status. The BCLC system offers treatment recommendations for each corresponding stage, which enhances its clinical feasibility. This system has been widely accepted in the Western and has been acknowledged by the European Association for the Study of the Liver (EASL) and the American Association for the Study of Liver Diseases (AASLD). The updated edition of the BCLC system provides guidance for the treatment of early and very early HCC. It also serves as a reference for the grouping of patients in clinical trials. However, this system is too stringent on the indication for surgery, which has been challenged by several liver centers throughout the world since its publication. The BCLC system plays down the significance of liver transplantation and local antitumor treatment to make clinical application easier. Due to safety concerns, the BCLC system only recommends TACE or targeted drug therapy for patients with intermediate and advanced-stage HCC who may benefit from surgical treatment. Based on current experience in China, much needs to be done to improve the BCLC system. First, the BCLC system does not consider tumor location, which is a fundamental factor for assessing the resectability of HCC. Data has shown that a favorable tumor location can still ensure R0 resection to provide long-term survival despite its large size. Second, the BCLC system only recommends hepatectomy for very early HCC or some early HCC. However,

Table 7.2 BCLC staging (1999)

Staging	ECOG performance status	Tumor burden	Liver function
A: Early stage			
A1	0	Single	No portal hypertension with normal total bilirubin
A2	0	Single	Portal hypertension with normal total bilirubin
A3	0	Single	Portal hypertension with abnormal total bilirubin
A4	0	Fewer than 3 tumors, each <3 cm	Child-Pugh class A or B
B: Intermediate-stage	0	Multiple tumors, each >3 cm	Child-Pugh class A or B
C: Advanced-stage	1–2	Presence of vascular invasion or extrahepatic distant metastases	Child-Pugh class A or B
D: Terminal-stage	3–4	Any other	Child-Pugh C

Note: *ECOG* Eastern Cooperative Oncology Group

growing data have demonstrated that hepatectomy may also result in better survival outcomes in some selected patients with intermediate and advanced-stage HCC. Third, some patients who are otherwise suitable for liver transplantation are classified as terminal stage. Finally, aside from surgical treatment, the BCLC guidelines do not include radiotherapy or some novel treatments, such as radioembolization with Yttrium-90 microspheres and ^{125}I particle implantation, which are considered to have ideal efficacy in some unresectable HCC. Therefore, the BCLC system is much criticized in Eastern centers, particularly in China.

7.3.5 HKLC Staging

The Hong Kong Liver Cancer (HKLC) staging system was proposed in 2014. Similar to the BCLC system, the HKLC system also incorporates liver function, performance status, and tumor burden. This system emphasizes the importance of performance status scores for staging and provides prognostic stratification for patients with intrahepatic and extrahepatic vascular invasion. In addition, it seeks to overcome the shortcomings of the limitied therapy options of BCLC system and expands the use of surgery and TACE in patients with intermediate or advanced HCC. The HKLC system highlights the role of performance status and recommends making treatment decisions based on performance status and liver function. However, for patients eligible for liver transplantation, performance status is not considered. Compared to the BCLC system, the HKLC system recommends more active treatments for intermediate and advanced HCC. This system assumes that, through rigorous screening, some patients with intermediate or advanced HCC can still benefit from liver resection, liver transplantation, or TACE, making the staging guideline potentially closer to real-world practice. In contrast, the BCLC system recommends only targeted therapy for HCC with portal vein tumor thrombosis (PVTT), and only supportive therapy for patients with terminal-stage disease and poor performance status. Another characteristic of the HKLC system is that it affirms the status of local therapy in the treatment of large or multiple HCCs, while the BCLC system completely denies the status of radiation therapy in HCC treatment. The HKLC system is developed based on single-center retrospective data, and the majority of included cases are hepatitis B-related HCC, thus, further external validation is required for the applicability of this system in other populations, especially Western populations. In addition, the complexity of this staging system affects its convenience for clinical use.

7.3.6 ITA. LI. CA Staging

Italian Liver Cancer (ITA. LI. CA) staging system was issued in 2016. This system was developed based on the data of an Italian multicenter cohort study on HCC and was externally validated in a cohort of more than 2000 patients with HCC from the Taiwan region in China. Although the ITA. LI. CA system was developed based on retrospective analysis, the collection of clinical data was prospective. Moreover, the system provides good prognostic stratification for both the Eastern and Western cohorts. The ITA. LI. CA system stratifies tumor factors by tumor diameter, number, vascular invasion, and extrahepatic metastasis, and also incorporates performance status score and AFP ($\leq$ or $>$1000 ng/mL). AFP is incorporated in the Okuda and the CLIP systems, but not in the BCLC and HKLC systems. Stages 0 and A in the ITA. LI. CA system corresponds to the BCLC stages 0 and A, respectively. Since BCLC stage B does not take into account heterogeneous tumor diameter and number, the ITA. LI. CA system further divides stage B into stages B1, B2, and B3 by tumor diameter and number. Although this makes the staging system relatively complicated, since many studies have confirmed that tumor diameter exceeding 5 cm and tumor number exceeding 3 predict poor prognosis, the subdivision of stage B may help to predict prognosis more accurately. ITA. LI. CA system is developed based on an Italian cohort of patients with HCC mostly caused by viral hepatitis C, and although it has been externally validated in a Taiwan cohort on HCC, the accuracy of its application in Asian patients has yet to be further validated.

7.3.7 Other Clinical Staging Systems for HCC

In addition to the above-mentioned staging systems, there are the French GETCH staging system, the CUPI staging system of the Chinese University of Hong Kong, the American MESIAH staging system, and the Japanese JIS staging system. Each staging system is developed by analyzing the clinicopathological data of the respective HCC population. Due to the heterogeneity of each cohort in terms of factors such as types of liver disease, race, environment, and the tumor itself, as well as the significant difference in treatment means, the variables incorporated in each system differ greatly. Although each staging system provides good prognostic stratification in the respective cohort, it underperforms in other cohorts, and there is not yet a generally recognized staging system worldwide.

7.3.8 Nomogram-Based Clinical Staging of HCC

The above-mentioned HCC staging systems have a common advantage in that patients can be divided into several prognostic subgroups, which is convenient for classification by disease condition. In fact, there is heterogeneity in the disease conditions of patients in each subgroup, and with the increase of treatment options for HCC, the therapies for patients in each subgroup also vary greatly, making it challenging to achieve individualized treatment based on traditional staging. Molecular typing-based prognostic prediction in patients with HCC is still too immature to guide clinical individualized treatment. In view of this, a new disease staging method—nomogram model has attracted great attention in recent years. Nomogram is designed based on modern statistical methods. The key variables affecting prognosis obtained from cohort studies with large sample sizes are quantified based on their weights on prognostic impact and then presented in the form of slide rule.

The advantage of nomogram is that the subgroups in traditional staging systems can be further re-classified, and the prognostic probability of an individual patient can be accurately calculated (Fig. 7.2). A team led by Prof. Feng Shen from the Eastern Hepatobiliary Surgery Hospital, based on the clinicopathological characteristics and tumor biomarkers of subgroup of HCC patients, first in the world, proposed the nomogram stages for predicting survival outcomes of

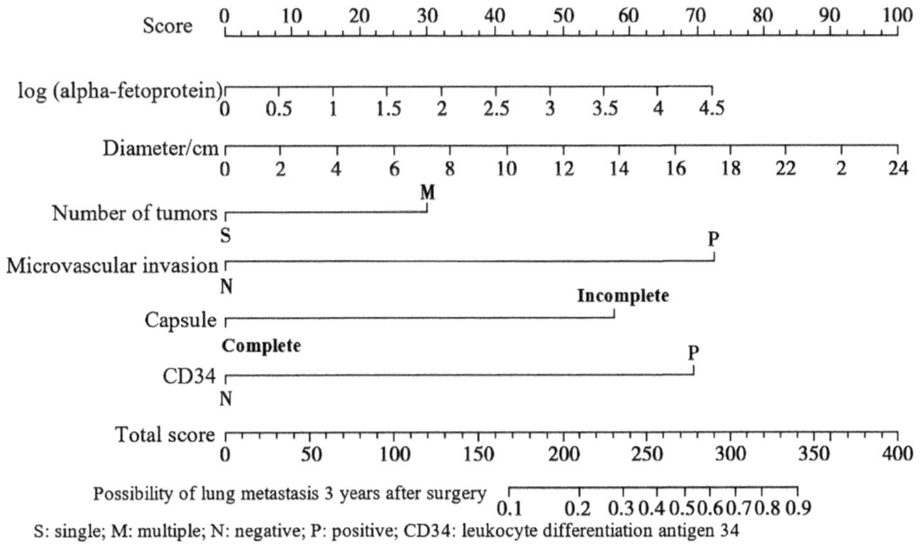

Fig. 7.2 Nomogram for predicting lung metastasis following surgical resection for HCC

patients with early stage HCC (within the Milan criteria), multiple tumors, giant tumors, or recurrent tumors following surgical treatment, guiding the decision that individuals with HCC who do benefit from a certain treatment can be selected for this therapy. In addition, a nomogram can be used to predict the risk probability of occurrence of certain events, such as lung metastasis from HCC, so as to facilitate clinical targeted prevention for individuals at high risk. Therefore, nomogram is an effective and practical staging method to guide individualized treatment for HCC.

7.4 Development of Clinical Staging Systems for HCC in China

7.4.1 Development of Clinical Staging Systems for HCC in China

China accounts for about 50% of the total new cases and deaths from HCC worldwide every year. HCC seriously endangers people's health and life. It is always an urgent task to establish a clinical staging system for HCC suitable for China's national conditions to guide clinical practice. As early as 1977, the National Collaborative Conference on Liver Cancer Prevention and Treatment proposed a clinical staging protocol to divide HCC into three stages: stage I HCC without symptoms or signs, stage III HCC with jaundice, ascites, extrahepatic metastasis or cachexia, and stage II HCC lying somewhere in between. This staging system is simple and easy to master by clinicians. Under the medical conditions at that time, it played a certain role in judging the stage of HCC. However, the staging protocol was only based on symptoms and signs, which is too crude, especially stage II, which has a too broad span. The disease conditions vary greatly in patients at the same stage, so it is difficult to accurately reflect the tumor burden and prognosis. The Society of Liver Cancer of China Anti-Cancer Association proposed clinical staging of HCC in 1998 and 1999. After extensive consultation, the "Criteria for Clinical Diagnosis and Staging of Primary Liver Cancer" was formally adopted at the eighth National Conference of Liver Cancer in 2001. These staging criteria were developed based on the Chinese HCC staging criteria in 1977, and in combination with the TNM staging system, modified Child-Pugh score for liver function and imaging examination results. The Eastern Hepatobiliary Surgery Hospital proposed the Eastern staging system for resectable HCC in 2011, incorporating variables such as tumor size, number, macrovascular invasion, microvascular invasion, extrahepatic metastasis, performance status score, and liver function, etc., which has certain clinical significance. During this period, the Chinese Guidelines for the Diagnosis and Treatment of Primary Liver Cancer (2011 Edition) were formulated, advocating multidisciplinary and comprehensive treatment focusing on surgery. However, the Guidelines did not put forward its own staging criteria for HCC but referred to the BCLC system and the TNM staging system. The Chinese staging protocol and corresponding treatment recommendations were put forward in the revised Guidelines for the Diagnosis and Treatment of Primary Liver Cancer in 2017 and 2019.

7.4.2 Staging System Proposed by the Guidelines for the Diagnosis and Treatment of Primary Liver Cancer (2019 Edition)

There are significant differences between Chinese and Western HCC patients in etiology, biological behavior of tumors, therapies, etc. Hepatitis B virus (HBV) remains the major etiology for HCC in China. Most patients have a history of HBV infection and cirrhosis, with poor liver functional reserve, and are diagnosed with intermediate or advanced-stage HCC. In addition, some regions are economically underdeveloped. All of these affect the choice of treatment and prognosis. Therefore, Western staging and treatment recommendations are not entirely suitable for the national conditions and clinical practice in China. For example, the BCLC staging system is too strict. Some patients with surgically resectable HCC can only receive palliative treatment such as intervention and chemotherapy. The TNM system is based on primary tumor, lymph node metastasis, and the status of distant metastasis, which is often used as postoperative pathological staging and of little use for guiding treatment decision-making. Based on the experience accumulated in clinical practice and the specific national conditions in China, and by referring to some critical clinical staging systems for HCC in the world, the Guidelines for the Diagnosis and Treatment of Primary Liver Cancer (2019 edition) stages HCC according to the patient's performance status, liver function, extrahepatic metastasis, vascular invasion, tumor number, tumor size, etc., and provides corresponding treatment recommendations for patients at different stages (see Fig. 4.3).

Compared with commonly used HCC staging systems in foreign countries, the remarkable features of the Chinese HCC staging system are its the corresponding relaxation of surgical resection and correspondingly relaxes the applicable conditions for liver transplantation. As such, Chinese system provides patients in relatively good general condition but with large tumors (>5 cm), multiple tumors (≥4), or even vascular invasion with the opportunity for curative treatment such as surgery or ablation, which is expected to improve the prognosis of such patients. The past decade has witnessed a spurt of progress in the comprehensive treatment for HCC. The 2019 staging system stresses the importance of multimodal and multidisciplinary comprehensive treatment for HCC, avoiding monotherapy or overtreatment. It forms a set of HCC staging and treatment option systems tailored for HCC patients in China, with good authority and operability, and will play a role in further improving the overall treatment outcome of HCC.

7.5 Prospects

Not only accuracy but also strong practicability and convenience are required for good cancer staging. The incorporation of multiple prognostic variables in a staging system can contribute to improved prediction accuracy, but overcomplicating the staging will impair clinical practicability. Conversely, a simple staging system is more convenient but less accurate. At present, there is no one HCC staging system that is widely accepted and applied at home and abroad. The reasons are that multiple factors, such as the type of liver disease, environment, lifestyle, and genetic background, cause high heterogeneity of HCC and differences in treatment, which further hurt the universality of clinical staging of HCC. In today's era of precision medicine and big data, the continuous emergence of new treatment concepts, technologies, and drugs, as well as more evidence on HCC treatment, will promote the continuous update of the clinical staging of HCC. In the future, domestic colleagues should actively participate in exchanges and cooperation, conduct multicenter randomized controlled studies and basic research, strengthen data sharing, and promote the continuous improvement of the HCC staging system in China. On this basis, and in combination with molecular typing, we can achieve individualized and accurate staging of HCC, finally further promoting the standardization and rationalization of HCC treatment and improving the efficacy in HCC patients.

Suggested Reading

1. Kuda K, Ohtsuki T, Obata H, et al. Natural history of hepatocellular carcinoma and prognosis in relation to treatment. Study of 850 patients. Cancer. 1985;56(4):918–28.
2. Sobin LH. International union against cancer (UICC). In: TNM classification of malignant tumors. 5th ed. New York: Wiley; 1997.
3. Llovet JM, Bru C, Bruix J. Prognosis of hepatocellular carcinoma: the BCLC staging classification. Semin Liver Dis. 1999;19(3):329–38.
4. Yau T, Tang VY, Yao TJ, et al. Development of Hong Kong liver cancer staging system with treatment stratification for patients with hepatocellular carcinoma. Gastroenterology. 2014;146(7):1691–700.e1693.
5. Farinati F, Vitale A, Spolverato G, et al. Development and validation of a new prognostic system for patients with hepatocellular carcinoma. PLoS Med. 2016;13(4):e1002006.

6. Li J, Liu Y, Yan Z, et al. A nomogram predicting pulmonary metastasis of hepatocellular carcinoma following partial hepatectomy. Br J Cancer. 2014;110(5):1110–7.
7. Yang T, Zhang J, Lu JH, et al. A new staging system for resectable hepatocellular carcinoma: comparison with six existing staging systems in a large Chinese cohort. J Cancer Res Clin Oncol. 2011;137(5):739–50.
8. Bureau of Medical Administration, National Health Commission of the People's Republic of China. Guidelines for the diagnosis and treatment of primary liver cancer (2017 edition). Chin J Hepatol. 2017;25(12):886–95.
9. Bureau of Medical Administration, National Health Commission of the People's Republic of China. Guidelines for the diagnosis and treatment of primary liver cancer (2019 edition). Chin J Pract Surg. 2020;40(2):121–38.
10. Li J, Zhou J, Yang PH, et al. Nomograms for survival prediction in patients undergoing liver resection for hepatitis B virus related early stage hepatocellular carcinoma. Eur J Cancer. 2016;62(5):86–95.
11. Li Y, Xia Y, Li J, et al. Prognostic nomograms for pre- and postoperative predictions of long-term survival for patients who underwent liver resection for huge hepatocellular carcinoma. J Am Coll Surg. 2015;221(5):962–74.
12. Yang P, Qiu J, Li J, et al. Nomograms for pre- and postoperative prediction of long-term survival for patients who underwent hepatectomy for multiple hepatocellular carcinomas. Ann Surg. 2016;263(4):778–86.

Liver Cancer Pathology in China

8

Wenming Cong, Yuan Ji, Guoping Wang, and Jia Chen

China is one of the countries with the highest incidence of HCC globally. The number of patients undergoing surgical resection or receiving pathological diagnoses ranks among the highest worldwide, leading to extensive expertise in HCC clinical-pathological diagnosis and research. Advances in hepatic surgical techniques and tumor molecular pathology have driven significant progress in HCC clinical-pathological studies. Especially in the past decade, the accuracy and standardization of pathological diagnosis of HCC have been significantly improved in China in terms of standardization of liver tumor specimen sampling protocol, regularization of histopathological diagnosis, modeling of immunopathological diagnosis, refinement of molecular pathology diagnosis, etc. The primary objectives of the ongoing development of HCC pathology in China are to address the requirements for individualized clinical treatment aimed at enhancing the long-term survival outcomes of HCC patients. Additionally, there is an emphasis on establishing a standardized pathological diagnosis system for HCC that incorporates Chinese characteristics and expertise. Furthermore, the promotion and implementation of Practice Guidelines for the Pathological Diagnosis of Liver Cancer are vital, underscoring the clinically oriented foundational development strategy and concepts guiding HCC pathology in China.

Based on the expert consensus on *Practice Guidelines for the Pathological Diagnosis of Primary Liver Cancer of China* (2010 edition), the experts in HCC pathology and clinical-related disciplines in China formulated the *Practice Guidelines for the Pathological Diagnosis of Primary Liver Cancer of China* (2015 edition) in 2015. The Practice Guidelines for the Pathological Diagnosis of Liver Cancer (2015 edition), published by the Institute for Hospital Management of the National Health Commission, and the Guidelines for the Diagnosis and Treatment of Primary Liver Cancer (2019/2022 edition) by the National Health Commission of China, incorporate new core pathological diagnostic indicators. These updates represent significant advancements in the establishment of pathological diagnostic criteria that reflect the specialized characteristics of HCC. This section aims to summarize the main advances in clinical pathology of HCC in China in the past decade from the following aspects.

W. Cong (✉) · J. Chen
Shanghai Eastern Hepatobiliary Surgery Hospital, Shanghai, China
e-mail: wmcong@smmu.edu.cn

Y. Ji
ZhongShan Hospital Fudan University, Shanghai, China

G. Wang
Tongji Hospital of Huazhong University of Science and Technology, Wuhan, China

X. Chen (ed.), *Diagnosis and Treatment of Liver Cancer in China*,
https://doi.org/10.1007/978-981-97-7969-7_8

8.1 Establishment of a New "7-Point" Baseline Sampling Protocol for HCC Specimens

For an extended period, there has been no consensus regarding standard criteria for the collection of gross specimens of HCC both domestically and internationally. There is significant inconsistency in the collection purpose of liver tumor specimens and great arbitrariness in the sampling method. For example, in 2003, Dr. Torbenson from the United States put forward a 3-point sample collection protocol for gross specimens, mainly aimed at qualitative diagnosis of HCC. However, it can no longer meet the current clinical needs to understand the biological invasive characteristics of HCC, such as the presence and distribution of microvascular invasion (MVI), which is an important pathological factor leading to postoperative recurrence and metastasis of HCC patients. In 2011, Fujita et al. from Japan introduced a methodology for representing the number of postoperative HCC specimens with 1–30 sections per case. The larger the tumor diameter is, the more sections will be taken. However, the authors did not explain whether sampling of the HCC tissue itself could meet the requirement for detecting the presence of MVI, nor did they make a correlation comparison with the MVI detection rate and the number of specimens. Therefore, the detection efficiency of this protocol for MVI is still unknown. In 2009, American scholar Roayaie et al. proposed to examine at least 10 sections from nontumor liver tissue for each case with HCC, but did not compare the correlation between the number of sections and the rate of MVI detection either. A significant advancement in the Chinese Practice Guidelines for the Pathological Diagnosis of Liver Cancer (2015 edition) is the application of the theory of heterogeneous biological behaviors of HCC to guide the collection of gross specimens. It proposes that the junction of cancer and peri-cancerous liver tissue is a representative region of heterogeneity of HCC, a dangerous region where highly invasive cell population are concentrated, a high-incidence region for MVI and satellite nodules, and a high-risk region that affects tumor metastasis, recurrence, and prognosis. Therefore, the junction of cancer and peri-cancerous liver tissue should be taken as a key region for specimen collection. Accordingly, the *Practice Guidelines for the Pathological Diagnosis of Liver Cancer* (2015 edition) introduced a significant update to the traditional pathological diagnostic framework for HCC, with more emphasis on the evaluation of biological behaviors such as the presence of MVI instead of excessive description of the common morphological characteristics of HCC tissue in the pathological diagnosis report, and more focus on sample collection on highly invasive region at the junction of cancer and peri-cancerous hepatic tissues instead of interior of cancer tissues, for improving the diagnostic accuracy of MVI.

According to a study on the correlation of the location and number of HCC specimens with the detection rate of MVI, the "7-point" baseline sampling protocol for HCC specimens has been identified as the most efficient method for MVI detection, with the following key points: (1) at 12, 3, 6, and 9 o'clock of tumor specimens should be collected from the junction of cancer and peri-cancerous hepatic tissues for observing tumor invasiveness, including capsule penetration, microvessel involvement, and infiltration into adjacent hepatic tissues (2) at least one specimen should be collected at the intratumoral region for molecular pathological examination; (3) at least one specimen should be collected at the adjacent peri-cancerous hepatic tissues (defined as ≤1 cm from the tumor capsule), as well as at distant peri-cancerous hepatic tissues (defined as >1 cm from the tumor capsule) for observing the microscopic lesions and background liver diseases (e.g., fibrosis and cirrhosis); (4) for small HCC nodule ≤3 cm in diameter, the entire tumor tissues can be collected for examination; (5) when collecting tumor specimens, the number and location of sections should be adjusted according to the tumor size, number, and the extent of lesions in the peri-cancerous hepatic tissues.

The main purpose of implementing the "7-point" baseline sampling protocol for HCC is to optimize the detection efficiency of MVI by carefully balancing interrelated constraints, including the number of sections, sampling points, time cost, and medical cost. Of note, the "7-point" sampling protocol is a baseline protocol, and the actual sampling point and number of sections can be adjusted based on the tumor diameter and number as well as the size of the peri-cancerous hepatic tissues. Since the detection rate of MVI and satellite nodes is closely related to the extent of surgical resection of peri-cancerous hepatic tissues, a certain range of resection should be preserved during surgery. However, it is important to note that the "7-point" sampling protocol and MVI examination are not applicable to HCC without obvious peri-cancerous hepatic tissues. One of the fundamental goal for designing the "7-point" sampling protocol is to optimize MVI detection efficiency with limited sections thereby reducing the workload for pathologists, minimizing costs for the pathology departments and avoiding significant increases in medical expenses. By focusing on key sampling points, this approach provides a deeper understanding of HCC's biological behavior and offers a robust pathological foundation for guiding postoperative adjuvant treatment.

It is evident that accurate and reliable detection of MVI in HCC can only be achieved when pathological diagnosis is based on standardized sampling protocols. It can be expected that the clinical studies on MVI of HCC will grow rapidly. In China, the Practice Guidelines for the Pathological Diagnosis of Liver Cancer (2015 edition) have played a pivotal role in standardizing liver tumor specimen collection. Since their promulgation in 2015, the Chinese liver tumor specimen collection standard has been widely implemented on a large scale, yielding encouraging preliminary results.

Notably, there is currently no internationally unified standard for the collection of gross specimens of HCC, with a certain degree of subjectivity and arbitrariness in the location and number of specimens. More than 700 research papers related to MVI of HCC are now available in PubMed, but almost none explicitly mentions the method for collecting gross specimens of HCC, which is an unavoidable problem to explain the MVI detection rate and the reliability of relevant study conclusions. An international multicenter STORM trial on HCC published in 2015 involved 900 surgical cases submitted by 202 medical centers across 28 countries between August 2008 and November 2010. Given no consensus on pathological diagnosis criteria for MVI and collection standards for gross specimens of HCC at that time, it could not be ruled out that this lack of standardization raises the possibility of baseline pathological data deviations among the included cases, which may have a significant influence on the negative research results. Therefore, high-quality clinical studies on HCC should be based on high-level pathological standards. Integrating HCC diagnosis and treatment standards with the molecular biological characteristics of tumors, particularly their metastatic and invasive behaviors, is essential for guiding individualized clinical practice. Therefore, the *Practice Guidelines for the Pathological Diagnosis of Liver Cancer of China* have aroused great attention since their publication. The National Health Commission has actively promoted the training and implementation of the *Practice Guidelines for the Pathological Diagnosis of Liver Cancer* in the pathology departments of hospitals nationwide. For pathology departments, early implementation of the "7-point" baseline sampling and MVI grading protocol for HCC contributes to the accumulation of valid and reliable pathological data as early as possible, which will provide valuable references for individualized HCC treatment. In addition, it is necessary to integrate pathology into clinical practice—such as initiative and detailed marking and description of the blood flow direction and the resection margin sites in gross specimens—enhances the accuracy of sampling and the precision of pathological diagnosis.

8.2 Establishment of a New Protocol for Pathological Diagnosis and Grading of Microvascular Invasion

The most fundamental feature of malignant tumor is metastasis. According to statistical data, cancer metastasis is to blame for 90% of cancer deaths. There are 841,000 new cases and 782,000 deaths of HCC in the world annually, while China accounts for more than 50% of both. As early as 2008, Prof. Zhaoyou Tang pointed out that the 5-year survival rate for small HCC resection in China had not significantly improved over the preceding 20 years, mainly due to the high rate of postoperative metastasis and recurrence. Studies on HCC from a biological point of view offer fresh clinical insights, as the 5-year cumulative recurrence rate of HCC after surgical resection exceeds 60%, which has become the "eye of the storm" that seriously decreases the HCC prognosis. Therefore, the biological characteristics of invasion and metastasis of HCC have become the most critical pathological factors of clinical concern. In the past, conventional pathology focused predominantly on the qualitative diagnosis of hepatic tumors, emphasizing tissue structure and cell morphology while paying less attention to pathological biological behaviors. As a result, the information on biological characteristics of HCC had failed to meet the clinical requirement for individualized treatment to a certain extent.

In view of this situation, in recent years, pathologists in China have actively explored the establishment of a standardized diagnostic indicator system for HCC, focusing on MVI as a major histological feature in specialized pathological diagnosis. As a hypervascular tumor with dual blood supply, HCC is highly prone to develop MVI, which is the most essential pathological basis for the occurrence of postoperative recurrence. However, the importance of MVI diagnosis in HCC has historically been underemphasized, with a long-standing lack of unified pathological diagnostic criteria both domestically and internationally. The World Health Organization (WHO) pathological classification of HCC and many international guidelines for the diagnosis and treatment of HCC did not include MVI as a routine indicator of pathological diagnosis either. The MVI grading protocol proposed by Sumie et al. mainly classifies MVI into no MVI, mild MVI (1–5 MVI), and severe MVI (>5 MVI) based on the number of MVI. However, this protocol failed to take into account the indicators of distribution distance or extent of MVI, nor is it based on standardized HCC sampling. As a result, it provides limited guidance for understanding the true degree of HCC invasion.

Fujita et al. proposed that classification should be based on cancer cell count. MVI cell count of more than 50 represents a high-risk state. However, cancer cell counting is inconvenient in routine pathological diagnosis. Roayaie et al. suggested that, for MVI grouping, at least 10 sections from nontumor hepatic tissues for each HCC case should be specially stained with trichrome to identify whether cancer has invaded the muscular layer of the blood vessel wall. If such invasion is detected, it should be further confirmed by immunohistochemical staining with anti-smooth muscle actin antibody, as one of the important indexes for predicting prognosis. However, special staining and immunohistochemical labeling of multiple tissue sections are labor-intensive and time-consuming, making this method impractical for routine pathological diagnosis. Moreover, a critical limitation of this method is that it may miss cases where the cancer has thoroughly destroyed the vascular wall. In a multicenter study on MVI by Hidaka et al., microportal invasion and microhepatic vein invasion were differentiated and grouped by experienced pathologists in each participating center. Since HCC often involves branches of portal vein and hepatic vein at the same time, these structures may be very similar in diameter, cell morphology, and distribution of vessels, making it quite difficult for even experienced hepatic pathologists to differentiate them. Therefore, this indicator is not suitable for routine pathological diagnosis.

One of the highlights of the *Practice Guidelines for the Pathological Diagnosis of Liver Cancer* of China is the provision of pathological diagnosis criteria and grading protocol of MVI of HCC based on the current research results and the practical experience in China, with the following key points: (1) MVI is defined as the presence of solid cancer cell clusterswithin endothelial-lined vascular spaces, primarily observed in portal vein branches in peri-cancerous liver tissues or vessels within the tumor capsule. (2) Pathological grading should be based on the number and distribution distance of

MVI. M0:no MVI; M1 (low-risk group): ≤5 MVI, located within the adjacent peri-cancerous hepatic tissues (≤1 cm away from the tumor capsule); M2 (high-risk group): >5 MVI, or any one located within the distant peri-cancerous hepatic tissues (beyond 1 cm away from the tumor capsule). (3) In cases where histological differentiation between MVI and satellite nodules is challenging, both entities may be interpreted as sequential manifestations of HCC metastasis and collectively classified as MVI. The tumor thrombus in bile duct, artery, and lymphatic vessel has different clinical significance, and should be described by classification, avoiding the use of the vague diagnosis description of "tumor thrombus in blood vessel."

More and more studies have shown that MVI is an independent risk factor of the prognosis of patients with HCC, an important predictor for evaluating the risk of postoperative recurrence of HCC, a momentous pathological indication for implementing postoperative adjuvant treatment for HCC, and also a crucial pathological basis for developing anti-recurrence treatment regimen for HCC. The *Practice Guidelines for the Pathological Diagnosis of Liver Cancer* of China provide simple, practical, and standardized diagnostic criteria and grading protocols for MVI, designed to enhance practicality and operability for pathologists. These guidelines aim to facilitate the accurate diagnosis and precise grading of MVI, enabling pathologists to integrate these assessments into routine and standardized pathological reporting. Clinicians should be able to objectively evaluate the prognosis and scientifically formulate individualized anti-recurrence and metastasis treatment regimen based on pathological grading of MVI.

A multicenter study using big pathological data of HCC in China is currently being carried out by the Liver Cancer Pathology Group of China, including 53,000 HCC patients who underwent surgical resection across 31 centers. The preliminary findings revealed that the overall detection rate of MVI has increased from 27.4% before using the *Practice Guidelines for the Pathological Diagnosis of Liver Cancer* of China to 38.3% after its application. Meanwhile, 74.2% of the centers have adopted both the "7-point" sampling and MVI grading protocol. Accordingly, it can be deduced that the overall level of standardized pathological diagnosis of HCC in China has been fundamentally improved.

8.3 Development of a New Strategy for Molecular Pathology Diagnosis of Clonal Origin in Multiple and Postoperative Recurrent HCC

The aggressive local spread and distant metastasis of HCC are the primary pathological mechanisms leading to high postoperative recurrence rate and poor long-term efficacy of HCC. Data have shown that metastasis is responsible for more than 90% of cancer deaths. The postoperative 5-year recurrence rate of HCC amounts to as high as 60–90%, which has become a bottleneck seriously restricting the long-term efficacy. According to incomplete statistics from the Department of Pathology of the Eastern Hepatobiliary Surgery Hospital, there was 830 surgically resected cases of recurrent HCC (RHCC) in the hospital from 1985 to 2011, including many patients receiving multiple resections due to repeated recurrences. The development of RHCC was previously considered an indication of metastasis and progress into advanced stage of HCC, often deemed no chance of radical treatment. However, with the evolving understanding of tumor cell clonal origin theory, more evidences have demonstrated that the origin of RHCC can be classified into two patterns: multicentric occurrence (MO)/polyclonal origin, and intrahepatic metastasis (IM)/monoclonal origin. However, the two patterns of clonal origin of RHCC are difficult to be distinguished by clinical manifestations and histomorphological observation. Therefore, the study of the clonal origin pattern of RHCC, the search for molecular markers for distinguishing tumor clones, and the establishment of the corresponding molecular pathology testing technique should be emphasized. These efforts are not only important theoretical issues, but also clinical practical problems that are essential for for understanding the characteristics of RHCC clonal origin, developing individualized treatment strategies scientifically, and improving the therapeutic level and long-term survival of RHCC patients.

A study from China revealed that at least 70–75% of RHCC had an IM/monoclonal origin, suggesting that it originated from tumor residue or intrahepatic metastasis after surgical resection. Conversely, 25–30% of RHCC had a MO/polyclonal origin, indicating that it originated from nascent tumor cell clones. These findings provide a valuable reference for clinical evaluation of the origin of RHCC. RHCC may originate from either a MO/polyclonal origin or a MI/monoclonal origin, with six molecular clonal subtypes, including type I, uninodular MO-RHCC; type II, uninodular IM-RHCC; type III, uninodular IM-RHCC with intrahepatic metastatic nodule; type IV, multinodular MO-RHCC; type V, uninodular MO-RHCC with intrahepatic metastatic nodule; and type VI, uninodular MO-RHCC combined with IM-RHCC nodules. The above results indicate the complexity and diversity of the origin of RHCC, so it is necessary to explore individualized treatment strategies.

Currently, recurrence of HCC within 2 years after surgical resection is clinically referred to as "early recurrence," which is considered as metastasis originating from the same clone as the primary tumor. Conversely, recurrence beyond 2 years of resection is defined as "late recurrence," which is deemed a nascent tumor. However, this understanding may need to be changed because residual cancer cells can remain dormant for years after leaving the primary tumor site, adapting to the new tumor microenvironment before reactivating and growing at metastatic sites. We found that a RHCC occurring at 8 years after surgery could still be of an IM-type origin, indicating that residual cancer cells can lurk at the metastatic site in a state of "dormancy" for a long time and recover under appropriate conditions. Therefore, attention should be paid to the development of a new approach to clinical individualized treatment based on the new molecular testing of the clonal origin patterns of RHCC.

At the 13th National Conference of Liver Cancer (2011), the Eastern Hepatobiliary Surgery Hospital reported five distinct clonal origin patterns in liver cancer tissue: (1) mixed HCC and ICC within a single nodule (monoclonal origin with bidirectional differentiation); (2) independent HCC and ICC in dual nodules (dual primary foci of dual clonal origins); (3) dual-phenotype HCC expressing both HCC and ICC markers (monoclonal origin); (4) tumors of different types or different tissue origins successively occur in the liver (epithelium + mesenchyme, polyclonal and polyembryonic origin); and (5) extrahepatic metastases accompany HCC (heterochronous multiple primary tumors). Chinese scholars have established a microsatellite-based detection technique of loss of heterozygosity for identifying the clonal pattern of HCC based on paraffin tissue microdissection. This technique can serve as a new detection method to clinically judge the origin pattern of RHCC and make individualized diagnosis and treatment strategy. At the 24th Conference of the Chinese Society of Pathology (2018), Dr. Jia Chen from the Eastern Hepatobiliary Surgery Hospital presented findings from 119 cases of binodular HCC, analyzed using polymerase chain reaction-single strand conformation polymorphism (PCR-SSCP) combined with capillary electrophoresis. The results demonstrated that MVI occurred in 71.2% of binodular HCC of monoclonal origin and 48.3% of binodular HCC of polyclonal origin. There was a significant correlation between clonal origin and MVI ($P = 0.038$). It is suggested that the analysis of the clonal origin pattern of multinodular HCC is conducive to prognostic evaluation and formulation of individualized treatment regimen.

As mentioned before, a study published by Chinese scholars in 2015 showed that RHCC can be classified into two major types: IM (25–30%) and MO (70–75%), with six molecular clonal subtypes. Further analysis revealed that the above six subtypes of clonal origin are applicable to both RHCC as well as multinodular HCC. Overall, the survival rate of MO-RHCC is significantly superior to that of IM-RHCC following re-resection. In principle, IM-RHCC results from the recurrence of residual tumor following the first resection of HCC and is often accompanied by formation of MVI or satellite node. Comprehensive treatment options including intervention therapies (e.g., radiofrequency ablation, hepatic arterial embolization/chemotherapy) and targeted drugs, are generally recommended for treating IM-RHCC. On the contrary, MO-RHCC is essentially a nascent tumor, and more suitable to be treated by re-operative resection or liver transplantation.

8.4 Recommended Scheme of Immunohistochemical Marker Profile in Diagnosis of HCC

The focus of immunohistochemical diagnosis has gradually transformed from auxiliary qualitative diagnosis (lesion nature: benign, malignant; tissue origin: hepatocyte/cholangiocyte/extrahepatic metastasis) to early diagnosis (high-grade dysplastic nodules/early well-differentiated small HCC) and stratified diagnosis (risk of metastasis and recurrence/evaluation of long-term prognosis).

8.4.1 International Marker Profile

The immunohistochemical markers for diagnosis of HCC proposed by the American Association for the Study of Liver Diseases include glypican-3 (GPC-3), heat shock protein 70 (Hsp70), and glutamine synthetase (GS). For small nodules in cirrhotic tissue, positive testing for at least two markers above is highly specific for the diagnosis of HCC.

8.4.2 Domestic Consensus

The immunohistochemical markers for diagnosis of HCC recommended in the *Practice Guidelines for the Pathological Diagnosis of Liver Cancer* in China mainly include: (1) hepatocyte antigen (Hep Par-1, hepatocyte-specific, with no ability to distinguish the nature of hepatocellular neoplasms); (2) glypican-3 (GPC-3); (3) CD34 (with the ability to mark tumor neovascularization); (4) polyclonal carcinoembryonic antigen (pCEA, hepatocyte-specific, with no ability to distinguish the nature of hepatocellular neoplasms); (5) CD10 (hepatocyte-specific, with no ability to distinguish the nature of hepatocellular neoplasms); (6) arginase-1 (hepatocyte-specific, with no ability to distinguish the nature of hepatocellular neoplasms); (7) HSP70; (8) GS; and (9) AFP. ICC: (1) cytokeratin CK19 and CK7; (2) mucin-1 (MUC-1). Hep Par-1, GPC-3, GS, and CD34 are recommended as the first-line antibodies are recommended for immunohistochemical diagnosis of HCC. CK19/CK7 and MUC-1 as the first-line antibodies are recommended for immunohistochemical diagnosis of ICC. The above profiles can basically solve the practical problems of routine pathological diagnosis of hepatic tumors.

It was reported overexpression of DUSP6 in HCC tissues could negatively regulate phosphorylated extracellular signal-regulated kinase (pERK), which may promote tumor proliferative activity. Kynurenine-3-monooxygenase (KMO) can serve as a new prognostic marker for HCC, as well as differential diagnosis from non hepatocellular tumors. The leukemia inhibitory factor receptor (LIFR) combined with CD34 can be used for differential diagnosis of well-differentiated HCC and high-grade dysplastic nodules. At present, these indicators have not yet been applied in clinical practice.

8.5 Establishment of a New Histopathological Classification System of Liver Tumors

The classic *Histologic Classification of Liver and Intrahepatic Bile Duct Cancers* formulated by WHO contains about 30 types of lesions, which cannot yet fully reflect the diversity and complexity of hepatobiliary tumors. Based on the large-scale cohort study on human hepatic tumors, Chinese pathologists put forward a new histological classification system of hepatobiliary tumors involving over 100 types of lesions, which are divided into "three types" (tumor-like lesions, benign tumors, and malignant tumors) and "six subtypes" (hepatocellular lesions; cholangiocellular lesions; muscular, fibrous and adipose tissues; vascular, lymphoid and hemopoietic tissues; neural and neuroendocrine tissues; and miscellaneous tissues). Among hepatic space-occupying lesions surgically resected in the Eastern Hepatobiliary Surgery Hospital, tumor-like lesions account for 4.3%, with the top three cases being focal nodular hyperplasia (51.5%), hepatic solitary necrotic nodules (19.6%), and hepatic inflammatory pseudotumor (12.0%); benign tumors account for 12.1%, with the top three cases being hepatic cavernous hemangioma (82.9%), hepatic angiomyolipoma (4.0%), and hepatocellular adenoma (3.9%); and malignant tumors account for 83.7%, with the top three cases being HCC (90.2%), ICC (8.2%), hepatoblastoma (0.1%), and undifferentiated (embryonal) sarcoma of the liver (0.1%).

Since hepatic angiomyolipoma (HAML) was first reported by the Department of Pathology of the Eastern Hepatobiliary Surgery Hospital in 1992, the total number of HAML diagnoses has exceeded that of HCA cases. Of the 189 surgically resected HCA cases demonstrated that 70% of HCA patients were middle-aged men, and 50% were overweight or obese. Notably, even female patients rarely had a history of long-term contraceptive drug use. Gene sequencing results showed that the mutation hotspots and frequency of HNF1 gene in HCA case in China were significantly different from those reported in European countries, and no β-catenin and gp130 gene mutations had been found. Based on these results, it is concluded that the population involved and pathogenesis of HCA in China are different from those in European countries. Given the diverse pathological types of liver tumors in China, China is well placed to conduct systematic large-scale cohort studies of liver tumors. In the future, emphasis should be placed on conducting studies on the integration of biological behavior, treatment mode, and clinical prognosis of HCC.

8.6 Research on New Markers for Molecular Pathological Diagnosis of HCC

8.6.1 Research on Prognostic Markers

Studies on prognostic markers related to HCC remain under way in recent years in China. Studies have shown that high expression of cofilin 1 is associated with postoperative recurrence and short survival time of patients with HCC, which made it an independent risk factor for postoperative recurrence and survival. In addition, a series of studies on prognosis-related molecular markers of HCC are in progress. Reportedly, the expression of such molecules as metadherin (MTDH), tumor necrosis factor alpha-induced protein 3 (TNFAIP 3), CDCA5, PKD3, and cathepsin B are all significantly associated with the prognosis of HCC. However, the actual clinical significance still needs further multicenter validation.

In addition to tumor cell-related molecular markers for predicting the prognosis of HCC by the expression level, the level of alpha B-crystallin phosphorylated at Ser59 is also an independent prognostic factor of HCC, associated with the malignant phenotype and prognosis of HCC. Moreover, researchers found that the cytoplasmic localization of HnRNPA-1 protein in HCC can also be used to predict the postoperative prognosis of patients with HCC, and some long noncoding RNAs such as SNHG20, have a certain correlation with the prognosis of HCC too. In addition, the tumor microenvironment can reflect the postoperative prognosis of patients with HCC to some extent. Some studies have demonstrated that the number of tumors infiltrating cells of HCC is significantly less in cancer nest than in peri-cancerous tissue. The tumor and peri-cancerous infiltrating cells are mainly $CD8^+$ cytotoxic T cells. The number of infiltrating CD8$^+$ T cells in tumor tissue is correlated with the prognosis.

8.6.2 Research on Recurrence Risk Markers

HCC is characterized by its aggressive local invasiveness and propensity for distant metastasis, which constitute the primary pathological mechanisms underlying the high postoperative recurrence rates and poor long-term survival outcomes observed in HCC patients. Data indicates that metastasis is responsible for more than 90% of cancer deaths. The 5-year recurrence rate of HCC reaches as high as 60–90%, which has become a bottleneck seriously restricting the long-term efficacy. Consequently, the scientific community has prioritized two critical areas of investigation in HCC research: elucidating the molecular mechanisms governing metastasis and recurrence, and developing comprehensive diagnostic and therapeutic strategies that integrate pathological evaluation with clinical individualized treatment approaches. In recent years, Chinese researchers have made substantial contributions to this field through extensive investigations. Emerging evidence has identified several molecular markers, including NUF2, AKIP1, and nuclear expression of SMARCA4/BRG1, as significant contributors to early HCC recurrence. Research on the malignant phenotype of HCC caused by these molecules will help to identify potential therapeutic targets.

In addition, by analyzing the clinicopathological features and protein expression of 29 biomarkers using immunohistochemistry, the prognosis and recurrence evaluation system was developed and validated using the maximum relevance minimum redundancy algorithm together with multivariate regression method. This system can divide patients with HCC into high survival group, low survival group, and recurrence group, which is very helpful for clinicians to judge whether postoperative adjuvant treatment is beneficial. Prof. Jian Zhou's team from Zhongshan Hospital, Fudan University carried out in-depth genomic analyses in a cohort of patients with HCC in China using the next-generation sequencing technology, thus characterizing the genomic profile of patients with HCC and identifying WNK2 as an important driver gene for early tumor recurrence after therapeutic resection.

8.6.3 Research on Diagnostic Markers

Significant progress has been made in the identification of pathological markers for the diagnosis of well-differentiated small HCC (≤3 cm in diameter). Through the application of isobaric tags for relative and absolute quantification (iTRAQ) proteomics technology coupled with two-dimensional liquid chromatography-tandem electrospray ionization mass spectrometry, researchers have successfully identified relevant immunomarkers, including ACY1, SQSTM1 and SUOX subsequently, three new immunohistochemical diagnostic marker profiles were proposed successively, namely, "ACY1+SQSTM1+CD34", "ACY1+SQSTM+GPC-3", and "SUOX+AKRIB10+CD34". "ACY1+SQSTM1+CD34" is mainly used for the differential diagnosis of dysplastic nodules and small HCC, with sensitivity and specificity of 96.1% and 98.0%, respectively. On this basis, the panel of "ACY1+SQSTM+GPC-3" was proposed for distinguishing between high-grade dysplastic nodules and well-differentiated small HCC. The study results showed that 95.2% of high-grade dysplastic nodules and 33.3% of well-differentiated small HCC tissues were positive for ACY1, while the positive rate was 19.0% and 84.4% for SQSTM, and 4.8% and 62.5% for GPC-3, respectively. The diagnostic sensitivity and specificity of the three combined were 93.8% and 95.2%, respectively.

8.7 Research on Drugs Targeting Molecular Markers

Glypican-3 (GPC-3), a carcinoembryonic proteoglycan anchored to the cell membrane, is usually detectable in fetal liver but not in normal adult liver. However, GPC-3 in patients with HCC is highly expressed at both the gene and protein levels, and its expression predicts a poor prognosis. So far, GPC-3-targeted magnetic resonance imaging, positron emission tomography, and near-infrared imaging have been used for early detection of HCC. Besides, many GPC-3-targeted immunotherapies have been developed, including the use of humanized anti-GPC-3 cytotoxic antibodies, peptide/DNA vaccine therapy, immunotoxic therapy, and gene therapy. GPC-3-targeted CAR-T cells can effectively kill GPC-3-positive HCC cells, providing a promising intervention option for GPC-3-positive HCC.

A study from Zhongshan Hospital, Fudan University demonstrated that patients with low miR-26 expression in HCC tissues were highly sensitive to interferon-alpha treatment, which could be an effective target for drug selection. A team led by Prof. Fuchu He from the Academy of Military Medical Sciences, Academy of Military Science of the Chinese People's Liberation Army, and Prof. Jia Fan from Zhongshan Hospital, Fudan University, achieved a milestone by mapping the proteomic and phospho-proteomic expression profiles of early-stage HCC. This study, based on the proteomic data of cancer tissue and paired peri-cancerous tissue samples of 101 early-stage HCC patients, classified these patients into three proteomic subtypes (S-I, S-II, and S-III). Patients with different subtypes have different prognostic characteristics and should adopt different treatment strategies after surgery. This study not only incorporates the proteome and phospho-proteome of more than 100 pairs of HCC tissues but also provides whole genome sequencing and RNA sequencing data, marking the first comprehensive molecular typing of early-stage HCC based on proteomics. In addition, a new therapeutic target, SOAT1, for S-III early stage HCC with the worst prognosis was identified, which has been validated in the patient-derived tumor xenograft (PDX) mouse model. In parallel, Prof. Weijie Zhou and his team from the Department of Pathology, Southern Medical University pointed out that capillarization of hepatic sinusoids promotes hepatic fibrosis, whereas angiogenesis in portal area inhibits hepatic fibrosis. In the treatment of liver fibrosis from the perspective of vascular intervention, it is necessary to distinguish the different roles of angiogenesis in portal area and capillarization of hepatic sinusoids in the progress of liver fibrosis, so as to achieve better results. Additionally, Prof. Wenxin Qin from the Shanghai Cancer Institute cooperated with a team from the Eastern Hepatobiliary Surgical Hospital and found that the expression of RCAN1. 4, a new tumor suppressor gene, was significantly down-regulated in HCC and associated with the poor prognosis of patients with HCC.

In the era of precision medicine, the latest breakthroughs in cancer immunotherapy revolutionize the treatment methods of cancer, including HCC, and the highly concerned immune checkpoint inhibitors of programmed death-1 (PD-1) receptor and PD-ligand-1 (PD-L1) have demonstrated good clinical efficacy in various solid tumors. Liiie MA et al. explored the genetic variation of PD-Ls using fluorescence in situ hybridization (FISH) technique and assessed their mRNA and protein levels through qPCR and immunofluorescence techniques. This investigation aimed to evaluate the clinical relevance and prognostic value of PD-1-localized 9p24.1 gene alterations in tissue samples from three independent cohorts comprising 578 HCC patients. The results showed that the amplification rate of 9p24.1 and multimer in the three cohorts of patients were 7.1–15.0% and 15.8–31.3%, respectively, which were similar to the objective response rate of PD-1 antibody in patients with HCC. Patients with 9p24.1 gene alteration had a poor outcome compared to those without 9p24.1 gene alterations. The results of FISH test and qPCR with immunofluorescence assay indicated that the 9p24.1 gene alteration greatly contributed to the upregulation of PD-L1 and PD-L2. In addition, through multivariate analysis, increased expression of PD-1 instead of PD-L2 predicted a low survival rate. The high infiltration of PD-1-positive immune cells also suggested a poor survival for patients with HCC. Accordingly, the amplification or high expression of PD-L1 was closely related to the poor survival of patients with HCC, proving that the PD-1/PD-L1 axis is a reasonable immunotherapeutic target for HCC.

In the field of HCC treatment, several clinical trials have demonstrated that PD-1/PD-L1 monoclonal antibody treatment can also bring some survival benefits to patients, and it has been approved by the Food and Drug Administration (FDA) for second-line treatment in HCC. Currently, five drugs targeting the PD-1/PD-L1 pathway have been approved and are available on the market, including two humanized IgG monoclonal antibodies against PD-1 (namely, nivolumab and pembrolizumab) and three humanized IgG monoclonal antibodies against PD-L1. Each of these antibody drugs is designed to target specific antigenic epitopes on PD-1 or PD-L1, which may influence their efficacy and clinical application. For the actual clinical application, corresponding tumor tissues need to be tested to determine whether patients can benefit from treatment with such drugs.

8.8 Prospects

Prof. Mengchao WU, an academician of the China Academy of Sciences, pointed out in 2008 that China had previously formulated guidelines for the diagnosis and treatment of HCC, but the guidelines failed to consider the molecular biological characteristics of tumors, especially their metastatic and invasive characteristics, thus providing limited guidance for individualized treatment. This oversight limited their ability to guide individualized treatment strategies. Standardized pathological diagnosis of HCC is not only crucial to the accuracy of pathological diagnosis but also greatly influences the results of clinical studies on HCC. For example, the "true" or "false" pathological diagnosis of MVI will obstruct the selection of clinical treatment regimen. As such, emphasis should be placed on standardizing the pathological diagnostic process, unifying the pathological diagnostic criteria, and promoting and applying the standardized pathological diagnostic system. Meanwhile, the pathology disciplines should strengthen the communication and contact with clinical disciplines through multidisciplinary teams (MDT) and other forms to understand the actual clinical needs, thus constantly updating and improving the standardized pathological diagnostic system and the level of standardized pathological diagnosis of HCC.

The biological characteristics of HCC, i.e., prone to metastasis and recurrence, are the main bottleneck for improving the long-term prognosis of patients with HCC, and also the focus of pathological diagnosis and clinical treatment. Molecular markers are at the core of molecular pathology diagnosis of HCC. Novel molecular markers for liver cancer are continually emerging but should be validated by scientific and meticulous multicenter clinical studies with a large sample size, so as to optimize the molecular pathological diagnostic marker profile with real practical clinical application and guiding value. China has advantages in the field of clinical and pathological research of HCC, leveraging its large patient population, advanced research infrastructure, and growing expertise in oncology. However, there is still a long way to go before the establishment of a practical and standardized technical system for molecular pathological diagnosis of HCC. Therefore, hepatic tumor pathologists should keep up with the major clinical needs, update the traditional concept of morphological diagnosis, and actively explore a new pathobiological diagnostic model of "morphology+biology." Furthermore, with the focus on improving long-term survival outcomes, new molecular pathological diagnostic markers should be developed, and emphasis should be attached to the establishment of a diagnostic indicator system related to biological characteristics including well-differentiated small HCC, precancerous lesion diagnosis, invasion and metastasis capability evaluation, recurrence risk prediction, clonal origin determination, molecular target screening, drug sensitivity analysis, and long-term prognosis evaluation. Simultaneously, attention should be paid to evaluation of the actual effect of clinical transformation and application. The joint clinical and pathological research should be further strengthened to provide more valuable molecular pathological evidence for improving the treatment level of HCC in China.

In the future, the pathology of hepatobiliary tumors should actively and positively adapt to the development trend of clinical hepatobiliary oncology and molecular biology of cancer, conduct multidisciplinary studies, and strengthen the research on developing diagnostic techniques of biological characteristics of tumor and molecular marker indicator system as well as on clinical transformation and application. At present, with special attention paid to systematic research on the occurrence mechanism, migration path, distribution characteristics, precise identification, and effective treatment of MVI, we should develop a new holistic pathological diagnostic model of "morphology + biology" through actively exploring new pathological diagnostic models and constantly expanding the connotation of clinical pathological diagnosis. Ultimately, these efforts will provide sufficient and more valuable information on the biological characteristics of tumor, enabling the formulat on of scientific clinical diagnosis and treatment regimen. This will not only improve treatment efficacy but also play a greater role in advancing clinical diagnosis and treatment, paving the way for more personalized and effective management of HCC.

Suggested Reading

1. Chinese Society of Liver Cancer, China Anti-Cancer Association, Chinese Society of Clinical Oncology, China Anti-Cancer Association, Liver Cancer Study Group, Chinese Society of Hepatology, Chinese Medical Association, et al. Expert consensus on practice guidelines for the pathological diagnosis of primary liver cancer. Natl Med J China. 2011;91(12):802–4.
2. Cong WM, Bu H, Chen J, et al. Practice guidelines for the pathological diagnosis of primary liver cancer: 2015 update. World J Gastroenterol. 2016;22(42):9279–87.
3. Fujita N, Aishima S, Iguchi T, et al. Histologic classification of microscopic portal venous invasion to predict prognosis in hepatocellular carcinoma. Hum Pathol. 2011;42(10):1531–8.
4. Roayaie S, Blume IN, Thung SN, et al. A system of classifying microvascular invasion to predict outcome after resection in patients with hepatocellular carcinoma. Gastroenterology. 2009;137(3):850–4.
5. Jemal A, Bray F, Center M, et al. Global cancer statistics. CA Cancer J Clin. 2011;61(2):69–90.
6. Global Burden of Disease Cancer Collaboration. Global, regional, and national cancer incidence, mortality, years of life lost, years lived with disability, and disability-adjusted life-years for 32 cancer groups, 1990 to 2015: a systematic analysis for the global burden of disease study. JAMA Oncol. 2017;3(4):524–48.
7. Zhou M, Wang H, Zeng X, et al. Mortality, morbidity, and risk factors in China and its provinces, 1990-2017: a systematic analysis for the global burden of disease study 2017. Lancet. 2019;394(10204):1145–58.
8. Tang ZY. Challenges and prospects of liver cancer metastasis research. Chin J Surg. 2008;46(21):1601.
9. Song P, Cai Y, Tang H, et al. The clinical management of hepatocellular carcinoma worldwide: a concise review and comparison of current guidelines from 2001 to 2017. Biosci Trends. 2017;11(4):389–98.
10. European Association for the Study of the Liver, European Organisation for Research and Treatment of Cancer. EASL-EORTC clinical practice guidelines: management of hepatocellular carcinoma. J Hepatol. 2012;56(4):908–43.
11. Sumie S, Nakashima O, Okuda K, et al. The significance of classifying microvascular invasion in patients with hepatocellular carcinoma. Ann Surg Oncol. 2014;21(3):1002–9.
12. Hidaka M, Eguchi S, Okuda K, et al. Impact of anatomical resection for hepatocellular carcinoma with microportal invasion (vp1): a multi-institutional study by the Kyushu study group of liver surgery. Ann Surg. 2020;271(2):339–46.
13. Rodriguez-Peralvarez M, Luong TV, Andreana L, et al. A systematic review of microvascular invasion in hepatocellular carcinoma: diagnostic and prognostic variability. Ann Surg Oncol. 2013;20(1):325–39.
14. Ferrer-Fàbrega AJ, Forner A, Liccion IA, et al. Prospective validation of ab initio liver transplantation in hepatocellular carcinoma upon detection of risk factors for recurrence after resection. Hepatology. 2016;63(3):839–49.
15. Meniconi RL, Komatsu S, Perdigao F, et al. Recurrent hepatocellular carcinoma: a western strategy that emphasizes the impact of pathologic profile of the first resection. Surgery. 2015;157(3):454–62.
16. Cong WM, Wu MC. New ideas for molecular pathological diagnosis and new strategies for clinical treatment of liver cancer. Natl Med J China. 2014;94(20):1521–3.
17. Wang B, Xia CY, Lau WY, et al. Determination of clonal origin of recurrent hepatocellular carcinoma for personalized therapy and outcome evaluation: a new strategy to hepatic surgery. J Am Coll Surg. 2013;217(6):1054–62.
18. Zhu Y, Gu YJ, Lu XY, et al. Analysis of clonal characteristics of two cases of late recurrence of hepatocellular carcinoma after surgery. Chin J Oncol. 2014;36(6):450–2.
19. Cong WM, Wu MC. New insights into molecular diagnostic pathology of primary liver cancer: advances and challenges. Cancer Lett. 2015;368(1):14–9.
20. Cong WM. Molecular mechanism and pathological evaluation strategies for recurrence and metastasis of liver cancer. Chin J Hepatol. 2016;24(5):324–6.

21. Yang B, Ji Y, Tan YS. Study on the relevance between DUSP6 expression in hepatocellular carcinoma and MARK signaling pathway and clinicopathological features. Chin J Clin Oncol. 2012;39(24):2085–90.
22. Jin H, Zhang Y, You H, et al. Prognostic significance of kynurenine 3-monooxygenase and effects on proliferation, migration, and invasion of human hepatocellular carcinoma. Sci Rep. 2015;23(5):10466.
23. Luo Q, Zhang Y, Wang N, et al. Leukemia inhibitory factor receptor is a novel immunomarker in distinction of well-differentiated HCC from dysplastic nodules. Oncotarget. 2015;6(9):6989–99.
24. Cong WM. Surgical pathology of hepatobiliary tumors. Beijing: People's Medical Publishing House; 2015.
25. Liu HP, Zhao Q, Jin GZ, et al. Unique genetic alterations and clinicopathological features of hepatocellular adenoma in Chinese population. Pathol Res Pract. 2015;211(12):918–24.
26. Zhao Y, Zhang CY, Guo YC, et al. Relevance between cofilin 1 expression level and prognosis of patients with primary hepatocellular carcinoma. Chin J Clin Med. 2018;25(2):256–61.
27. Zhu K, Zhan H, Zhou J, et al. Expression changes and clinical significance of metadherin in hepatocellular carcinoma tissue. Chin J Clin Med. 2017;24(3):334–6.
28. Qiao P, Gao XM, Yu X, et al. Expression of A20 gene in hepatocellular carcinoma and its prognostic significance. Tumor. 2015;35(6):639–45.
29. Tian Y, Wu J, Chagas C, et al. CDCA5 overexpression is an indicator of poor prognosis in patients with hepatocellular carcinoma (HCC). BMC Cancer. 2018;18(1):1187–97.
30. Yang H, Xu M, Chi X, et al. Higher PKD3 expression in hepatocellular carcinoma (HCC) tissues predicts poorer prognosis for HCC patients. Clin Res Hepatol Gastroenterol. 2017;41(5):554–63.
31. Ruan J, Zheng H, Rong X, et al. Over-expression of cathepsin B in hepatocellular carcinomas predicts poor prognosis of HCC patients. Mol Cancer. 2016;15:17.
32. Huang XY, Ke AW, Shi GM, et al. Significance of alpha B-crystallin phosphorylated at Ser59 in hepatocellular carcinoma. Chin J Clin Med. 2015;22(6):734–7.
33. Zhou ZJ, Wang XY, Chen EB, et al. Localization and clinical significance of heterogeneous nuclear ribonucleoprotein A1 in primary hepatocellular carcinoma. Chin J Clin Med. 2016;23(6):720–4.
34. Liu J, Lu C, Xiao M, et al. Long non-coding RNA SNHG20 predicts a poor prognosis for HCC and promotes cell invasion by regulating the epithelial-to-mesenchymal transition. Biomed Pharmacother. 2017;89:857–63.
35. Shi J, Dong QZ, Qin LX, et al. Study on the phenotype and distribution of tumor-infiltrating lymphocytes in hepatocellular carcinoma. Chin J Clin Oncol. 2015;42(11):559–63.
36. Wang Y, Tan PY, Handoko YA, et al. NUF2 is a valuable prognostic biomarker to predict early recurrence of hepatocellular carcinoma after surgical resection. Int J Cancer. 2019;145(3):662–70.
37. Cui Y, Wu X, Lin C, et al. AKIP1 promotes early recurrence of hepatocellular carcinoma through activating the Wnt/β-catenin/CBP signaling pathway. Oncogene. 2019;38(27):5516–29.
38. Chen Z, Lu X, Jia D, et al. Hepatic SMARCA4 predicts HCC recurrence and promotes tumour cell proliferation by regulating SMAD6 expression. Cell Death Dis. 2018;9(2):59.
39. Zhou SL, Zhou ZJ, Hu ZQ, et al. Genomic sequencing identifies WNK2 as a driver in hepatocellular carcinoma and a risk factor for early recurrence. J Hepatol. 2019;71(6):1152–63.
40. Jin GZ, Li Y, Cong WM, et al. iTRAQ-2DLC-ESI-MS/MS based identification of a new set of immunohistochemical biomarkers for classification of dysplastic nodules and small hepatocellular carcinoma. J Proteome Res. 2011;10(8):3418–28.
41. Zhou F, Shang W, Yu X, et al. Glypican-3: a promising biomarker for hepatocellular carcinoma diagnosis and treatment. Med Res Rev. 2018;38(2):741–67.
42. Gao H, Li K, Tu H, et al. Development of T cells redirected to glypican-3 for the treatment of hepatocellular carcinoma. Clin Cancer Res. 2014;20(24):6418–28.
43. Ji J, Yu L, Yu Z. Development of a miR-26 companion diagnostic test for adjuvant interferon-alpha therapy in hepatocellular carcinoma. Int J Biol Sci. 2013;9(3):303–12.
44. Jiang Y, Sun A, Zhao Y, et al. Proteomics identifies new therapeutic targets of early-stage hepatocellular carcinoma. Nature. 2019;567(7747):257–61.
45. Xu M, Xu H, Lin Y. LECT2, a ligand for Tie1, plays a crucial role in liver fibrogenesis. Cell. 2019;178(6):1478–92.
46. Jin H, Wang C, Jin G, et al. Regulator of calcineurin 1 gene isoform 4, down-regulated in hepatocellular carcinoma, prevents proliferation, migration, and invasive activity of cancer cells and metastasis of orthotopic tumors by inhibiting nuclear translocation of NFAT1. Gastroenterology. 2017;153(3):799–811.
47. Ma LJ, Feng FL, Dong LQ, et al. Clinical significance of PD-1/PD-Ls gene amplification and overexpression in patients with hepatocellular carcinoma. Theranostics. 2018;8(20):5690–702.
48. Chen XP, Zhang ZW. Setting and working of multidisciplinary team for liver cancer. Chin J Pract Surgery. 2014;34(8):685–7.
49. Cong WM, Wu MC. Efforts to improve the fine diagnosis and individualized treatment of microvascular invasion in liver cancer in China. Chin J Hepatobiliary Surg. 2019;25(10):721–4.
50. Sheng X, Ji Y, Ren GP, et al. A standardized pathological proposal for evaluating microvascular invasion of hepatocellular carcinoma: a multicenter study by LCPG. Hepatol Int. 2020;14(6):1034–47.

Part III

Surgical Treatment for Liver Cancer

Overview and Classification of Local Treatment Options for Liver Cancer

9

Wanguang Zhang

Back in October 2001, the earliest *Selection of Surgical Treatments for Primary Liver Cancer* in China was prepared by the Section of Hepatic Surgery, Branch of Surgery, Chinese Medical Association in Wuhan. These guidelines clarified that a surgical treatment-based comprehensive treatment model should be adopted for primary liver cancer, and detailed the indications of surgical treatment and local treatment for primary liver cancer. Most patients are already in the intermediate or advanced stages at the time of diagnosis, with a high proportion of with a high proportion of concurrent liver cirrhosis and a low surgical resection rate; meanwhile, the problem of high postoperative recurrence rate of liver cancer also poses a challenge to surgical treatment. Local treatment is minimally invasive and cost-effective with good repeatability and efficacy. Therefore, its application in liver cancer treatment has become increasingly widespread. This section provides an overview and classification of current local therapies for liver cancer.

Local treatment can be classified into two broad categories: local physical therapy and chemotherapy. Local physical therapies mainly include percutaneous radiofrequency ablation (PRFA), percutaneous microwave coagulation therapy (PMCT), high-intensity focused ultrasound (HIFU), cryotherapy, external beam radiotherapy (EBRT), etc. Local chemotherapy works mainly through the hepatic vascular approach, which mainly includes transcatheter arterial embolization (TAE), transcatheter arterial chemoembolization (TACE), drug-eluting bead transcatheter arterial chemoembolization (DEB-TACE), transcatheter arterial radioembolization (TARE) with yttrium-90 microspheres, implantable chemotherapy pump infusion chemotherapy, and percutaneous ethanol injection (PEI). Additionally, combined physical and chemotherapy may be recommended for certain tumors.

9.1 Transarterial Interventional Therapy

Transarterial interventional therapy is a minimally invasive treatment approach that kills the tumor cells by blocking the tumor blood supply through the selective infusion of particulate matters into the hepatic artery supplying nutrients to the tumor with a catheter. This therapy is feasible because the liver is an organ with a dual blood supply from the hepatic artery and portal vein. Normally, 25% of the blood flowing to the liver is from the hepatic artery, and 75% is from the portal vein, while the blood supply to a liver tumor is mainly from the hepatic artery. Infusion of embolic agents and

W. Zhang (✉)
Tongji Hospital Affiliated to Tongji Medical College, Huazhong University of Science & Technology, Wuhan, China
e-mail: wgzhang@tjh.tjmu.edu.cn

X. Chen (ed.), *Diagnosis and Treatment of Liver Cancer in China*,
https://doi.org/10.1007/978-981-97-7969-7_9

chemotherapeutic drugs through the hepatic artery not only reduces and blocks blood flow to the tumor to induce ischemic changes in the tumor but also prolongs the duration of action of chemotherapeutic drugs, which increases the drug concentration inside the tumor while significantly reducing the side effects of systemic chemotherapy. The complementary application of both greatly improves the treatment effect.

Currently, the clinically applied transarterial interventional therapies mainly include TAE, TACE, DEB-TACE, and TARE with yttrium-90 microspheres. TACE, DEB-TACE, and TARE are all developed from TAE, with the addition of chemotherapeutics, drug-eluting beads, or radioactive elements into the embolic agents.

In 1953, Seldinger invented the percutaneous arteriography method. In 1983, Konno T et al. first reported the administration of lipiodol mixed with anticancer drugs via the hepatic artery to treat liver cancer. In 1987, scholars from China published the first study in China on the diagnosis and treatment of liver cancer with abdominal angiography and embolic agents. With the advances in imaging technology, Zhaoyou Tang, Han Chen, et al. performed the second-stage surgery after the liver cancer shrank following interventional therapy, opened up new possibilities for improving the efficacy of hepatectomy for the treatment of liver cancer. During the seventh National Conference on Liver Surgery in 2003, Wu Mengchao proposed that TACE is the preferred treatment for unresectable liver cancer. However, many studies have shown that the disadvantages of preoperative TACE outweigh the advantages for patients with resectable liver cancer.

The 2018 European Association for the Study of the Liver (EASL) Clinical Practice Guidelines point out that: (1) TACE is recommended for use in BCLC stage B patients (with a high level of evidence and strong recommendation); (2) DEB-TACE has comparable efficacy to conventional TACE (with a high level of evidence and strong recommendation); (3) TACE is prohibited for use in patients with decompensation of liver function, progressive hepatic insufficiency and renal insufficiency (with a high level of evidence and strong recommendation); and (4) TARE is used for bridging liver transplantation in BCLC stage A patients and the treatment of BCLC stage B patients and may be an alternative to TACE. The existing data showed that TARE is safe and feasible with an excellent local control effect. Still, its overall survival (OS) is lower than that of BCLC stage B and stage C patients treated with sorafenib (with a middle level of evidence).

The 2019 Guidelines for the Diagnosis and Treatment of Primary Liver Cancer in China make the following recommendations: (1) In most cases, the efficacy of TACE and other non-surgical treatments is not inferior to that of surgical resection for the treatment of China Liver Cancer Staging (CNLC) stage IIb liver cancer patients; (2) The efficacy of TACE or external beam radiotherapy may be comparable to that of surgical treatment for CNLC stage IIa patients with (type III) tumor thrombus in the main trunk of the portal vein (with a level 3 of evidence); and (3) Comprehensive treatment by combining TACE with local ablation, surgical procedure, radiotherapy, molecular targeted drugs, immunotherapy, and antiviral therapy is recommended to improve the efficacy of TACE further.

As liver cancer has a high postoperative recurrence rate, the earliest prophylactic measures against postoperative intrahepatic recurrence primarily rely on systemic chemotherapy, but it has strong side effects and poor treatment effects. The implantable chemotherapy pump infusion chemotherapy supplies drugs directly to the liver via catheterization of the hepatic artery and portal vein. At the same time, chemotherapeutic drugs flow at a slow rate in the low-pressure, low-flow portal vein system, which increases the contact duration of chemotherapeutic drugs with tumors and is conducive to killing cancer cells. This method has the advantages of a slight systemic reaction, high local drug concentration, significant efficacy, and simple operation, serving as a new approach for postoperative adjuvant chemotherapy. Current studies showed that the infusion of oxaliplatin, calcium folinate, and fluorouracil via the hepatic artery significantly improves the survival and tumor response rate with tolerable adverse reactions. Compared with

TACE, the FOLFOX infusion regimen via the hepatic artery has a better objective response rate, progression-free survival (PFS), and fewer adverse reactions. Infusion chemotherapy for liver cancer has many medication regimens and has achieved a certain effect. The adjuvant infusion chemotherapy through an implantable chemotherapy pump allows the administration of chemotherapeutic drugs via the portal vein, which can prevent cancer cells from spreading through the portal vein and thus complement the shortcomings of TACE to a certain degree.

9.2 Ablation Therapy

Ablation therapy is a treatment option that utilizes chemicals, cold, or heat to necrotize tumors directly and has the advantages of minimal invasiveness, cost-effectiveness, and good repeatability. It includes chemical ablation (injection of ethanol, acetic acid, etc.), cryoablation, and thermal ablation (radiofrequency and microwave ablation). Ablation therapy can be performed via percutaneous, laparoscopic, or open approaches. Among them, microwave ablation (MWA), radiofrequency ablation (RFA), and percutaneous ethanol injection (PEI) are the most common ablation methods, and the percutaneous procedure is a common surgical approach.

The *Selection of Surgical Treatments for Primary Liver Cancer* outlined the principles for selecting suitable patients for radiofrequency, cryoablation, absolute ethanol injection, and microwave ablation. In the interpretation of the *Expert Consensus on the Selection of Surgical Treatments for Hepatocellular Carcinoma* in 2017, the indications of ultrasound or CT-guided local ablation therapy (RFA, cryoablation, MWA, and ethanol injection) were redefined as follows:

1. Requirements for general conditions: (1) The general condition of the patient is good (with a PST score of 0–2); (2) Vital organs such as the heart, lung, kidney, and brain have no apparent organic lesions, with good or only slightly impaired functions; (3) Liver function is normal or only slightly impaired, with a class A or class B Child-Pugh score; and (4) Hepatic functional reserve is good or slightly impaired.
2. Local condition requirements: (1) With a single tumor, or lesions <5, with the maximum diameter of a single tumor <5 cm; (2) Liver cancer relapsed shortly after hepatectomy, for which the patient is unsuitable or unwilling to undergo another hepatectomy; and (3) Absolute ethanol injection is mainly used in combination with RFA, cryoablation, and MWA for the treatment of liver cancer in privileged sites (close to the first hepatic hilum, gallbladder, stomach, colon, and diaphragm) to reduce the injury to corresponding organs or vessels.
3. Intraoperative application: Local ablation therapy may be performed for the hepatic tissue with suspected residual tumor cells on the incision margin. After resection of the main lesion, local ablation therapy can be applied if residual lesions in the liver are detected by intraoperative ultrasound examination. Laparoscope can be used for local ablation therapy of liver cancer in privileged sites (close to the first hepatic hilum, gallbladder, stomach, colon, and diaphragm). For an unresectable massive hepatocellular carcinoma, local ablation therapy can be combined intraoperatively following TACE; Local ablation therapy can also be applied to treat the bleeding area after hepatectomy.

9.2.1 Microwave Ablation

Microwave ablation (MWA) involves placing the microwave electrode inside the tumor parenchyma. Electromagnetic waves at a particular frequency are emitted to agitate many charged particles, proteins, and other polar molecules in intracellular fluid and tissue fluid, producing friction and heat. MWA can cause protein denaturation and nuclear coagulation through thermal agglomerate, eventually leading to the death of tumor cells and thus fulfilling the function of killing tumors directly.

In 1986, Tabuse et al. from Japan developed the small-diameter coaxial microwave system. In 1990, the MWA technique was used to treat liver cancer for the first time. In 1995, a study of microwave tissue coagulation techniques for treating rupture and bleeding of liver cancer was first reported in China.

For hepatocellular carcinoma (HCC) meeting the Milan Criteria (a single tumor ≤5 cm in diameter, or no more than 3 lesions, each ≤3 cm in diameter or smaller), MWA has a lower incidence rate of postoperative complications and similar treatment effects compared to surgery, especially for patients with a relatively low albumin level. There is no significant difference in the treatment effect and incidence of complications between RFA and MWA, but the latter requires a significantly lower operation time.

9.2.2 Radiofrequency Ablation

Radiofrequency ablation (RFA) has basically the same working principles as MWA, the difference being that the frequency range of electromagnetic waves adopted by RFA is usually lower than that adopted by MWA. This difference leads to different frequencies of high-speed vibration of charged ions in the tumor and different levels of heat generated by friction between molecules in unit time, leading to different rates of protein denaturation and irreversible coagulation necrosis of tumor tissues surrounding the probe, which means that the efficiency of RFA is lower than that of MWA. Its indications and contraindications are consistent with those of MWA.

In 1990, the MWA technique was used to treat liver cancer, and in the same year, McGahan, Rossi, et al. proposed the application of RFA for liver cancer and published the study of PRFA for the treatment of small liver cancer in 1995. In 2001, Tongji Hospital, Affiliated with Tongji Medical College of Huazhong University of Science & Technology of China, introduced the first cool-tip RFA instrument in the Asia-Pacific region for the treatment of recurrent liver cancer and liver cancer with cirrhosis that is unsuitable for surgical resection and published an article on the study of ultrasound-guided cool-tip RFA for the treatment of liver tumor in 2005. In the article, it was considered that ultrasound-guided cooled RFA is applicable to patients with multiple separate masses unsuitable for surgery, hepatic insufficiency, other concomitant diseases intolerable to surgery, postoperative recurrence, and those who are unwilling to undergo surgery, and this method has definite treatment effects for liver tumor <5 cm in size, with few complications.

RFA is superior to PEI regarding overall survival rate, recurrence-free survival, and recurrence rate. A study comparing RFA with surgery in treating single small liver cancer showed that patients in the RFA group had a higher incidence of recurrence but less severe complications and shorter hospital stays than those in the surgery group.

9.2.3 Percutaneous Ethanol Injection

PEI is a type of chemical ablation and has the advantages of simple operation, cost – effectiveness, and less complications. Ethanol can injure the intrahepatic microvascular intima and denature proteins, causing chronic microvascular embolism; Absolute ethanol can directly cause the coagulation, denaturation, and necrosis of tumor tissues. The efficacy of PEI depends on whether the injection volume is adequate and whether the ethanol can uniformly infiltrate into the entire tumor. Ethanol thoroughly diffuses and produces good efficacy if the tumor tissue composition is simple containing less connective tissue. If there are fibrous spaces inside the tumor tissue, ethanol does not fully diffuse, leading to poor efficacy.

In 1986, Livraghi et al. from Italy first reported the investigation of ultrasound-guided PEI to treat small liver cancer and small abdominal tumors. In 1987, the preliminary report on treating primary liver cancer by intratumoral injection of absolute ethanol was published in China.

Multiple studies revealed that PEI achieved a complete ablation rate of 90% for tumors <2 cm in diameter. While complete ablation is hard to achieve for a great majority of tumors >2 cm in diameter, which thus leading to an increased local recurrence rate after surgery. However, there is insufficient evidence that RFA is superior to PEI in HCC patients with cirrhosis.

9.2.4 Acetic Acid Injection

The mechanism of action of acetic acid injection therapy is that acetic acid at a concentration of 50% causes denaturation and coagulation necrosis of cellular protein and cell death by directly injuring or changing various membranous structures of the cell and disrupting the stability of the intracellular environment. Compared with absolute ethanol, acetic acid has a stronger infiltration ability, and can easily penetrate through the fibrous septa inside tumor tissue to get uniform diffusion, thereby exhibiting a stronger ability to kill tumor cells. Acetic acid at 50% has an ablation efficacy of 1:3 against tissue protein, with the advantages of less total injection volume and treatment sessions.

In 1994, Ohnishi et al. from Japan published the first study of ultrasound-guided acetic acid injection to treat small liver cancer. In 1997, Chinese researchers published the first study of percutaneous acetic acid injection (PAI) for small hepatocellular carcinoma.

The currently existing clinical studies showed that the efficacy of PAI is not superior to that of PEI. There are no significant differences between PAI and PEI concerning benefits and hazards in treating patients with early HCC. Neither is there sufficient evidence proving a better treatment effect of PEI against surgery (partial hepatectomy).

9.2.5 Cryoablation

Argon-helium cryoablation (argon-helium knife) is a treatment modality that destroys the tumor tissue maximally through a few repeated cycles of rapid discharge of high-pressure argon to generate an ultra-low temperature of −140 °C, followed by the generation of a heating effect of about 30 °C with high-pressure helium. More and more evidence shows that cryoablation is a safe and effective alternative treatment for liver cancer.

In 1970, German scholars Stucke et al. first reported the study of cryotherapy for malignant liver tumors. In 1979, Chinese scholars Xinda Zhou, Zhaoyou Tang, et al. published the experimental and clinical study article on cryotherapy for liver cancer.

The clinical studies confirmed that cryoablation exhibits a similar safety and efficacy profile to RFA and may have a lower local tumor progression rate compared with RFA.

9.3 External Beam Radiotherapy

External beam radiotherapy (EBRT) is a treatment that administers high-dose radiotherapy into a liver tumor without injuring the surrounding liver tissues. External beam radiotherapies applied in liver cancer treatment mainly include three-dimensional conformal radiotherapy (3D-CRT), stereotactic body radiotherapy (SBRT), and proton and heavy-ion radiotherapy.

EBRT is mainly applicable to patients with unresectable lesions or those medically inoperable to surgery due to comorbidities. Meanwhile, it can also be used as an alternative or adjunct for ablation or arterial interventional procedures. Generally speaking, the effect of radiotherapy on the tumor is closely related to factors such as radiation dose and fraction dose, and within the tolerance range of the liver, the higher the radiation dose, the better the efficacy. 3D-CRT is an effective treatment method for liver cancer with tumor thrombus. SBRT mainly treats smaller liver cancers, with relatively significant treatment effects in recent years. Proton and heavy-ion radiotherapy is limited to a few centers only and is expensive, and its wide application within a foreseeable future is impractical. Therefore, it is unlikely to become a conventional therapy.

Currently, 3D-CRT is an important measure for adjuvant therapy of liver cancer. The operation of 3D-CRT is basically not restricted by the adjacent tissues of liver cancer, with an extensive operation range, good adaptability, and minimal damage to patients. A study of SBRT for liver tumors by Tongji Hospital Affiliated with Tongji Medical College of Huazhong University of Science & Technology in 2000 showed that stereotactic radiotherapy is a safe and effective method for treating liver tumors, with a relatively high complete response rate.

SBRT is a special type of 3D-CRT. The accuracy of SBRT in targeting the lesion was significantly improved while the radiation dose on the surrounding normal tissues was able to be substantially reduced. Compared to conventional radiotherapy, the advantages of SBRT lie in that the way it tracks tumors reduces injuries to the surrounding normal liver or surrounding gastrointestinal tract and other organs and avoids the impact of respiratory motility on radiotherapy as far as possible.

Proton and heavy-ion radiotherapy allow the delivery of sufficient radiation dose into the tumor at deeper sites within the body to release its maximum energy to kill tumor cells while protecting the normal tissues surrounding the tumor to the greatest extent. Theoretically, it is a promising liver treatment option. A prospective, randomized, and controlled trial showed that proton beam radiotherapy achieved a better local tumor control effect of tumor and PFS than TACE for patients meeting the Milan Criteria.

9.4 High-Intensity Focused Ultrasound

HIFU is capable of focusing a high-intensity ultrasound wave onto a specific target region inside the body to damage the target region through thermal effects while maintaining the surrounding normal tissues outside the target region undamaged or minimally damaged due to non-increased temperature. With the development of modern imaging technology, this new technique has attracted more attention for the treatment of liver cancer. In an animal experiment, a pathological biopsy of the target region after multiple times of HIFU treatments still indicated the presence of a viable tumor, which suggesting that improvement can still be made in technical equipment, standard operating procedures, and other aspects. At present, there is still a paucity of large-scale of cases for evaluating the efficacy of HIFU in clinical patients with liver cancer worldwide. A recent retrospective study revealed that HIFU therapy has a similar treatment effect to TACE in liver cancer patients and does not increase the risks of treatment, which may provide a new strategy for clinical treatment, especially for patients with HCC smaller in diameter.

9.5 Combination of Local Therapies

To precisely and reliably improve the effectiveness and thoroughness of treatment, multidisciplinary comprehensive treatment is essential for most liver cancers, and different local therapies can be combined. Combined local therapies commonly used at present mainly include TACE + ablation, ablation + radiotherapy, TACE + ablation + radiotherapy, etc. In general, combining local therapies can further improve the treatment efficacy.

9.6 Summary and Outlook

Surgery (resection and liver transplantation) still plays a dominant role in liver cancer treatment. Local treatments (single and combined) are essential treatment measures for patients who cannot undergo surgery, and systemic therapies (chemotherapy and molecular targeted therapy) have a certain efficacy. An appropriate combination of multiple treatment modalities can exert synergistic effects and improve efficacy. In addition, continued efforts shall be made to improve equipment further, develop better therapeutic drugs, optimize treatment methods, and formulate related standards to completely remove the tumor, decrease tissue injury, improve clinical efficacy, and even achieve a radical cure of surgery, thereby benefiting more patients with tumor.

Suggested Reading

1. Chen X, Chen H. Selection of surgical treatments for primary liver cancer. Chin J Gen Surg. 2001;23(10):762–3.
2. Konno T, Tashiro S, Maeda H, et al. Intra arterial injection of an oily antineoplastic agent in hepatic cancer. Gan To Kagaku Ryoho. 1983;10(2 Pt 2):351–7.
3. Sun Z. Abdominal angiography and embolic agent treatment in 68 patients. Mod Med J. 1987;15(4):198.
4. Chen X. Development and outlook of liver surgery. Chin J Dig Surg. 2015;14(1):9–10.
5. Li X, Zhang Z, Chen X. Summary of the 7th national conference on liver surgery. J Abdom Surg. 2003;16(1):64–5.
6. Galle PR, Forner A, Llovet JM, et al. EASL clinical practice guidelines: management of hepatocellular carcinoma. J Hepatol. 2018;69:S0168827818302150.
7. Bureau of Medical Administration, National Health Commission of the People's Republic of China. Guidelines for the diagnosis and treatment of primary liver cancer (2019 edition). J Clin Hepatol. 2020;36(2):277–92.
8. He M, Li Q, Zou R, et al. Potential areas of interest in a trial of sorafenib plus hepatic arterial infusion of oxaliplatin, fluorouracil, and leucovorin vs. sorafenib alone for hepatocellular carcinoma with portal vein invasion: a randomized clinical trial. JAMA Oncol. 2019;5(7):953–60.
9. He MK, Le Y, Li QJ, et al. Hepatic artery infusion chemotherapy using mFOLFOX versus transarterial chemoembolization for massive unresectable hepatocellular carcinoma: a prospective non randomized study. Chin J Cancer. 2017;36(1):83.
10. Chen X, Zhang Z. Interpretation of expert consensus on the selection of surgical treatments for hepatocellular carcinoma. Chin J Surg. 2017;55(1):7–10.
11. Liu X, Xia Z. Application of microwave tissue coagulation technique for rupture and bleeding of liver cancer. Chin J Gen Surg. 1995;10(4):193–5.
12. Zhang QB, Zhang XG, Jiang RD, et al. Microwave ablation versus hepatic resection for the treatment of hepatocellular carcinoma and oesophageal variceal bleeding in cirrhotic patients. Int J Hyperth. 2017;33(3):255–62.
13. Kamal A, Elomety A, Rostom Y, et al. Percutaneous radiofrequency versus microwave ablation for management of hepatocellular carcinoma: a randomized controlled trial. J Gastrointest Oncol. 2019;10(3):562–71.
14. Rossi S, Di Stasi M, Buscarini E, et al. Percutaneous radiofrequency interstitial thermal ablation in the treatment of small hepatocellular carcinoma. Cancer J Sci Am. 1995;1(1):73–81.
15. Qiao S, Chen X. Ultrasound-guided cool-tip radiofrequency ablation for the treatment of liver tumor. Shandong Med J. 2005;45(21):62–3.
16. Germani G, Pleguezuelo M, Gurusamy K, et al. Clinical outcomes of radiofrequency ablation, percutaneous alcohol and acetic acid injection for hepatocelullar carcinoma: a meta analysis. J Hepatol. 2010;52(3):380–8.
17. Cho YK, Kim JK, Kim MY, et al. Systematic review of randomized trials for hepatocellular carcinoma treated with percutaneous ablation therapies. Hepatology. 2010;49(2):453–9.
18. Orlando A, Leandro G, Olivo M, et al. Radiofrequency thermal ablation vs. percutaneous ethanol injection for small hepatocellular carcinoma in cirrhosis: meta analysis of randomized controlled trials. Am J Gastroenterol. 2009;104(2):514–24.
19. Chen Y, Hu G, Huang H. Recent efficacy of stereotactic radiotherapy for live tumor. Acta Med Univ Sci Technol Huazhong. 2000;29(6):578–80.
20. Livraghi T, Festi D, Monti F, et al. US guided percutaneous alcohol injection of small hepatic and abdominal tumors. Radiology. 1986;161(2):309–12.
21. Dai S, Fang Z, Liu S. Preliminary report on the treatment of primary liver cancer by intratumoral injection of absolute ethanol. Shanghai Med J. 1987;10(3):161–2.
22. Livraghi T, Giorgio A, Marin G, et al. Hepatocellular carcinoma and cirrhosis in 746 patients: long term results of percutaneous ethanol injection. Radiology. 1995;197(1):101–8.
23. Sala M, Llovet JM, Vilana R, et al. Initial response to percutaneous ablation predicts survival in patients with hepatocellular carcinoma. Hepatology. 2005;40(6):1352–60.
24. De Matthaeis N, Saviano A, De Sio I, et al. Single hepatocellular carcinoma smaller than 2 cm: are ethanol injection and radiofrequency ablation equally effective? Anticancer Res. 2013;58:S108–9.
25. Yang B, Zan RY, Wang SY, et al. Radiofrequency ablation versus percutaneous ethanol injection for hepatocellular carcinoma: a meta analysis of randomized controlled trials. World J Surg Oncol. 2015;8(13):96–8.
26. Ohnishi K, Ohyama N, Ito S, et al. Small hepatocellular carcinoma: treatment with US guided intratumoral injection of acetic acid. Radiology. 1994;193(3):747–52.
27. Ren S. Prognostic study of percutaneous acetic acid injection for the treatment of small hepatocellular carcinoma. Foreign Med Sci (Cancer Sect). 1997;24(2):123.
28. Huo TI, Huang YH, Wu JC, et al. Comparison of percutaneous acetic acid injection and percutaneous ethanol injection for hepatocellular carcinoma in cirrhotic patients: a prospective study. Scand J Gastroenterol. 2003;38(7):770–8.
29. Schoppmeyer K, Weis S, Mssner J, et al. Percutaneous ethanol injection or percutaneous acetic acid injection for early hepatocellular carcinoma. Cochrane Database Syst Rev (Online). 2009;1(3):CD006745.

30. Stucke K, Hirte D. Cryosurgery of malignant liver tumors. Acta Hepatosplenol. 1970;17(6):416.
31. Zhou X. Experimental and clinical study of cryotherapy for liver cancer. Chin J Surg. 1979;17(6):480–3.
32. Wang C, Wang H, Yang W, et al. Multicenter randomized controlled trial of percutaneous cryoablation versus radiofrequency ablation in hepatocellular carcinoma. Hepatology. 2015;61(5):1579–90.
33. Bush DA, Smith JC, Slater JD, et al. Chemoembolization for hepatocellular carcinoma: results of an interim analysis. Int J Radiat Oncol Biol Phys. 2016;95(1):477–82.
34. Huang L, Zhou K, Zhang J, et al. Efficacy and safety of high intensity focused ultrasound ablation for hepatocellular carcinoma by changing the acoustic environment: microbubble contrast agent (SonoVue) and transcatheter arterial chemoembolization. Int J Hyperth. 2019;36(1):244–52.

10 Innovations and Breakthroughs in Surgical Techniques for Liver Cancer in China

Peng Zhu and Xiaoping Chen

Surgery-based multimodality therapy is currently the primary treatment for liver cancer. In 1958, the Second Affiliated Hospital of Wuhan Medical College (now Tongji Hospital Affiliated to Tongji Medical College of Huazhong University of Science & Technology) reported the first case of hepatectomy for liver cancer, marking the beginning of surgical treatment of liver cancer in China. The continuous advancements in liver surgery techniques has brought tremendous benefits to liver cancer patients. An epidemiological study was conducted by the Tongji Hospital Affiliated to Tongji Medical College of Huazhong University of Science & Technology and the Liver Surgery Group of the Chinese Surgical Society, Chinese Medical Association on 42,573 patients who underwent hepatectomy (67% of whom had hepatocellular carcinoma; Fig. 10.1). The data collected from 112 medical institutions in China showed that the median overall survival time after hepatectomy was 631 days, and the 3- and 5-year overall survival rates were 28.8% and 19.6%, respectively (Fig. 10.2). The joint efforts of liver surgeons in the past decade have led to remarkable achievements in the surgical treatment of liver cancer in China.

P. Zhu · X. Chen (✉)
Tongji Hospital Affiliated to Tongji Medical College,
Huazhong University of Science & Technology,
Wuhan, China

X. Chen (ed.), *Diagnosis and Treatment of Liver Cancer in China*,
https://doi.org/10.1007/978-981-97-7969-7_10

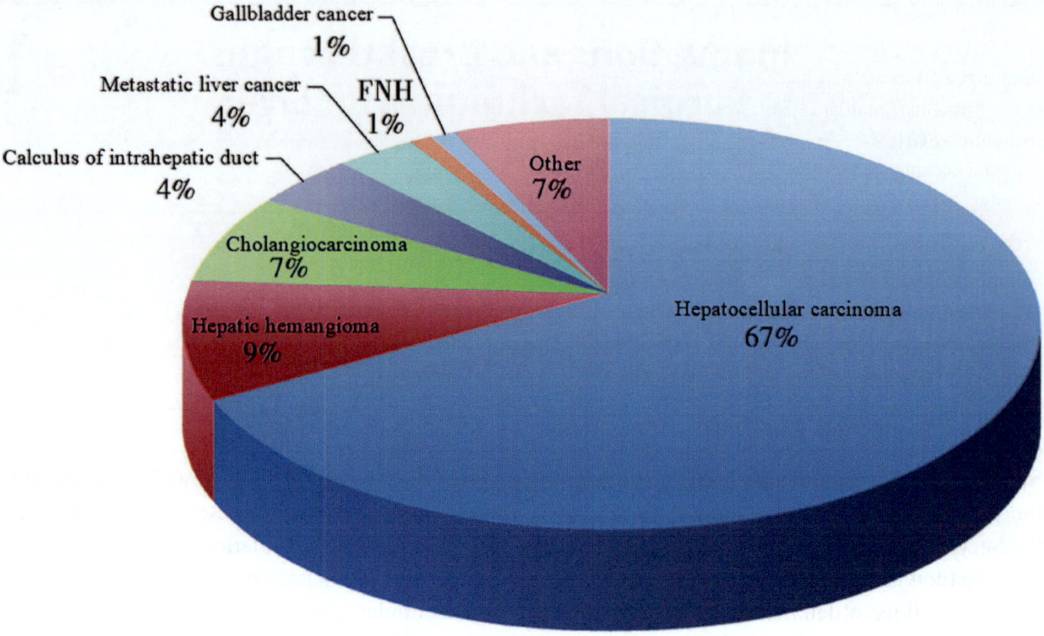

Fig. 10.1 Distribution of diseases among the 42,573 patients who underwent hepatectomy in the multicenter national study. Note: *FNH* focal nodular hyperplasia of the liver

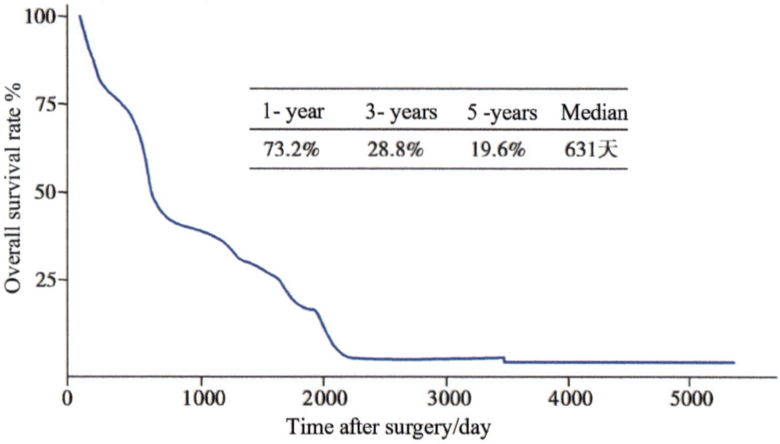

Fig. 10.2 Overall survival of the 18,275 patients with hepatocellular carcinoma in the multicenter national study

10.1 Precise Preoperative Assessment

During clinical practice, an adequate and precise preoperative assessment is crucial for the patient's safety as it ensures both the radical resection of the tumor and adequate remnant liver function. The *Expert Consensus on Preoperative Assessment of Hepatic Functional Reserve for Hepatectomy (2011 edition)*, which combines the experiences in hepatic functional reserve assessment from multiple centers nationwide, points out that precise preoperative assessment of hepatic functional reserve is important for selecting reasonable treatment methods, determining the safe range of liver resection, and reducing the incidence of postoperative liver failure in patients. At present, the most commonly used liver func-

Table 10.1 Modified Child-Pugh scoring system

Clinical and biochemical indicators	1 point	2 points	3 points
Prolonged prothrombin time/s	1–3	4–6	>6
Total bilirubin/(μmol/L)	<34	34–51	>51
Albumin/(g/L)	>35	28–35	<28
Hepatic encephalopathy/grade	None	1–2	3–4
Ascites	None	Mild	Moderate/severe

Note: Grade A: 5–6 points; Grade B: 7–9 points; Grade C: 10–15 points

tion scoring system is still the modified Child-Pugh scoring system (Table 10.1). On the other hand, the indocyanine green (ICG) excretion test is an accurate method for the quantitative assessment of hepatic functional reserve and has been widely used in multiple centers across China.

As imaging techniques continue to advance in recent years, ultrasound, computed tomography (CT), and magnetic resonance imaging (MRI) have allowed us to determine with greater precision the extent of lesions and their spatial relationship with important intrahepatic ductal structures, and hence better select surgical protocols and other treatment regimens. Furthermore, the advancement in digital medicine has also allowed us to reconstruct 3D models and even virtual reality from 2D image data. The *Expert Consensus on the Selection of Surgical Treatment for Hepatocellular Carcinoma (3rd Revision in 2016)*, *Expert Consensus on Perioperative Management of Hepatectomy*, *Guidelines on the Diagnosis and Treatment of Primary Liver Cancer (2019 Edition)*, and *Expert Consensus on Precise Hepatectomy* all stated that 3D visualization technique could clearly display the spatial structures of intrahepatic lesions and vascular system, and preoperative surgical planning can be improved with liver transparency and local magnification techniques. Moreover, quantitative assessment of liver volume derived from 3D reconstruction can accurately determine the postoperative liver volume to be reserved, which greatly ensures the patient's safety.

However, the experience and knowledge in preoperative patient assessment vary across hepatobiliary surgery centers both in China and abroad. The current assessment criteria at Tongji Hospital, Affiliated to Tongji Medical College of Huazhong University of Science & Technology, are Preoperative modified Child-Pugh score <7 points; ICGR15 <10% for major hepatectomy; and remnant liver mass >1% of the body mass after liver resection. These precise preoperative assessments have significantly reduced the risk of post-hepatectomy complications in several large liver surgery centers in China and decreased the mortality rate to less than 1%. According to recent statistics on 140 cases of robotic hepatectomy, perioperative mortality was observed in 0 out of 79 liver cancer patients, and grades 3 and 4 Clavier-Dindo complications were observed in 8.6% of patients. In general, these preoperative quantitative assessments have greatly ensured the patient's safety during surgery.

10.2 Minimally Invasive Hepatectomy

With the development of surgical techniques in the past decade, laparoscopic techniques has also made significant progress in hepatectomy. According to a survey conducted in 2015, over 1,640 (43.6%) of the 3,765 patients who underwent laparoscopic hepatectomy at 27 liver surgery centers from 2008 to 2013 had hepatocellular carcinoma. At present, laparoscopic hepatectomy has been performed on over 1,000 liver cancer patients in several large liver surgery centers in China.

Current evidence shows that the advantages of laparoscopic hepatectomy include small incision, less blood loss during operation, rapid recovery of gastrointestinal function after surgery, short average hospitalization time, and rapid overall recovery. A large-cohort retrospective study by Parks and Cheung et al. showed that the long-term survival benefits of laparoscopic hepatectomy were similar to those of open hepatectomy. In addition, a prospective cohort study by Zheng et al. showed that the 1- and 3-year overall survival rates of liver cancer patients were not significantly different between the laparoscopic hepatectomy group (94.4% and 81.4%, respectively) and open hepatectomy group (93.6% and 82.2%, respectively).

It is important to note that the selection of surgical indications and the learning curve are also important issues to be considered in the clinical practice of laparoscopic hepatectomy. Therefore, the Morioka Consensus Statement formed at the International Conference on Laparoscopic Liver Resection proposes that while minor laparoscopic hepatectomy can be used as a standard surgical procedure, the feasibility and safety of major hepatectomy deserve further exploration. Laparoscopic hepatectomy should also be considered with care by clinicians for some patients who cannot tolerate pneumoperitoneum, suffer from dense intraabdominal adhesions, have lesions that are in close proximity to or directly invade large vessels, have lesions that affect the exposure and separation of the first and second hepatic portals, have other medical conditions that render safe operation under laparoscope impossible or invade the hepatic portal region, or have portal vein tumor thrombus. In 2016, the Asia-Pacific Consensus Statement on Laparoscopic Liver Resection for Hepatocellular Carcinoma shared a similar attitude. Apart from the advantage of less blood loss, laparoscopic hepatectomy should be the preferred surgical method for minor liver resection, including left lateral lobectomy. Furthermore, laparoscopic hepatectomy has superior efficacy to radiofrequency ablation in removing surrounding small liver tumors and is thus worthy of promotion. However, major liver resection involving more than three liver segments is only recommended in a few experienced laparoscopy centers due to technical limitations.

With the gradual introduction of the da Vinci robotic system into China over the past decade, more and more institutions have also begun to apply robotic hepatectomy to treat liver cancer. Compared with traditional laparoscopy, the robotic system has significant advantages in clinical application, including high-definition 3D vision, multi-degree-of-freedom instrument design, and delicate operation. Since the first robotic hepatectomy in February 2015, Tongji Hospital, Affiliated to Tongji Medical College of Huazhong University of Science & Technology, has performed over 300 robotic laparoscopic hepatectomies involving different parts of the liver such as the hemiliver, right posterior lobe, and caudate lobe. Moreover, the experiences of Tongji Hospital, Affiliated to Tongji Medical College of Huazhong University of Science & Technology, suggest that robotic hepatectomy has a shorter learning curve than conventional laparoscopy and requires only about 30 cases for the surgeon to become proficient in the procedure. A study by Eric Lai (Hong Kong, China) compared liver cancer patients who underwent robotic hepatectomy (n = 100) with those who underwent conventional laparoscopic surgery (n = 35). Aside from a longer operative time in the robotic group, no statistically significant differences were observed in intraoperative blood loss, complication rate, R0 resection rate, tumor-free survival rate, and 5-year survival rate between the two groups. However, since the sample size was substantially different and tumor volume, location, and extent of hepatectomy were incomparable between the two groups, further research is required to confirm the above conclusion. We also conducted a prospective cohort study comparing robotic and conventional laparoscopic hepatectomy for liver cancer, which is currently in the follow-up phase. Preliminary results showed comparable short- and long-term efficacy between the two groups. However, the da Vinci robotic system also has disadvantages such as expensive systems, costly equipment, and an oversized robotic arm system. These problems hinder the wide application of this system in the short term.

10.3 Standardization of Hepatectomy Principles

Over the past decade, some progress has been made in the principles of hepatectomy for liver cancer.

10.3.1 Controversy on Anatomic Resection Versus Nonanatomic Resection

Moris et al. analyzed 12,429 liver cancer patients who underwent liver resection, including 6,839 cases of anatomic liver resection and 5,590 cases of nonanatomic resection. The results showed that patients in the anatomic resection group had significantly improved 1-, 3-, and 5-year tumor-free survival after surgery but no significant difference in overall survival rate compared with the nonanatomic resection group. Eguchi from Japan reported that among the three single tumor groups (<2 cm diameter group, 2–5 cm diameter group, and >5 cm diameter group), only the patients who underwent anatomic liver resection in the 2–5 cm group had significantly improved tumor-free survival. The 2015 Morioka Consensus Statement on Laparoscopic Liver Resection explicitly pointed out that liver cancer should be treated by anatomic liver resection. However, the 2018 "Guidelines for liver cancer" by the European Association for the Study of the Liver (EASL) state that anatomic and nonanatomic hepatectomy are optional based on current findings. Furthermore, for a single liver tumor <2 cm in diameter, both resection and ablation can be used as first-line treatments, which to some extent acknowledges the application of nonanatomic liver resection.

Therefore, both the *Expert Consensus on Selection of Surgical Treatments for Hepatocellular Carcinoma* and *Guidelines for Diagnosis and Treatment of Primary Liver Cancer (2019 Edition)* have clarified the general principles for liver cancer hepatectomy: (i) Thoroughness: Complete resection of tumor with negative margin; (ii) Safety: Retainment of adequate functional liver tissues and reduction of surgical mortality and complications.

Both intraoperative and postoperative criteria should be considered when determining the use of radical resection for liver cancer:

1. Intraoperative judgment criteria: (i) No tumor thrombus visible in the vessels; (ii) No invasion of adjacent organs or hilar lymph nodes or distant metastases; and (iii) >1 cm incisional margin or incisional margin <1 cm but is confirmed as negative incisional margin by histology.
2. Postoperative judgment criteria: (i) No tumor lesions observed by imaging 2 months after surgery; and (ii) If preoperative alpha-fetoprotein (AFP) was positive, the AFP level has returned to normal range 2 months after surgery.

As long as the above criteria are met, any treatment option can be considered appropriate for liver cancer. Both anatomic resection and nonanatomic resection are common surgical treatments for liver cancer, and there is currently no preferential recommendation for either procedure. More than 80% of liver cancer cases in China have underlying hepatitis B or C, and more than half of these patients also have cirrhosis. Therefore, the decision to perform anatomical resection is sometimes not based on just the physician's will, as the extent of liver resection also depends on the patient's liver function, degree of cirrhosis, and tumor-related factors. The current practice at Tongji Hospital, Affiliated to Tongji Medical College of Huazhong University of Science & Technology, employs both hepatectomy strategies with a preference for anatomic hepatectomy. However, patient safety should always be a priority, especially for those with single liver tumors measuring 2–5 cm in diameter. For example, among the 121 liver cancer patients who underwent robotic hepatectomy in the early stage of the disease, 84 cases underwent anatomic hepatectomy, and the remaining 37 cases underwent nonanatomic hepatectomy.

10.3.2 Vascular Inflow Occlusion During Hepatectomy

In recent years, some researchers in China believe that vascular inflow occlusion is unnecessary during liver resection, as this can reduce ischemia-reperfusion injury of liver tissues. Accumulating clinical evidence shows that hepatic vascular inflow occlusion (i.e., Pringle maneuver,

Fig. 10.3) during hepatectomy, even when performed many times, has no significant effect on postoperative liver function recovery provided that certain principles are followed (15 min occlusion followed by 5 min reperfusion, which can be changed to 10 min occlusion and 5 min reperfusion for cirrhotic livers). For this reason, the Hepatic Surgery Team of the Surgery Branch of the Chinese Medical Association (CMA) has made a consensus statement on some commonly used vascular inflow occlusion techniques and selection principles. We believe that rational vascular inflow occlusion techniques and the application of intraoperative controlled low central venous pressure can make the surgical view clearer and guarantee patient safety. There are currently two available methods for lowering the central venous pressure. One is the traditional low central venous pressure technique controlled by anesthesiologists, which requires drugs such as nitroglycerin and furosemide. The other is the subhepatic inferior vena cava occlusion technique proposed by the Hepatic Surgery Center of Tongji Hospital, Affiliated to Tongji Medical College of Huazhong University of Science & Technology, which can reduce venous return by 60–70% by occluding the subhepatic inferior vena cava (Fig. 10.3), resulting in a rapid decrease in central venous pressure. However, not all patients need to undergo these procedures. As pointed out by the Hepatic Surgery Team of the Surgery Branch of CMA on intraoperative bleeding control methods and selection principles, the bleeding control method during hepatectomy depends on the patient's age, general conditions, degree of cirrhosis, hepatic functional reserve, tumor size and site, the extent of liver resection, and surgical procedure. It should be flexibly selected considering various factors such as the surgeon's experience and the operating room and equipment conditions. Nonetheless, patient safety should be the priority of all principles and premises.

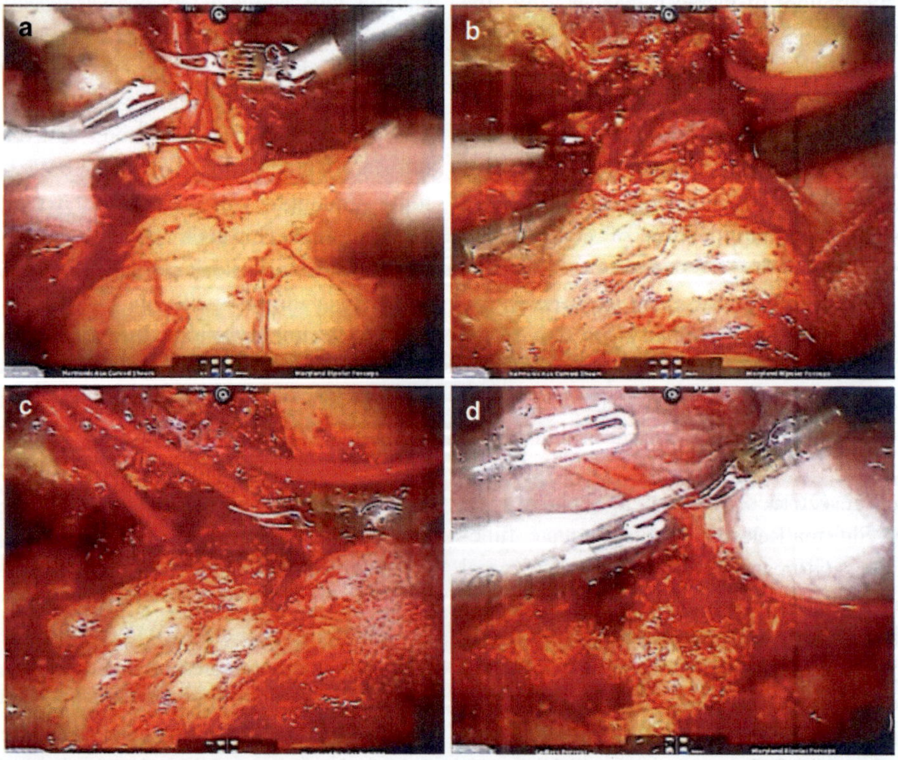

Fig. 10.3 Application of the Pringle maneuver combined with subhepatic inferior vena cava occlusion in robotic hepatectomy. (**a**) Pringle maneuver; (**b**) Subhepatic inferior vena cava; (**c**) Occlusion band around subhepatic inferior vena cava; (**d**) Subhepatic inferior vena cava occlusion

10.3.3 Application of Navigation Techniques (Ultrasound, ICG, and Mixed Reality Technique) in Hepatectomy

Visualization techniques can render liver resection much safer. Professor Makuuchi was the first to apply the ultrasound navigation technique during hepatectomy in Japan starting as early as the 1980s. Intraoperative ultrasound has unique advantages in tumor localization, liver resection planning, catheter injection/puncture, and ablation guiding. In recent years, with the widespread application of laparoscopic hepatectomy, the use of laparoscopic ultrasound has also become more common. The high image resolution of laparoscopic ultrasound allows for the detection of many tiny satellite and metastatic foci, marking important ductal structures, confirmation of incision margins, and puncture guiding. Acting as the hepatobiliary surgeons' "third eye," laparoscopic ultrasound overcomes some exploration and discrimination obstacles caused by the loss of tactile sensation in laparoscopic hepatectomy, thus effectively improving the safety and efficacy of the procedure.

With the continuous application of robotic laparoscopic hepatectomy, Tongji Hospital Affiliated to Tongji Medical College of Huazhong University of Science & Technology proposed a four-stage ultrasound procedure for robotic hepatectomy based on their experience in intraoperative ultrasound application. This procedure involves exploration, identification, navigation, and confirmation. Among the 110 patients who underwent robotic hepatectomy in our previous study, unexpected small lesions were found in 10% of the patients, including 6 patients with liver cancer. Of these six patients, one had an unexpected small lesion located outside the intended resection area and five required surgical plan adjustment. These data highlight the importance of intraoperative ultrasound during hepatectomy, especially during robot-assisted laparoscopic hepatectomy, since this surgical technique lacks direct tactile feedback.

At present, ICG fluorescence imaging is a hot technique that has been widely used in traditional laparoscopic hepatectomy. This technique has demonstrated outstanding advantages in tumor labeling and staining liver lobes or segments. However, ICG staining also has some obvious shortcomings, such as poor fluorescence penetration, high false-positive rate, and difficulty in controlling ICG injection time and concentration due to factors such as cirrhosis. As techniques and equipment continue to upgrade, the application of some of the above real-time imaging techniques in hepatectomy will become increasingly common.

10.3.4 Application of Associating Liver Partition and Portal Vein Ligation (ALPPS) for Two-Stage Hepatectomy in Liver Cancer

This technique has emerged in recent years and is intended for patients whose expected remnant liver volume is less than 30–40% of the standard liver volume. After stage 1 portal vein ligation and liver parenchyma dissection, the remnant liver on the healthy side can generally proliferate by 30–70% after 1–2 weeks, reaching at least 30% of the standard liver volume, hence allowing for safe stage 2 hepatectomy. Patients should be carefully selected for this type of surgery according to the degree of cirrhosis, age, ability to tolerate two surgeries in a short time, and the risk of rapid tumor progression during the waiting period. Some improvements have been made in ablation and binding instead of liver parenchyma dissection and laparoscopic surgery to reduce surgical trauma. The *Guidelines for Diagnosis and Treatment of Primary Liver Cancer (2019 Edition)* lists some contraindications for this type of surgery: (i) Presence of unresectable extrahepatic metastatic lesions; (ii) Patients with concurrent severe portal hypertension; (iii) High-risk patients with general conditions who cannot tolerate major surgery and other anesthesia; and (iv) Patients with visible hepatocellular nodules in the remnant liver during stage 1 surgery. Most researchers think that ALPPS has high complication and mortality rates and is thus not suitable for patients with large liver cancers accompanied by significant cirrhosis.

10.4 Expansion of Indications for Liver Transplant

Liver transplantation is also a surgical treatment choice for liver cancer. At present, the Milan criteria are still the most widely used criteria for selecting liver transplant recipients with liver cancer, i.e., single tumor ≤5 cm or up to 3 tumors each ≤3 cm in diameter without large vessel invasion or extrahepatic metastases. After a liver transplant, the 4-year overall survival rate and recurrence-free survival rate in liver cancer patients who meet this criterion are 85% and 92%, respectively. However, due to the tight conditions of this treatment, many patients who do not meet the Milan criteria cannot benefit from liver transplantation. Therefore, foreign researchers proposed using the Pittsburgh criteria, UCSF criteria, and Up-to-7 criteria, all of which (Table 10.2) have expanded indications for liver transplant recipient selection and have demonstrated satisfactory patient outcomes.

Chinese liver transplantation scholars have also made continuous efforts to explore the selection criteria. Fan Jia et al. put forward the Shanghai Fudan criteria for liver transplant recipient selection, and the indications are expanded to the following: (i) Single tumor ≤9 cm in diameter; (ii) Up to 3 tumors each ≤5 cm in diameter; and (iii) Total diameter of all tumors ≤9 cm. The follow-up results showed that the survival rate was comparable between patients who meet the Fudan criteria and those who meet the Milan criteria, with a 5-year postoperative survival rate up to 78.1%. Zheng Shusen et al. put forward the Hangzhou criteria: (i) No large vessel invasion or extrahepatic metastasis; and (ii) Cumulative lesion diameter of ≤8 cm, or cumulative lesion diameter >8 cm, preoperative AFP ≤400 ng/mL, and well or moderately differentiated determined by histopathological grading. This criterion innovatively introduced biological indicators such as AFP and histological grading as one of the criteria, and the validation results showed a 51.5% increase in the beneficiary population and similar long-term survival compared to the Milan criteria. Other similar criteria in China include the West China criteria and Sanya Consensus. The latest guidelines recommend the UCSF criteria. As donors are still in short supply today, we think that the selection criteria for liver transplant recipients with liver cancer should be stringent rather than relaxed, and more caution should be placed in the selection of living liver transplant recipients.

Table 10.2 Selection criteria for liver transplant recipients with liver cancer

Selection criteria	Specific contents
Milan criteria	Single tumor ≤5 cm in diameter or up to 3 tumors ≤3 cm in maximum diameter without vascular invasion or lymph node metastases
Pittsburgh criteria	Large vessel invasion, lymph node involvement, and distant metastases are all contraindications for transplant, while tumor size, number, and distribution are not used as the exclusion criteria
UCSF criteria	Single tumor ≤6.5 cm in diameter or up to 3 tumors each ≤4.5 cm in diameter with a total diameter of ≤8 cm
Up-to-7 criteria	Sum of maximum tumor diameter and number of tumors ≤7, without large vessel invasion, lymph node metastases, and extrahepatic metastases
Hangzhou criteria	No large vessel invasion, cumulative tumor diameter ≤8 cm, or cumulative tumor diameter >8 cm, and preoperative AFP ≤400 ng/mL and well or moderately differentiated determined by histopathological grading
Shanghai Fudan criteria	Single tumor ≤9 cm in diameter or up to 3 tumors each ≤5 cm in diameter with a total diameter of ≤9 cm, without large vessel invasion, lymph node metastases, and extrahepatic metastases

Suggested Reading

1. Xia SH. Partial liver resection. J Wuhan Med Coll. 1958;1:9.
2. Zhang B, Zhang B, Zhang Z, et al. 42,573 cases of hepatectomy in China: a multicenter retrospective investigation. Sci China Life Sci. 2018;61(6):660–70.
3. Dong JH, Zheng S, Chen XP, et al. Expert consensus on evaluation of hepatic functional reserve before liver resection (2011 edition). Chin J Dig Surg. 2011;10(1):20–5.
4. Section of Hepatic Surgery, Branch of Surgery, Chinese Medical Association. Expert consensus on selection of surgical treatments for hepatocellular carcinoma (2016 3rd edition). Chin J Dig Surg. 2017;16(2):113–5.
5. Chen XP, Mao YL, Qiu YD, et al. Expert consensus on perioperative management of liver resection. Chin J Pract Surg. 2017;37(5):525–30.
6. Bureau of Medical Administration, National Health and Family Planning Commission of the People's Republic of China. Guidelines for diagnosis and treatment of primary liver cancer (2019 edition). Chin J Dig Surg. 2020;19(1):1–20.
7. Professional Committee of Hepatobiliary and Pancreatic Surgery, Chinese Research Hospital Association. Expert consensus on precise hepatectomy. Chin J Dig Surg. 2017;6(9):883–93.
8. Wakabayashi G, Cherqui D, Geller DA, et al. Recommendations for laparoscopic liver resection: a report from the second international consensus conference held in Morioka. Ann Surg. 2015;261(4):619–29.
9. Cheung T, Han HS, She WH, et al. The Asia Pacific consensus statement on laparoscopic liver resection for hepatocellular carcinoma: a report from the 7th Asia-pacific primary liver cancer expert meeting held in Hong Kong. Liver Cancer. 2018;7(1):28–39.
10. European Association for the Study of the Liver. EASL clinical practice guidelines: management of hepatocellular carcinoma. J Hepatol. 2018;69(1):182–236.
11. Hepatic Surgery Team, Surgery Branch, Chinese Medical Association. Nomenclature for liver anatomy and hepatectomy, and bleeding control methods and selection principles during liver resection (2017 1st revision, 2nd edition). J Abdom Surg. 2017;30(2):75–8.

11 Advances in Small Liver Cancer Treatment and the Establishment of an Early Diagnosis and Treatment System for Small Liver Cancer

Wei Zhang and Xiaoping Chen

11.1 Definition

In recent years, the level of early diagnosis of liver cancer has rapidly improved due to the continuous development of diagnostic imaging technologies, and there are more clinical cases of small liver cancer. The early detection of small liver cancer has dramatically improved the efficacy of resection for liver cancer, thus significantly improving its prognosis and changing liver cancer from an "incurable disease" to a "partially curable disease."

To date, there is no universally accepted international definition of small liver cancer. In 1983, small liver cancer was defined as a lesion with a diameter of less than 2 cm in the *General Rules for the Clinical and Pathological Study of Primary Liver Cancer* published by the Liver Cancer Study Group of Japan. The Milan Criteria for liver transplantation in liver cancer patients specify a single lesion less than 5 cm in size or up to three lesions, each less than 3 cm in size, with no vascular invasion or distant metastasis. In the BCLC staging system proposed by Llovet et al. in 1999, liver cancer ≤3 cm was defined as early-stage cancer; in the amended BCLC system proposed in 2004, liver cancer ≤2 cm in diameter was defined as very early-stage cancer. The T stage was updated in the eighth AJCC/UICC staging system for liver cancer. A study of 1019 patients with liver cancer showed that patients with a single tumor <2 cm in diameter experienced prolonged survival, regardless of vascular invasion or histological grade. In the eighth AJCC staging system for liver cancer, T1 is divided into T1a and T1b according to tumor size and the presence of vascular invasion, Specifically, T1a refers to a solitary tumor ≤2 cm in diameter, irrespective of vascular invasion, and T1b refers to a solitary tumor >2 cm in diameter and no vascular invasion. According to the *Practice Guidelines for the Pathological Diagnosis of Primary Liver Cancer* (2015 edition) and *Guidelines for Diagnosis and Treatment of Primary Liver Cancer* (2011 edition), small liver cancer was defined as a single tumor ≤3 cm in diameter, or multiple tumor nodules, no more than 2, and the sum of the maximum diameters of ≤3 cm. The Liver Cancer Institute of Fudan University, however, defines small liver cancer as a single tumor nodule <5 cm in diameter or two tumor nodules with a combined diameter <5 cm. Research indicates that when small liver cancer reaches a diameter of 3 cm, it marks a critical transition in the tumor's biological behavior, shifting from relatively benign to highly malignant. For a liver cancer >3 cm in diameter, the risks of microvascular invasion, satellite nodules, and poor prognosis increase significantly. Therefore, using the diameter ≤3 cm as the criterion for small liver

W. Zhang · X. Chen (✉)
Tongji Hospital Affiliated to Tongji Medical College, Huazhong University of Science & Technology, Wuhan, China

X. Chen (ed.), *Diagnosis and Treatment of Liver Cancer in China*,
https://doi.org/10.1007/978-981-97-7969-7_11

cancer can better reflect the biological characteristics of early-stage liver cancer.

11.2 Treatment Methods

Surgical resection has always been regarded as the gold standard for treating small liver cancer. However, in recent years, with the rapid development of minimally invasive techniques and a deeper understanding of the concept of minimally invasive treatment, the clinical treatment of small liver cancer has evolved from the traditional "surgical resection alone" to a more comprehensive strategy. This modern approach integrates surgical resection, local regional therapy, and liver transplantation, complemented by biotherapy and immunotherapy. Commonly used treatment methods in clinical practice include surgical resection, liver transplantation, radiofrequency ablation (RFA), microwave ablation (MWA), transarterial chemoembolization (TACE), percutaneous ethanol injection (PEI), and stereotactic body radiotherapy (SBRT). Among them, surgical resection, liver transplantation, and local ablation therapy are radical treatments. The choice of treatment modality depends on tumor size, number, location, and liver function classification, and controversy still exists on selecting the optimal treatment strategy for small liver cancer.

11.2.1 Surgical Resection

Surgical resection is the preferred treatment option for small liver cancer and is essential for achieving long-term survival for patient. A study conducted by the Liver Cancer Institute of Fudan University reported a 5-year survival rate of 62.7% and a 10-year survival rate of 46.3% among 1,000 patients with small liver cancer who underwent surgical resection. Similarly, a study from the Sun Yat-Sen University Cancer Center, which examined 380 patients treated with nonanatomical and simplified hepatectomy for small liver cancer between 1964 and 1999, found a postoperative 5-year survival rate of 57.13%. Rongping Guo et al. retrospectively analyzed the outcomes of 406 patients with small liver cancer treated by surgical resection. The overall 3-year survival rate was 72.11%, with a rate of 73.13% for 262 patients whose liver tumors were smaller than 3 cm in diameter, and 70.15% for 144 patients with tumors between 3 and 5 cm in diameter. In all groups, the postoperative 2- and 3-year recurrence rates were 29.19% and 39.18%, respectively. Scholars from Japan evaluated the efficacy of surgical resection for liver cancer in 12,118 Japanese patients across Japan from 1990 to 1999. Among them, 2,320 patients had small liver cancer (≤2.0 cm in diameter) with a postoperative 5-year survival rate of 66%, while another 2,320 patients had tumors measuring 2.1–5.0 cm in diameter, achieving a 5-year survival rate of 53%.

The methods of liver resection include anatomical resection (AR) and nonanatomical resection (NAR). NAR preserves a significant portion of functional liver parenchyma and ensures a tumor-free margin of more than 1 cm. n contrast, AR involves removing a segment of the liver along with its associated portal vein system, which can help minimize tumor cell metastasis and reduce postoperative recurrence, making it a theoretically reasonable approach. However, since most patients with primary liver cancer also suffer from liver cirrhosis, AR can severely compromise hepatic functional reserve due to the extensive removal of liver tissue. This may result in postoperative liver failure and even death, despite its potential therapeutic benefits. The necessity of AR for small liver cancer remains a topic of debate. A Japanese multicenter study demonstrated that AR only provided survival benefits for liver cancers measuring 2–5 cm in diameter, while offering no significant advantage over NAR for tumors smaller than 2 cm. A recent South Korean study involving 1,572 patients with single liver cancers of 2–5 cm in diameter established an ADV score based on AFP levels, Des-gamma-carboxy prothrombin (DCP) levels, and tumor size to assess tumor invasiveness. The results showed that patients with ADV ≤4 logs or no microvascular invasion (MVI) can obtain more survival benefits from AR. In a study by Shin S et al., which included 116 patients with small liver cancers (<3 cm in diameter), no significant differences in overall survival (OS) or recurrence-free survival (RFS) rates were observed between AR and NAR. There was no significant difference between AR and NAR in OS rate and RFS rate. For patients with suspected MVI, a wide resection margin (>1 cm) is recommended to reduce postoperative recurrence. A study conducted by Yamashita et al. found that AR yielded better OS and RFS rates compared to NAR and radiofrequency ablation (RFA) in patients with small liver cancer and suspected MVI. Similarly, a study conducted by Cucchetti A et al. discovered that AR significantly reduced early recurrence rates in cirrhotic patients with poorly differentiated liver cancer and MVI. A meta-analysis conducted by Shuangxi Han et al. revealed that AR had better 3- and 5-year survival rates and 1-, 3- and 5-year tumor-free survival rates than NAR. The authors concluded that AR should be preferred option for patients with a adequate hepatic functional reserve who are suitable for AR, Conversely, NAR is recommended for patients with compromised liver function to avoid the risk of postoperative liver failure.

With the advances in laparoscopic techniques and the development of new technological equipment, an increasing number of hepatobiliary surgery centers have adopted laparoscopic liver resection for the treatment of small liver cancer. The 2008 "Louisville Declaration" established the indications for laparoscopic liver resection, which include: superficial localized lesions located within liver segments 2–6; benign tumor ≤5 cm in diameter (except exogenous tumor); malignant tumor ≤3 cm in diameter, without invading major vessels or bile ducts. As laparoscopic liver resection techniques have progressed, along with improvements in equipment and instruments, and the application of intercostal puncture, transthoracic, and retroperitoneal approaches, the range of resectable tumor sites has gradually expanded to include previously considered non-laparoscopic liver segments, or upper posterior segments, specifically segments 1, 4a, 7, and 8. Additionally, the size limitation for tumors has been extended to 8 cm. In 2012, Prof. Xiaoping Chen advocated and organized liver surgeons in China to develop the first Expert Consensus and *Operation Guidelines for Laparoscopic Liver Resection* (2013 edition). Subsequently, in 2015, the Asia Pacific and China expert committee for the promotion and development of laparoscopic liver resection technology was established, playing a pivotal role in the promotion and development of laparoscopic liver resection in the Asia-Pacific Region and China.

Studies have shown that laparoscopic hepatectomy has advantages over traditional open hepatectomy in terms of improved tumor margin, reduced intraoperative bleeding, lower rates of hematogenous metastasis, decreased postoperative mortality, fewer postoperative complications, and shorter hospital stays. Moreover, there is also no statistical difference in the OS and RFS rates between the two approaches. Therefore, laparoscopic liver resection has attracted more attention as a viable treatment option for small liver cancers. When considering laparoscopic liver resection for small HCC, strict adherence to indication criteria is essential to ensure both safety and efficacy. The resectability of the tumor should be carefully evaluated, taking into account its location and anatomical relationship with critical vascular and bile duct structures. Small liver cancer located in the peripheral area of liver is a good indication of laparoscopic liver resection. However, for tumors situated in challenging locations, such as the posterosuperior segments of the liver, treatment should be conducted at experienced hepatobiliary surgery centers with specialized expertise. Due to the inherent limitations of laparoscopy in controlling major bleeding and accurately assessing surgical margins, small liver cancers located deep within the liver—especially those in close proximity to major vessels or bile ducts—are better managed through open surgery or ablation therapy.

A comprehensive disease assessment is the premise and key in the reasonable selection of treatment strategies for small liver cancer patients with portal hypertension and hypersplenism. Not only HCC itself, but also portal hypertension, hypersplenism, and liver function status are pivotal determinants of patient prognosis. (1) For patients with resectable HCC and preserved liver function, the following approaches are recommended: In cases of severe gastroesophageal varices, a history of hemorrhage, or a hemorrhagic tendency, hepatectomy combined with splenectomy and pericardial devascularization is a suitable option. If varices are not severe but hypersplenism is present, hepatectomy with splenectomy can be performed. This combined procedure not only removes HCC but also mitigates the risk of hemorrhage and corrects hypersplenism, making it an optimal therapeutic strategy. (2) For patients with poor liver functions who can not tolerate surgery and present with severe hypersplenism, a comprehensive treatment approach for HCC combined with splenic artery embolization is advisable. Additionally, for patients with severe gastroesophageal varices, a history of bleeding, or bleeding tendency, esophageal vein ligation or injection of sclerosing agents can be performed. (3) For patients with mild to moderate varicose veins and insignificant hypersplenism, treatment targeting the varices or spleen is generally unnecessary. Instead, the focus should be on managing the small liver cancer in accordance with standard HCC treatment principles.

Theoretically, liver transplantation (LT) represents the optimal treatment for small liver cancer. LT not only removes the cirrhotic liver but also addresses the tumor, effectively reducing the risk of cancer recurrence and reversing liver failure. However, the acute shortage of organ donors poses a significant challenge. Each year, 20% of patients on the transplant waiting list die due to prolonged waiting time, highlighting the urgent need to allocate limited donor organs to those most likely to derive the greatest survival benefit from transplantation. The most widely accepted selection criteria for LT in liver cancer patients are the Milan Criteria proposed by Mazzaferro et al. in 1996. Extended criteria such as the UCSF criteria are also generally considered suitable for LT in selected patients, as they demonstrate comparable long-term survival outcomes. While most LT criteria for liver cancer are based on imaging findings, recent studies have incorporated tumor biomarkers to refine patient selection for transplantation. One of the most common biomarkers is the pretransplant AFP level. Hameed et al. reported that AFP level >1000 ng/mL as the only significant predictor of HCC recurrence and proposed it as a cutoff value. Excluding 4.7% of patients with AFP levels beyond this cut-off point from LT would reduce the post-transplant HCC recurrence rate by 20%. In some Asian LT centers, other biomarkers (e.g., DCP or PIVKA-II) are commonly applied in patients with liver cancer. Chaiteerakij R et al. found that the risk of liver cancer recurrence after LT could be predicted using a combination of three biomarkers: AFP, AFP-L3, and DCP. Integrating these tumor markers with the Milan Criteria may further optimize the selection of liver cancer patients for LT. In summary, there is growing recognition that the Milan Criteria may be too restrictive, and several alternative LT criteria for liver cancer have been proposed, However, a consensus on the optimal selection criteria has yet to be established.

Studies reported that 20–30% of liver cancer patients waiting for transplantation were removed from the waiting list due to tumor progression. In order to delay tumor progression and reduce the possibility of liver cancer patients being deprived of the opportunity for LT during the waiting period due to tumor progression, bridging therapy has been introduced. In 2012, an international consensus conference recommended that LT patients with an estimated waiting time of more than 6 months should receive bridging therapy. A recent retrospective study by Mehta et al. identified several high-risk factors associated with the removal of liver cancer patients from the waiting list. These factors include: solitary tumor with a diameter of 3–5 cm (compared to ≤3 cm), the presence of two or three tumors, lack of complete response after initial locoregional therapy, and elevated alpha-fetoprotein (AFP) levels. The choice of bridging therapy depends on tumor size, number, and liver function. For small tumor ≤3 cm in diameter, ablation is the optimal method. For larger and multiple lesions, TACE or TARE therapy is recommended. In recent years, SBRT has emerged as a viable bridging therapy for patients with compromised liver function, offering a promising alternative therapy for these patients. While systemic chemotherapy has been explored, it remains experimental and is not recommended as a standard therapy at present.

Salvage liver transplantation (SLT) is a treatment strategy that involves initial liver resection for resectable small liver cancer in patients with good liver function, followed by LT in cases of intrahepatic recurrence or liver failure after liver resection. Curative treatments for small liver cancer include partial hepatectomy and LT. Studies have demonstrated that hepatectomy yields comparable OS rates to LT in early-stage liver cancer. However, due to the invasive and metastatic characteristics of HCC, hepatectomy is associated with a higher risk of tumor recurrence or liver function deterioration. Studies also revealed that approximately 70% of patients would experience intrahepatic recurrence within 5 years after hepatectomy. Nevertheless, it is encouraging that 80% of patients with recurrent HCC following radical resection remain eligible for LT. Most experts consider patients with resectable and recurrent small liver cancer, good liver function (Child-Pugh class A), and who meet LT inclusion criteria as suitable candidates for the SLT strategy. Recently, Wang et al. performed a meta-analysis comparing SLT with curative locoregional therapy for recurrent liver cancer, including 840 patients from seven retrospective studies. The results showed that SLT was superior to curative loco-regional therapy in 5-year OS rate and 1-, 3-, and 5-year DFS rates, indicating that the SLT strategy can further improve the treatment effect of recurrent small liver cancer.

11.2.2 Ablation Therapy

Ablation therapy currently applied in clinical practice involve different mechanisms of cell injury. These therapeutic approaches can be broadly categorized into: thermal ablation techniques utilizing high temperatures (radiofrequency and microwave energy, ultrasound or laser energy), cryoablation employing extremely low temperatures, chemical ablation through cytotoxic agents (e.g., ethanol or acetic acid injection) or nonthermal energy (e.g., irreversible electroporation). Among these, radiofrequency ablation (RFA) and microwave ablation (MWA) represent the most widely utilized ablation modalities in clinical practice at present. Both techniques induce tissue temperature elevation to levels sufficient to cause irreversible cellular damage. When tissue temperatures exceed 60 °C, immediate and irreversible thermal denaturation of cellular proteins occurs, resulting in coagulative necrosis and consequent cell death.

While ethanol-based chemical ablation has the longest history of clinical application, comparative studies have demonstrated the superior efficacy of RFA. Lencioni et al. conducted a randomized controlled trial comparing RFA with absolute ethanol ablation in patients with Child-Pugh grade A or B cirrhosis and single early-stage HCC (≤3 cm), revealing significantly improved 2-year RFS rates for RFA (96% vs. 62%). The study conducted by Livraghi et al. also showed that higher rates of complete necrosis with RFA compared to ethanol ablation. Consequently, ethanol ablation is primarily reserved for cases where thermal ablation is contraindicated, such as when lesions are adjacent to critical vascular structures (posing thermal injury risks) or when cost considerations are paramount. Regardless of ablation method chosen, the optimal ablation result is closely related to the experience of the operators. This relationship was quantitatively demonstrated in a recent study by Lee et al., which revealed that early-stage HCC patients treated by experienced operators (>70 cases) had significantly lower 2-year recurrence rates compared to those treated by less experienced practitioners (<10 cases).

Early studies demonstrated that RFA was most effective in treating HCCs smaller than 2 cm in diameter (very early HCC) and 3 cm in diameter (early HCC), achieving a complete necrosis rate of 90%; for tumors ≤3 cm in diameter with preserved liver function (Child-Pugh class A), the 5-year OS rate ranges from 61% to 86%. for tumors ≤2 cm in diameter, RFA and MWA exhibit comparable long-term efficacy, with no significant differences in OS, RFS, or time to tumor progression. However, evidence suggests that MWA may be more effective than RFA for ablating lesions adjacent to larger vessels due to its reduced heat-sink effect. For larger liver cancers (>3 cm in diameter), RFA demonstrates suboptimal local tumor control and poorer long-term outcomes. Specifically, the complete necrosis rate declines to approximately 70% for lesions measuring 3–5 cm and drops further to 24% for lesions >5 cm, with even lower rates observed in invasive tumors. Among patients with tumors ≤3 cm, local tumor progression at the ablation margin occurs in approximately 10% of cases within 12–18 months post-treatment. While residual tumors at the ablation margin can be managed with repeated ablation, these patients typically experience inferior long-term survival compared to those achieving complete ablation. Notably, aggressive tumor characteristics in small liver cancers, such as MVI, high level of tumor markers, and poor differentiation, are closely associated with high local tumor progression rates and poor OS rates.

The choice between surgical resection and ablation therapy for small liver cancer remains a subject of debate. A retrospective cohort study conducted by Livraghi et al. in 2008 demonstrated that for a small liver cancer ≤2 cm in diameter, RFA could be an alternative to surgical resection due to a comparable survival outcomes. The study reported a sustained complete response rate of 97.2% and a 5-year survival rate of 68.5% in the RFA group, which was similar to the 62–70% 5-year survival rate observed with surgical resection. However, surgical resection demonstrated superior long-term outcomes as tumor size increased, particularly for tumors larger than 4–5 cm. To date, five prospective randomized controlled studies have compared the efficacy of ablation therapy with surgical resection. In 2006, a study by Minshan Chen et al. involving patients with a single small liver cancer ≤5 cm in diameter found no significant difference in the 1-, 2-, 3-, and 4-year OS and DFS between the RFA group ($n = 71$) and surgical resection group ($n = 90$), and the incidence of complications was higher in the surgical resection group. In 2010, Huang et al. included 230 patients with small liver cancer meeting the Milan Criteria. Both the OS and DFS were significantly worse in the RFA group than in the surgical resection group. The investigator concluded that surgical resection had a better outcome for small liver cancer within the Milan Criteria. In 2012, Feng et al. studied 168 patients with small liver cancers (maximum tumor diameter ≤4 cm and no more than two lesions) and found no significant differences in OS and RFS between the surgical resection and RFA groups. Similarly, In 2014, Fang et al. included 120 patients with a single small liver cancer ≤3 cm in diameter. There was no significant difference in the 1-, 2-, and 3-year OS and RFS between the RFA group and surgical resection group. The complication rates and length of hospital stay were lower in the RFA group. More recently, in a 2018 study by Lee et al. involving 63 patients with a single small liver cancer (2–4 cm in diameter) found no significant difference in 5-year OS between the two groups, but the surgical resection group had significantly better 3- and 5-year DFS and a lower intrahepatic recurrence rate. The discrepancies in these findings can be attributed to variations in inclusion criteria for small liver cancer across studies, as well as the influence of operator experience and equipment on RFA efficacy. A recent meta-analysis of the above five prospective, randomized, and controlled studies showed RFA had comparable 1- and 3-year OS to surgical resection, but the 5-year OS in the RFA group was significantly lower than that in the surgical resection group, and the overall recurrence rate was higher.

11.2.3 TACE

The principles of transarterial chemoembolization (TACE) involve the selective delivery of embolic agents and chemotherapeutic drugs into the tumor through a catheter inserted into the tumor's feeding artery. This dual-action approach achieves two key objectives: (1) reducing blood supply to the tumor, leading to ischemic necrosis, and (2) minimizing systemic drug loss while maximizing the local concentration and contact time of chemotherapeutic agents with tumor cells. By combining chemotherapy and embolization, TACE effectively targets and destroys tumor cells. TACE is primarily indicated for patients with multifocal small liver cancers who are ineligible for or decline surgical resection or RFA. Ideal candidates typically have preserved liver function, absence of vascular invasion or extrahepatic metastasis, and are unable or unwilling to undergo more invasive treatments.

Bargellini et al. compared first-line treatment outcomes of RFA (n = 315) and TACE (n = 215) in HCC patients who met Milan criteria. Univariate analysis showed that the RFA group had a longer survival time than the TACE group, however, after propensity score matching, no statistically significant difference in OS was observed between the two groups. In contrast, another similar study found that for patients with small liver cancer who met the Milan Criteria, patients treated with TACE experienced a significantly poorer long-term survival rate than those treated with RFA. A study conducted by Kim JW et al. revealed that there was no significant difference in 5-year OS between TACE and RFA for patients with BCLC stage 0 small liver cancer, that TACE may serve as an alternative treatment for patients unsuitable for surgery or RFA. For patients with BCLC stage A liver cancer, TACE has been shown to reduce long-term local tumor progression rates. A study conducted by Martin AN et al. discovered that TACE, RFA, or combination of TACE and RFA had a similar 1-year RFS rate and 5-year OS rate for single small liver cancers ≤3 cm in diameter.

Traditional TACE uses iodinated oil as embolic materials but is associated with limitations such as suboptimal long-term embolic efficacy and significant systemic toxicity. These drawbacks have prompted extensive research into alternative embolic materials. Drug-eluting beads (DEB), a novel embolic agent for liver cancer therapy, have garnered considerable attention due to their enhanced embolic effect and reduced systemic toxicity, offering promising clinical applications. Recently, Lee IJ et al. compared the efficacy of traditional TACE and DEB-TACE in patients with a single small liver cancer ≤5 cm in diameter. The results demonstrated comparable OS rates between the two groups; however, traditional TACE had a longer PFS rate than DEB-TACE. This study also showed the tumor response following DEB-TACE was significantly poorer for small liver cancer with a diameter of 1.0–2.0 cm than for liver cancer with a diameter of 2.1–5.0 cm. Manini MA et al. treated 55 liver cancer patients meeting the Milan Criteria with DEB-TACE; Complete response was achieved in 53% of patients after the first TACE session, with 1-, 2-, and 3-year tumor-free survival (TFS) rates of 29%, 21%, and 9%, respectively. The investigators concluded that DEB-TACE could effectively control tumor progression for liver cancer patients while waiting for LT.

11.2.4 Radiotherapy

With the rapid development of precise radiotherapy technology, the clinical application of radiotherapy for liver cancer has gradually increased. Many studies have confirmed the clinical benefits of radiotherapy for patients across early, intermediate, and advanced stages of liver cancer. The National Cancer Comprehensive Network (NCCN) Guidelines stand as one of the most comprehensive and widely recognized international clinical oncology practice guidelines currently available. The expert team made special recommendations for SBRT as an alternative for ablation/TACE and other treatments, as an option after failure of ablation/TACE and other treatments, or as a treatment option for patients with contraindications to ablation/TACE. It is generally accepted that SBRT is most suitable for small tumors with a diameter of ≤4–5 cm. In 2016, a consensus on SBRT for small liver cancer was developed during the annual meeting of the seventh Asia-Pacific Primary Liver Cancer Expert (APPLE). This consensus delineated the definition, indications, radiotherapy effect and toxic and side effects, optimal radiation dosage, radiotherapy technology and imaging follow-up protocols for SBRT in treating small liver cancer. The consensus considers SBRT to be an effective treatment option for early liver cancers (a single lesion ≤5 cm in diameter or up to 3 tumor foci, each ≤3 cm in diameter). Furthermore, the *Consensus on Radiation Therapy for Primary Liver Cancer in 2016* in China recommends that for patients with small liver cancer who are not suitable for surgical resection, SBRT, like RFA, can be used as an alternative treatment option for inoperable small liver caner.

Sanuki et al. from Japan reported 185 patients with hepatocellular carcinoma <5 cm in diameter treated by SBRT. The 3-year local control rate and OS rate were 91% and 70%, respectively. The 5-year OS rate reported in China is 64%, which is comparable to the survival rates reported in the literature for surgical resection or LT. In another study, Wahl et al. analyzed 224 patients with unresectable small HCC, of whom 161 underwent RFA and 63 received SBRT. The retrospective analysis showed no significant differences in 1- and 2-year OS rates between RFA and SBRT groups. A single-center study comparing the outcomes of TACE and SBRT in 209 patients with small liver cancer found no significant difference in the OS rate between the two groups. However, the 2-year local control rate was significantly higher in the SBRT group than that in the TACE group. SBRT has also been identified as an effective bridging therapy for patients with HCC awaiting LT. Katz AW et al. retrospectively analyzed 18 patients with liver cancer who received SBRT treatment; 11 of whom successfully underwent orthotopic liver transplants.

11.2.5 Combination Therapy

11.2.5.1 TACE Combined with Ablation

TACE combined with ablation is the most widely applied combination therapy approach at present. However, the optimal sequence and timing of TACE relative to RFA remain subjects of debate. Performing TACE prior to RFA can embolize the tumor's arterial blood supply, leading to tumor ischemia, necrosis, and shrinkage. Additionally, this approach reduces the heat-sink effect during RFA, enabling a more extensive and thorough ablation. Conversely, if ablation therapy is performed first, TACE can target the residual region of the tumor margin that has not been completely ablated. Studies showed that combination therapy could achieve complete response in lesions larger than 3 cm. In a prospective randomized controlled trial, Peng et al. compared the efficacy of TACE combined with RFA versus RFA alone in patients with single liver cancer ≤7 cm in diameter and found that the combination therapy group had significantly better OS rates (4-year OS: 62% vs. 45%) and RFS rates (4-year DFS: 55% vs. 39%) compared to the RFA-alone group. The effect of TACE combined with ablation for tumors <3 cm in diameter remains controversial, some studies have suggested that combination therapy does not offer significant advantages over ablation monotherapy for smaller lesions. A study evaluating TACE combined with RFA or Microwave Ablation (MWA) in patients with liver cancer ≤5 cm in diameter and Child-Pugh class A or B cirrhosis found that for tumors measuring 3–5 cm, TACE combined with MWA achieved a higher complete response rate compared to TACE combined with RFA. However, for smaller lesions, there were no inter-group and intra-group differences in response rate and survival rate. Similarly, a prospective study by Japanese scholar Shibata et al., involving 89 patients with small liver cancer ≤3 cm in diameter, compared the efficacy of RFA combined with TACE versus RFA monotherapy. The study found no significant differences in 1-, 2-, 3-, and 4-year local tumor progression, OS, PFS, or RFS rates between the two groups. Therefore, combination therapy may be unnecessary for small liver cancer.

11.2.5.2 Ablation Combined with Systemic Treatment

In some studies. RFA was combined with sorafenib, a multi-kinase inhibitor that inhibits angiogenesis and improved the survival rate of patients with advanced liver cancer. Preliminary small-sample studies have suggested that RFA combined with sorafenib may reduce tumor recurrence rates and improve OS in patients with early-stage HCC compared to RFA monotherapy. However, the recent STORM study, which evaluated the efficacy and safety of sorafenib as adjuvant therapy following liver resection or RFA, found no improvement in RFS rates compared to placebo. Other studies have explored the combination of liposomal doxorubicin with ablation therapy, demonstrating that this approach can enhance cellular cytotoxicity in local tumor cells and expand the extent of ablation. A recent prospective randomized phase III study, including 701 patients with unresectable HCC 3–7 cm in diameter, showed that RFA combined with thermosensitive liposomal doxorubicin did not improve the 3-year OS rate compared with RFA monotherapy. However, the subgroup analysis of 285 patients who received prolonged ablation (>45 min) revealed an improved OS rate in the combination therapy group. The combination of ablation therapy with immunotherapy has emerged as a promising area of research. Focal tumor ablation can release tumor antigens through cellular injury, triggering local tissue responses such as inflammation, changes in vascular permeability, and the recruitment of immune cells, which may enhance the efficacy of immunotherapy. In a recent experimental study, 21 patients with advanced multiple liver cancers were treated with CTLA-4 inhibitors for 4 weeks, followed by RFA or cryoablation and subsequent continuous immunotherapy. Partial response was observed in 26% of patients, and tumor biopsy during the follow-up visits showed an increased level of cytotoxic $CD8^+$ T cells, indicating a potential immune-mediated antitumor effect.

Suggested Reading

1. Bruix J, Takayama T, Mazzaferro V, et al. Adjuvant sorafenib for hepatocellular carcinoma after resection or ablation (STORM): a phase 3, randomised, double blind, placebo controlled trial. Lancet Oncol. 2015;16(13):1344–54.
2. Duffy AG, Ulahannan SV, Makorova Rusher O, et al. Tremelimumab in combination with ablation in patients with advanced hepatocellular carcinoma. J Hepatol. 2017;66(3):545–51.
3. Liver Cancer Study Group of Japan. Classification of primary liver cancer. 1st English ed. Tokyo: Kanehara Press Co; 1997.
4. Mazzaferro V, Regalia E, Doci R, et al. Liver transplantation for the treatment of small hepatocellular carcinomas in patients with cirrhosis. N Engl J Med. 1996;334(11):693–9.
5. Llovet JM, Brú C, Bruix J. Prognosis of hepatocellular carcinoma: the BCLC staging classification. Semin Liver Dis. 1999;19(3):329–38.
6. Amin MB, Edge SB, Greene FL, et al. AJCC cancer staging manual. 8th ed. New York: Springer; 2016.
7. Shindoh J, Andreou A, Aloia TA, et al. Microvascular invasion does not predict long term survival in hepatocellular carcinoma up to 2 cm: reappraisal of the staging system for solitary tumors. Ann Surg Oncol. 2013;20(4):1223–9.
8. Wu M, Tang Z, Liu T, et al. Evidence-based practice guidelines for the pathological diagnosis of primary liver cancer (2015 update). J Clin Hepatol. 2015;31(3):241–6.
9. Ministry of Health of the People's Republic of China. Guidelines for the diagnosis and treatment of primary liver cancer (2011 edition). J Clin Oncol. 2011;16(10):929–46.
10. Zhou X, Tang Z, Yang B, et al. Experience in one thousand hepatectomy for small hepatocellular carcinomas. Chin J Pract Surg. 2001;21(1):41–4.
11. Cong W, Wu M. Progress in study on biopathological characteristics of small hepatocellular carcinoma. Oncol Sect Foreign Med Sci. 1989;4:198–9.
12. Tak WY, Lin SM, Wang Y, et al. Phase III heat study adding lyso-thermosensitive liposomal doxorubicin to radiofrequency ablation in patients with unresectable hepatocellular carcinoma lesions. Clin Cancer Res. 2018;24(1):73–83.
13. Zhang Y, Chen M. Treatment strategies for management of small hepatocellular carcinoma. Chin J Oncol Prev Treat. 2017;9(6):423–6.
14. Guo R, Li J, Li G, et al. Clinical treatment of small hepatocellular carcinoma. Acta Acad Med Sin. 2006;28(3):318–21.
15. Ikai I, Arii S, Kojiro M, et al. Reevaluation of prognostic factors for survival after liver resection in patients with hepatocellular carcinoma in a Japanese nationwide survey. Cancer. 2004;101(4):796–802.
16. Eguchi S, Kanematsu T, Arii S, et al. Comparison of the outcomes between an anatomical subsegmentectomy and a non anatomical minor hepatectomy for single hepatocellular carcinomas based on a Japanese nationwide survey. Surgery. 2008;143(4):469–75.
17. Jung DH, Hwang S, Lee YJ, et al. Small hepatocellular carcinoma with low tumor marker expression benefits more from anatomical resection than tumors with aggressive biology. Ann Surg. 2019;269(3):511–9.
18. Shin S, Kim TS, Lee JW, et al. Is the anatomical resection necessary for single hepatocellular carcinoma smaller than 3 cm: single center experience of liver resection for a small HCC. Ann Hepatobil Pancreat Surg. 2018;22(4):326–34.
19. Yamashita YI, Imai K, Yusa T, et al. Microvascular invasion of single small hepatocellular carcinoma ≤3 cm: predictors and optimal treatments. Ann Gastroenterol Surg. 2018;2(3):197–203.
20. Cucchetti A, Qiao GL, Cescon M, et al. Anatomic versus nonanatomic resection in cirrhotic patients with early hepatocellular carcinoma. Surgery. 2014;155(3):512–21.
21. Han S, Wu D. A meta-analysis of the efficacy of anatomical verses non-anatomical resection for a single small hepatocellular carcinoma. Chin J Gen Surg. 2011;26(10):864–5.

22. Buell JF, Cherqui D, Geller DA, et al. The international position on laparoscopic liver surgery: the Louisville statement, 2008. Ann Surg. 2009;250(5):825–30.
23. Chen X. Expert consensus and operation guidelines for laparoscopic liver resection (2013 edition). Chin J Surg. 2013;51(4):289–92.
24. Jiang S, Wang Z, Ou M, et al. Laparoscopic versus open hepatectomy in short and long term outcomes of the hepatocellular carcinoma patients with cirrhosis: a systematic review and meta analysis. J Laparoendosc Adv Surg Tech A. 2019;29(5):643–54.
25. Chen X, Cao Z. Surgical treatment for hepatocellular carcinoma with portal hypertension and hypersplenism. Chin J Pract Surg. 2004;24(12):716–8.
26. Yao FY, Ferrell L, Bass NM, et al. Liver transplantation for hepatocellular carcinoma: expansion of the tumor size limits does not adversely impact survival. Hepatology. 2001;33(6):1394–403.
27. Hameed B, Mehta N, Sapisochin G, et al. Alpha fetoprotein level >1,000 ng/mL as an exclusion criterion for liver transplantation in patients with hepatocellular carcinoma meeting the Milan criteria. Liver Transpl. 2014;20(8):945–51.
28. Chaiteerakij R, Zhang X, Addissie BD, et al. Combinations of biomarkers and Milan criteria for predicting hepatocellular carcinoma recurrence after liver transplantation. Liver Transpl. 2015;21(5):599–606.
29. Clavien PA, Lesurtel M, Bossuyt PM, et al. Recommendations for liver transplantation for hepatocellular carcinoma: an international consensus conference report. Lancet Oncol. 2012;13(1):e11–22.
30. Mehta N, Dodge JL, Goel A, et al. Identification of liver transplant candidates with hepatocellular carcinoma and a very low dropout risk: implications for the current organ allocation policy. Liver Transpl. 2013;19(12):1343–53.
31. Chen J, Li X. Surgery for early-stage hepatocellular carcinoma: resection versus transplantation. Chin J Hepatobiliary Surg. 2010;16(10):794–7.
32. Margarit C, Escartin A, Castells L, et al. Resection for hepatocellular carcinoma is a good option in Child Turcotte Pugh class A patients with cirrhosis who are eligible for liver transplantation. Liver Transpl. 2005;11(10):1242–51.
33. Kamiyama T, Nakanishi K, Yokoo H, et al. Recurrence patterns after hepatectomy of hepatocellular carcinoma: implication of Milan criteria utilization. Ann Surg Oncol. 2009;16(6):1560–71.
34. Poon RT, Fan ST, Lo CM, et al. Long term survival and pattern of recurrence after resection of small hepatocellular carcinoma in patients with preserved liver function: implications for a strategy of salvage transplantation. Ann Surg. 2002;235(3):373–82.
35. Wang HL, Mo DC, Zhong JH, et al. Systematic review of treatment strategy for recurrent hepatocellular carcinoma: salvage liver transplantation or curative locoregional therapy. Medicine (Baltimore). 2019;98(8):e14498.
36. Lencioni RA, Allgaier HP, Cioni D, et al. Small hepatocellular carcinoma in cirrhosis: randomized comparison of radio frequency thermal ablation versus percutaneous ethanol injection. Radiology. 2003;228(1):235–40.
37. Livraghi T, Goldberg SN, Lazzaroni S, et al. Small hepatocellular carcinoma: treatment with radio frequency ablation versus ethanol injection. Radiology. 1999;210(3):655–61.
38. Lee TY, Lin JT, Ho HJ, et al. Evaluation of the effect of cumulative operator experience on hepatocellular carcinoma recurrence after primary treatment with radiofrequency ablation. Radiology. 2015;276(1):294–301.
39. Brunello F, Cantamessa A, Gaia S, et al. Radiofrequency ablation: technical and clinical long term outcomes for single hepatocellular carcinoma up to 30 mm. Eur J Gastroenterol Hepatol. 2013;25(7):842–9.
40. Francica G, Saviano A, De Sio I, et al. Long term effectiveness of radiofrequency ablation for solitary small hepatocellular carcinoma: a retrospective analysis of 363 patients. Dig Liver Dis. 2013;45(4):336–41.
41. Xu Y, Shen Q, Wang N, et al. Microwave ablation is as effective as radiofrequency ablation for very early stage hepatocellular carcinoma. Chin J Cancer. 2017;36(1):14.
42. Lucchina N, Tsetis D, Ierardi AM, et al. Current role of microwave ablation in the treatment of small hepatocellular carcinomas. Ann Gastroenterol. 2016;29(4):460–5.
43. Livraghi T, Goldberg SN, Lazzaroni S, et al. Hepatocellular carcinoma: radio frequency ablation of medium and large lesions. Radiology. 2000;214(3):761–8.
44. Lencioni R, Cioni D, Crocetti L, et al. Early stage hepatocellular carcinoma in patients with cirrhosis: long term results of percutaneous image guided radiofrequency ablation. Radiology. 2005;234(3):961–7.
45. Yin XY, Xie XY, Lu MD, et al. Percutaneous thermal ablation of medium and large hepatocellular carcinoma: long term outcome and prognostic factors. Cancer. 2009;115(9):1914–23.
46. Livraghi T, Meloni F, Di Stasi M, et al. Sustained complete response and complications rates after radiofrequency ablation of very early hepatocellular carcinoma in cirrhosis: is resection still the treatment of choice. Hepatology. 2008;47(1):82–9.
47. Liu H, Wang ZG, Fu SY, et al. Randomized clinical trial of chemoembolization plus radiofrequency ablation versus partial hepatectomy for hepatocellular carcinoma within the Milan criteria. Br J Surg. 2016;103(4):348–56.
48. Chen MS, Li JQ, Zheng Y, et al. A prospective randomized trial comparing percutaneous local ablative therapy and partial hepatectomy for small hepatocellular carcinoma. Ann Surg. 2006;243(3):321–8.
49. Huang J, Yan L, Cheng Z, et al. A randomized trial comparing radiofrequency ablation and surgical resection for HCC conforming to the Milan criteria. Ann Surg. 2011;254(5):838–9.

50. Feng K, Yan J, Li X, et al. A randomized controlled trial of radiofrequency ablation and surgical resection in the treatment of small hepatocellular carcinoma. J Hepatol. 2012;57(4):794–802.
51. Fang Y, Chen W, Liang X, et al. Comparison of long term effectiveness and complications of radiofrequency ablation with hepatectomy for small hepatocellular carcinoma. J Gastroenterol Hepatol. 2014;29(1):193–200.
52. Lee HW, Lee JM, Yoon JH, et al. A prospective randomized study comparing radiofrequency ablation and hepatic resection for hepatocellular carcinoma. Ann Surg Treat Res. 2018;94(2):74–82.
53. Xu XL, Liu XD, Liang M, et al. Radiofrequency ablation versus hepatic resection for small hepatocellular carcinoma: systematic review of randomized controlled trials with meta analysis and trial sequential analysis. Radiology. 2018;287(2):461–72.
54. Bargellini I, Sacco R, Bozzi E, et al. Transarterial chemoembolization in very early and early stage hepatocellular carcinoma patients excluded from curative treatment: a prospective cohort study. Eur J Radiol. 2012;81(6):1173–8.
55. Liu PH, Lee YH, Hsu CY, et al. Survival advantage of radiofrequency ablation over transarterial chemoembolization for patients with hepatocellular carcinoma and good performance status within the Milan criteria. Ann Surg Oncol. 2014;21(12):3835–44.
56. Kim JW, Kim JH, Sung KB, et al. Transarterial chemoembolization vs. radiofrequency ablation for the treatment of single hepatocellular carcinoma 2 cm or smaller. Am J Gastroenterol. 2014;109(8):1234–40.
57. Martin AN, Wilkins LR, Das D, et al. Efficacy of radiofrequency ablation versus transarterial chemoembolization for patients with solitary hepatocellular carcinoma ≤3 cm. Am Surg. 2019;85(2):150–5.
58. Lee IJ, Lee H, Lee YB, et al. Effectiveness of drug eluting bead transarterial chemoembolization versus conventional transarterial chemoembolization for small hepatocellular carcinoma in Child Pugh class A patients. Ther Adv Med Oncol. 2019;11:1–4.
59. Manini MA, Sangiovanni A, Martinetti L, et al. Transarterial chemoembolization with drug eluting beads is effective for the maintenance of the Milan in status in patients with a small hepatocellular carcinoma. Liver Transpl. 2015;21(10):1259–69.
60. Yang Y, Tian Y. A review of updated guidelines for radiotherapy for primary liver cancer. Chin J Radiat Oncol. 2018;27(5):538–41.
61. Zeng ZC, Seong J, Yoon SM, et al. Consensus on stereotactic body radiation therapy for small sized hepatocellular carcinoma at the 7th Asia Pacific primary liver cancer expert meeting. Liver Cancer. 2017;6(4):264–74.
62. Radiation Oncology Branch of the Chinese Medical Association, Expert Committee on Liver Cancer and Digestive System of China Institute of Biomedical Engineering, et al. Consensus on radiation therapy for primary liver cancer in 2016. Chin J Radiat Oncol. 2016;25(11):1141–50.
63. Sanuki N, Takeda A, Oku Y, et al. Stereotactic body radiotherapy for small hepatocellular carcinoma: a retrospective outcome analysis in 185 patients. Acta Oncol. 2014;53(3):399–404.
64. Su TS, Liang P, Lu HZ, et al. Stereotactic body radiation therapy for small primary or recurrent hepatocellular carcinoma in 132 Chinese patients. J Surg Oncol. 2016;113(2):181–7.
65. Wahl DR, Stenmark MH, Tao Y, et al. Outcomes after stereotactic body radiotherapy or radiofrequency ablation for hepatocellular carcinoma. J Clin Oncol. 2016;34(5):452–9.
66. Sapir E, Tao Y, Schipper MJ, et al. Stereotactic body radiation therapy as an alternative to transarterial chemoembolization for hepatocellular carcinoma. Int J Radiat Oncol Biol Phys. 2018;100(1):122–30.
67. Katz AW, Chawla S, Qu ZH, et al. Stereotactic hypofractionated radiation therapy as a bridge to transplantation for hepatocellular carcinoma: clinical outcome and pathologic correlation. Int J Radiat Oncol Biol Phys. 2012;83(3):895–900.
68. Peng ZW, Zhang YJ, Chen MS, et al. Radiofrequency ablation with or without transcatheter arterial chemoembolization in the treatment of hepatocellular carcinoma: a prospective randomized trial. J Clin Oncol. 2013;31(4):426–32.
69. Lu Z, Wen F, Guo Q, et al. Radiofrequency ablation plus chemoembolization versus radiofrequency ablation alone for hepatocellular carcinoma: a meta analysis of randomized controlled trials. Eur J Gastroenterol Hepatol. 2013;25(2):187–94.
70. Abdelaziz AO, Abdelmaksoud AH, Nabeel M, et al. Transarterial chemoembolization combined with either radiofrequency or microwave ablation in management of hepatocellular carcinoma. Asian Pac J Cancer Prev. 2017;18(1):189–94.
71. Shibata T, Isoda H, Hirokawa Y, et al. Small hepatocellular carcinoma: is radiofrequency ablation combined with transcatheter arterial chemoembolization more effective than radiofrequency ablation alone for treatment. Radiology. 2009;252(3):905–13.
72. Llovet JM, Ricci S, Mazzaferro V, et al. Sorafenib in advanced hepatocellular carcinoma. N Engl J Med. 2008;359(4):378–90.
73. Feng X, Xu R, Du X, et al. Combination therapy with sorafenib and radiofrequency ablation for BCLC stage 0 B1 hepatocellular carcinoma: a multicenter retrospective cohort study. Am J Gastroenterol. 2014;109(12):1891–9.
74. Kan X, Jing Y, Wan QY, et al. Sorafenib combined with percutaneous radiofrequency ablation for the treatment of medium sized hepatocellular carcinoma. Eur Rev Med Pharmacol Sci. 2015;19(2):247–55.

Multimodality Treatments for Large and Giant Liver Cancers

12

Zhiwei Zhang

12.1 Overview

In China, liver cancer has two notable features: more than 80% of the patients with liver cancer have varying degrees of cirrhosis; the tumors of 80% of the patients have already grown large and are in the intermediate to advanced stage at the time of the hospital visit. Traditionally, liver cancers are categorized into large and small liver cancers, with a maximum tumor diameter of 5 cm as the boundary. However, with the increase in surgical cases and the accumulation of experience, this classification method is far from meeting the clinical needs. Therefore, Xiaoping Chen et al. proposed in 1994 that liver cancers can be divided into the following classes according to the tumor size: micro-liver cancer (maximum tumor diameter ≤2.0 cm); small liver cancer (2.0 cm <maximum tumor diameter ≤5.0 cm); large liver cancer (5.0 cm <maximum tumor diameter ≤10.0 cm); giant liver cancer (maximum tumor diameter >10.0 cm). Hepatectomy is the preferred treatment option for micro and small liver cancer if the patient's condition permits. However, the overwhelming majority of liver cancer patients present with intermediate to advanced-stage disease with large or giant liver cancer during the hospital visit, and 80% of patients have liver cirrhosis. The mortality and morbidity of postoperative complications of surgical resection are relatively high in these patients, and therefore, many physicians do not recommend surgical treatment. But, in clinical practice, a good few patients with giant liver cancer treated by surgical resection do obtain long-term survival. If surgery is quickly abandoned, these patients will lose the opportunity to achieve long-term survival.

In 1994, we found through clinical studies that for large liver cancer and giant liver cancer, the actual remnant volume of viable liver tissues on the lesion side was very small due to compression or direct damage by the cancer. At the same time, the liver volume of the uninvolved side was compensatory enlarged. The results were that the smaller the tumor, the larger the volume of tumor-free liver tissue resected; the larger the cancer, the smaller the resected volume of tumor-free liver tissue (Fig. 12.1). That is to say, for right hemihepatectomy of cancer >10 cm in diameter versus cancer <5 cm, the volume of tumor-free liver tissue resected of the latter is more than that of the former based on a pro-rata calculation. Hence, the volume of liver parenchyma resected and the extent of damage to hepatic functional reserve vary between the two. The surgical results of a study of 171 patients with giant liver cancer by Tongji Hospital Affiliated to Tongji Medical College of Huazhong University of Science &

Z. Zhang (✉)
Tongji Hospital Affiliated to Tongji Medical College, Huazhong University of Science & Technology, Wuhan, China
e-mail: zwzhang@tjh.tjmu.edu.cn

X. Chen (ed.), *Diagnosis and Treatment of Liver Cancer in China*,
https://doi.org/10.1007/978-981-97-7969-7_12

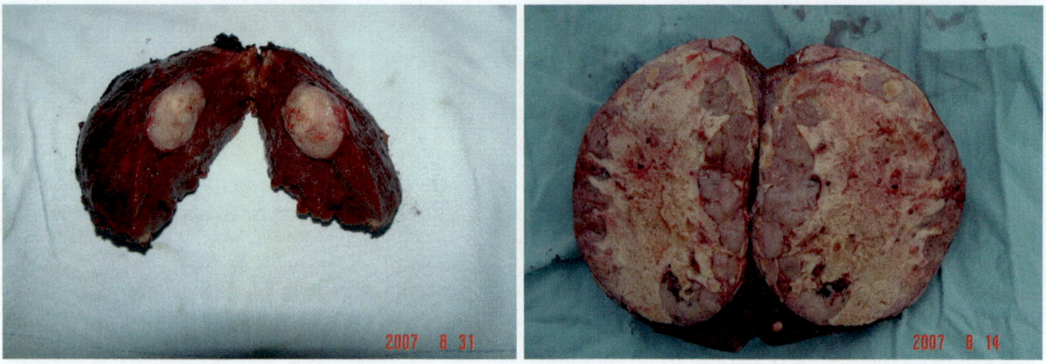

Fig. 12.1 The volume of tumor-free liver tissue resected for giant liver cancer (left) is significantly smaller than that of tumor-free liver tissue resected for small liver cancer (right)

Technology showed that intraoperative death did not occur in the entire group. In total, 2 patients died after surgery; the postoperative 1-, 2-, 3-, 5- and 10-year survival rates were 66.1%, 42.1%, 32.7%, 12.2%, and 2.3%, respectively, and 2 patients had a survival time of more than 20 years. So, it can be seen that hepatectomy is safe and feasible for the treatment of giant liver cancer and can significantly improve the patients' survival rate.

12.2 Surgical Treatment

At present, the main measures for surgical treatment of large liver cancer and giant liver cancer include surgical resection, ablation therapy (RFA, MWA, cryoablation), and LT. Surgical resection should be preferred, but not all large liver cancers and giant liver cancers are suitable for liver resection treatment. Surgery can only be considered when the following conditions are met: (1) The patient has a good general condition, with performance status test (PST) of 0–1 and no significant organic lesion of vital organs such as the heart, lungs, kidneys, and brain. (2) Liver function is normal or only slightly impaired, with a class A Child-Pugh score. (3) Hepatic functional reserve is good, such as a normal indocyanine green retention rate at 15 min (ICGR15). (4) The tumor-free liver has a significant compensatory enlargement, accounting for >50% of total liver volume. (5) There is no extrahepatic metastatic tumor.

Surgical resection for large liver cancer and giant liver cancer is a relatively complex procedure, and proficiency in surgical techniques for resection of large liver cancer is essential to avoid surgical risks and improve surgical efficacy. During the surgical procedure, the following points should be mastered:

1. Fully expose the surgical field and free the perihepatic ligament as completely as possible. An oblique incision under the right costal margin supplemented by an automatic frame-type retractor can meet the requirements of most hepatectomies for large liver cancers. In the case of giant liver cancer, a herringbone incision under bilateral costal margins is more conducive to exposing the operating field. Prior to resection, the liver should be freed as completely as possible so that it can be held to the incision for easy operation under direct vision. But for giant tumors located in the right liver, freeing or moving the liver by force may cause injury and hemorrhage of proximal hepatic veins or spreading of cancer cells as a result of tumor squeezing, and therefore, freeing the ligaments of the right liver can be deferred at the moment. Instead, liver resection via the anterior approach can be performed. Due care should be exercised for patients who had undergone TACE leading to severe local adhesion when freeing the liver to prevent injuring the diaphragm and adjacent organs. Once an injury occurs, it should be repaired.

2. Appropriate application of the hepatic vascular occlusion technique. Regarding large and giant liver cancer, hepatectomy can be cautiously performed under the conditions of not occluding the hepatic blood inflow only for some patients with severe liver cirrhosis whose tumor is located in the left lateral lobe of the liver or in the right liver where the tumor can be successfully held and moved to the incision for the operation. For other patients, various hepatic vascular inflow occlusion techniques should be applied. For patients with giant liver cancer <10 cm in diameter with a distance to the first and second hepatic hila that is easier to resect and good liver function, intermittent occlusion of the first hepatic hilum is preferred and can significantly reduce intraoperative bleeding of hepatectomy. For patients with relatively severe liver cirrhosis or great operative difficulty as estimated preoperatively requiring a long time of hepatic vascular inflow occlusion, hepatectomy can be performed under the condition of only occluding the hepatic blood inflow of the diseased side to avoid injuries to the uninvolved liver. However, when the tumor is closely attached to or invading the main hepatic veins or the inferior vena cava, or hemorrhage of the hepatic vein branches needs to be further controlled, hepatectomy can be performed under total hepatic vascular occlusion (THVO). Conventional THVO is complex to perform and may cause uncontrollable hemorrhage of the vena cava, especially when it is difficult to free the suprahepatic inferior vena cava. Therefore, an improved THVO method (i.e., hepatectomy is performed under the occlusion of the hepatic blood inflow and subhepatic inferior vena cava only) was adopted by our center since 1989 and has been used to complete more than 2000 cases of open and laparoscopic liver resection. The clinical outcomes prove that this technique is easy to perform and significantly reduces hemorrhage.
3. Proficiency in surgical techniques of hepatectomy. For patients with large and giant liver cancer, especially those with liver cirrhosis, anatomical hepatectomy is not strictly required, and the width of resection margin of the tumor from normal liver tissue is no longer than 1–2 cm. With regard to large liver cancers closely attached to the first, second, or third hepatic hilum, the tumor often can only be removed close to the tumor capsule. Many liver parenchyma transection instruments can be used when transecting the liver parenchyma, including cavitron ultrasound surgical aspirator (CUSA), Biclamp, etc. During transection of liver parenchyma, appropriate hemostatic measures should be taken for the section through electrocoagulation, titanium clip, or suturing. In case of injury of the important ducts of the remnant liver, delicate repair shall be performed to ensure the functions of the remnant liver. In the case of giant liver cancer, presence of extensive adhesion with or even invasion into the adjacent gastrointestinal tract where conventional hepatectomy is complex, exposure is poor, and uncontrollable major bleeding may easily be caused, it is better to perform hepatectomy via the anterior approach, which has been adopted by Tongji Hospital Affiliated to Tongji Medical College of Huazhong University of Science & Technology since 1987. This procedure directly cuts liver parenchyma from the diaphragmatic surface along the predefined incision line to the anterior inferior vena cava after occluding (or not occluding) the hepatic blood inflow, followed by freeing and ligation of the hepatic veins and short hepatic veins, then freeing of the ligaments of liver and eventually removing the resected liver. This reduces the risk of cancer cell spreading and injuries to proximal hepatic veins caused by inverting the liver and squeezing the tumor. However, the application of this procedure for liver resection requires the surgeon to be extremely familiar with liver anatomy and highly proficient in surgical techniques. For some patients suitable for right hemihepatectomy, left hemihepatectomy, or left lateral sectionectomy, we adopt a technical hepatectomy without occluding the hilar vessels (referred to as bloodless hepatec-

tomy) by direct ligation of the inflow and outflow vessels of the diseased liver. This method not only complies with the principles of oncology management but also has a minimal impact on hemodynamics as only the blood flow of the diseased liver is completely occluded; moreover, this method also has the advantages of convenience and time efficiency and less hemorrhage during liver transection. For large and giant liver cancer patients with portal vein tumor thrombosis (PVTT), if the tumor thrombus is within the portal vein branches of the liver segment or liver lobe where the liver cancer is located, lobectomy of the liver, including the tumor and the tumor thrombus may be performed. For patients whose tumor thrombus cannot be completely resected, the thrombus can be removed through the broken end of portal vein branches of the liver section after resection of the tumor. If the tumor thrombus is located in the main trunk or branch of the portal vein, a portal vein incision can be performed to remove the thrombus concurrently with liver cancer resection. In the case of liver cancer with inferior vena cava (IVC) thrombus, THVO is required to cut the IVC directly to remove the thrombus. Among the 171 patients with giant liver cancer reported by us, 49 had a concomitant tumor thrombus in the main trunk or a branch of the portal vein, and they were treated by hepatectomy plus tumor thrombectomy, the postoperative 1-, 2- and 3-year survival rates were 38.8%, 22.4%, and 4.1%, respectively, and these results were significantly superior to those of nonsurgical treatment method. As large and giant liver cancers are often adjacent to or even pressing important vascular structures, intraoperative ultrasound can be applied to understand the anatomical relationship of tumors with portal veins, hepatic duct, hepatic veins, and their main branches during hepatectomy to avoid accidental injuries. In case of doubt about the biliary anatomy during operation, intraoperative cholangiography can also be performed to determine the transportation and distribution of bile ducts to avoid accidental injuries.

4. Hepatectomy for large and giant liver cancer usually involves hepatic veins, short hepatic veins, and IVC, and once there are injuries to these veins, an unmanageable massive hemorrhage and sometimes, an air embolism may occur. So, the surgeon should avoid excessive traction and inversion of the liver and be patient and meticulous when dissecting and freeing the short hepatic veins by ligating before cutting. In the event of an injury, handle it calmly. For a minor injury, immediately press the rupture with your fingertip, suck up the outflowing blood, and then suture and repair with an atraumatic suture. If there is an injury to hepatic veins close to the second hepatic hilum, part of the liver tissues near the rupture site can also be sutured together during repair to avoid further tearing. If the injured vein has already had a certain width of exposure, the rupture can be squeezed by fingers at the two sides or clamped with Satinsky forceps, followed by careful repair. For a small IVC rupture in the deep wound site after hepatectomy, if there still are liver tissues on both sides, the two sides of liver tissues can be directly closed together to achieve the goal of hemostasis. It is safer to use an endovascular stapler to treat the hepatic veins, especially the shorter right hepatic veins. If the liver cancer involves the second hepatic hilum or invades the hepatic veins and cannot be separated, atraumatic vascular forceps may be employed to clamp the hepatic veins or IVC, followed by repair after tumor resection.

In most cases, horizontal mattress suture plus an interrupted suture can be used to close the liver section after resection of the tumor. Closure of the wound edges is not required if it produces excessive tension on the entire wound surface, but measures must be taken to ensure hemostasis and prevent bile leakage by covering the wound with greater omentum, hemostatic gauze, and hemostatic glue.

Most surgeons propose that a surgical resection margin of at least 1 cm should be retained. But for most patients with giant liver cancer, it is almost impossible to retain the surrounding surgical resection margin of 1 cm to the tumor. For many patients, the tumor can often only be removed close to the tumor capsule to retain sufficient liver parenchyma. If a surgical resction margin of 1 cm is to be retained when transecting the liver parenchyma at the first, second, or third hepatic hilum, the major blood vessels or bile ducts of the corresponding site may be injured, leading to ischemia and necrosis of remnant liver tissues of the corresponding region. Experience proves that complete tumor removal close to the tumor capsule can also achieve good efficacy. Yoshida et al. also consider that a surgical resction margin of 1 cm cannot prevent postoperative early intrahepatic recurrence because there may be the presence of undetectable micro-lesions beyond 1 cm from the boundary of the primary tumor for some patients. Among the factors affecting the surgical effect, we place more emphasis on the pathological and histological characteristics of the tumor, the presence of satellite nodules, PVTT, etc.

When performing hepatectomy for large and giant liver cancer, intraoperative bleeding should be particularly controlled to reduce intraoperative bleeding and blood transfusion volume, which can help improve the success rate of hepatectomy for the treatment of giant liver cancer. For patients with liver cirrhosis, massive blood loss may cause a disorder of the coagulation mechanism: in case of massive blood loss, to maintain stable blood circulation, a large amount of banked blood needs to be transfused, which further aggravates the coagulation disorder, eventually leading to uncontrollable extensive bleeding or even death as a result of severe hemorrhagic shock. Moreover, massive blood transfusion has a risk of causing the spread of cancer and infectious diseases. Therefore, we particularly stress that intraoperative bleeding and transfusion should be reduced as far as possible when performing hepatectomy for liver cancer patients. The causes of major bleeding during hepatectomy for giant liver cancer lie in many aspects: Many patients have concomitant liver cirrhosis and portal hypertension, or there is a tumor thrombus inside the main trunk of the portal vein, and more collateral circulations are established in the hilar region. During dissection of the hilar region, these small collateral vessels are easily injured to cause major bleeding. If the tumor is giant and difficult to expose, the liver needs to be freed for conventional hepatectomy. In the process of freeing the liver, excessive traction and squeezing can cause bleeding due to rupture of the tumor capsule; major bleeding may also occur due to tearing the short hepatic veins, right adrenal gland, and its vessels.

12.3 Nonsurgical Treatment

For patients with unresectable large and giant liver cancer, one of the treatment principles is to try second-stage surgical resection and prolong the tumor-bearing survival time following nonsurgical comprehensive treatment. Another principle is to perform palliative care to alleviate the patient's pain and prolong survival. For large or even giant liver cancers that are intolerable to surgical resection, TACE therapy may be selected as long as the liver function is generally good. Some patients may have a reduced tumor and compensatory enlargement of the uninvolved liver tissue after treatment to obtain an opportunity for second-stage surgery. As TACE has a certain limitation, surgery should be performed as soon as possible for large and giant liver cancer as long as the surgical requirements are met after TACE therapy. Shuguang Chen et al. reported 21 surgically unresectable large liver cancer patients who obtained the opportunity of second-stage surgical exploration after TACE therapy; 13 cases underwent surgical resection, and 8 cases received cryotherapy for liver cancer. The 1-, 3- and 5-year survival rates of second-stage surgical resection were 84.6%, 72.7%, and 63.5%, respectively. It should be noted that TACE can achieve an exact effect for unresectable liver cancer. For resectable liver cancer, the value of TACE should be re-evaluated, and most literature considers preoperative TACE harmful rather than helpful. Preoperative application of TACE has a significantly decreased 5-year survival rate despite a relatively low short-term recurrence rate, and the 5-year survival rate of patients treated by TACE is 24%, whereas that of patients not treated by TACE is 63%. Other studies also confirmed that preoperative application of TACE is an independent risk factor for a poor prognosis of resectable liver cancer. Mengchao Wu emphasized that preoperative TACE delayed the timing of surgery and increased the surgical difficulty and the probability of tumor invading adjacent organs and extrahepatic recurrence for resectable large liver cancer or giant liver cancer. The Tongji Hospital Affiliated to Tongji Medical College of Huazhong University of Science & Technology reported 68 patients with large HCC treated by TACE only, and the 1-, 2- and 3-year survival rates were 30.9%, 19.1%, and 7.4%, respectively, and there were no 5- and 10-year survivors, indicating a significantly poorer outcome compared with the hepatectomy group ($P < 0.05$). Therefore, the preoperative interventional procedure is not performed in principle for resectable large and giant liver cancer.

TACE is necessary as adjuvant therapy after resection of large and giant liver cancer; it has multiple purposes of monitoring, preventing, and treating recurrence and is expected to improve the surgical effect further. For surgically unresectable large liver cancer and giant liver cancer, ablation therapy (RFA, MWA, and cryoablation) can be used as a part of comprehensive treatment to alleviate patients' pain and prolong survival time. CT or ultrasound-guided percutaneous ablation therapy has minimal invasiveness, reliable tumor-killing effect, and relatively high clinical application value. Ultrasound-guided percutaneous ablation has the advantages of real-time imaging and good accuracy. But, if the tumor is shielded by pulmonary and intestinal gas or close to the hila and visceral surface, which affects paracentesis positioning or impedes the entry of puncture needle, laparoscopy-guided ablation may also be performed. For large liver cancer or giant liver cancer, both TACE and ablation therapy have their limitations. As a giant tumor is often accompanied by the formation of collateral circulation and arteriovenous fistula, a good treatment effect often cannot be achieved by TACE alone. Ablation alone also inevitably leaves some viable tumor cells due to the large size of the tumor, which can rapidly lead to recurrence within the short term.

In contrast, combining the two therapies can compensate for the shortcomings of monotherapy to enhance the treatment effect. From 2003 to 2005, the Tongji Hospital Affiliated to Tongji Medical College of Huazhong University of Science & Technology, used intraoperative cryotherapy combined with TACE for the treatment of 10 patients with giant liver cancer combined with moderate to severe liver cirrhosis, and the results showed there was no operative death and the 6-month survival rate was 80%. Among them, two cases had a survival of more than 1 year, and one case had more than 2 years. The above results demonstrated that combining the above two options is superior to monotherapy by either of them.

With the improvement of LT techniques and the update of antirejection drugs, LT for liver cancer has gradually become one of the important options for treating liver cancer. Theoretically, LT for liver cancer treatment can remove the lesion and the soil (cirrhotic tissue) for liver cancer growth, showing an attractive prospect. However, practical experience proves a high recurrence rate and undesirable outcome of LT for large liver cancer, and its indications should be strictly master. At present, most scholars believe that: when the tumor can only be resected by total hepatectomy due to a large size, LT may also be considered, and for surgically resectable large liver cancer, LT is not suitable.

12.4 Treatment of Postoperative Recurrence

Over the recent 10 years, the treatment effect of liver cancer has been improved, but the long-term efficacy is still unsatisfactory, and the main cause is the high postoperative recurrence rate. It is reported that the 5-year recurrence rate reaches up to 80% after resection of large liver cancer, and most recurrences are within 2 years after surgery. In practice, recurrence after resection of large liver cancer includes the following three situations: (1) the primary tumor was not completely removed, or satellite lesions near the main tumor were missed, and the recurrent lesion is located in the same or adjacent hepatic segment of the primary tumor; (2) multiple intrahepatic micrometastases existed preoperatively, or there was intrahepatic spreading of cancer cells due to intraoperative tumor squeezing, and the recurrent lesion is diffusely distributed in the liver; (3) the liver cancer is multicentric, the recurrent lesion is often not necessarily located in the same hepatic segment or lobe, and the biological characteristics of the recurrent tumor can be the same with or different from those of the primary cancer. To date, it has been realized that recurrent liver cancer can still achieve a good outcome after treatment, and therefore, active treatment is now performed for recurrent liver cancer instead of the old practice of palliative care. From 1997 to 2003, hepatectomy was performed for a total of 1143 patients in the Tongji Hospital Affiliated to Tongji Medical College of Huazhong University of Science & Technology (named Tongji Hospital Affiliated to Tongji Medical University from 1997 to 2000, and Tongji Hospital Affiliated to Tongji Medical College of Huazhong University of Science & Technology from 2001 to 2003), and 885 recurrent cases were found during follow-up. Treatment measures after recurrence included re-hepatectomy (n = 61), RFA and MWA (n = 358), TACE therapy (n = 519), intratumoral injection of ethanol (n = 189), and hepatic artery infusion chemotherapy (n = 12). The abovementioned treatments improved the postoperative 5-year survival rate to 38.7% for large liver cancer. A large volume of tumor tissues is removed during the initial surgery for large liver cancer, so the subsequent surgery is mainly based on local resection.

Local resection should be performed 1 cm to the tumor margin for a single lesion. For multiple lesions restricted to one lobe, if the volume of the remnant liver is relatively large, irregular lobectomy can be performed. It should be noted that for a large recurrent liver cancer adjacent to the second hepatic hilum, CT or MRI findings may consider it unresectable; however, the opportunity of re-hepatectomy should not be quickly abandoned if the patient is in good condition with no or mild liver cirrhosis. As adhesions caused by initial surgery may displace the tumor and change the anatomical relationship, lesions may be misjudged based on imaging examination findings. After intraoperative releasing adhesions, the relationship between the lesion and vessels can be visualized clearly, and it is still possible to resect the tumor. With the continuous progress in liver surgery, it is not uncommon for patients to undergo two to three surgeries after resection of the large primary liver cancer due to recurrence. As the preferred treatment for recurrent liver cancer, the efficacy of re-resection is far better than other treatment options. To sum up, for recurrence after resection of large liver cancer, re-resection should be preferred; for recurrent liver cancer <3 cm in diameter, RFA, MWA, and other ablation therapy may also be considered; for unresectable recurrent large liver cancer or diffuse recurrence, TACE is selected; for patients with multiple nodule recurrence, single nodule recurrence with poor liver function, or severe liver cirrhosis, LT may be considered.

From the perspective of tumor biology, a malignant tumor is a systemic disease, while a primary tumor is just the local manifestation of systemic diseases. Therefore, the treatment of large liver cancer includes not only local therapies such as surgical resection and ablation therapy but also systemic therapies such as systemic chemotherapy, targeted therapy, and treatment of preexisting diseases (antiviral and antifibrotic therapies), adjustment of the internal environment (immunotherapy and traditional Chinese medicine (TCM) treatment), rehabilitation, etc. The comprehensive treatment with the above multiple measures has a complementary and synergistic effect on killing the tumor to improve the overall efficacy for large and giant liver cancer.

Finally, it should be emphasized that when formulating the treatment regimens for large liver cancer at the current stage, the selection of surgical resection, LT, ablation, TACE, and other treatments or combination therapy is mainly based on the number of tumors, the presence of vascular tumor thrombus visible to naked eyes, tumor envelope, and distant metastasis, classification of the liver function and hepatic functional reserve. But strictly speaking, the biological characteristics of an individual with liver cancer should be used as the premise for the formulation of treatment regimens for large liver cancer, which also determines the prognosis of large liver cancer. In the future, the treatment of large liver cancer should be based on molecular subtyping of liver cancer, which allows detection at a molecular and cellular level through direct acquisition of tissue samples from an individual with liver cancer, such as detection of circulating tumor cells, chemosensitivity test and identification of activation targets required for targeted therapy to provide a basis or reference for clinical decision making.

Suggested Reading

1. Chen X, Zhang Z. Surgical treatment strategies for large hepatocellular carcinoma and giant hepatocellular carcinoma. Chin J Operat Proced Gen Surg (Electronic Ed). 2009;3(4):702–6.
2. Chen XP, Qiu FZ, Wu ZD, et al. Longterm outcome of resection of large hepatocellular carcinoma. Br J Surg. 2006;93(5):600–6.
3. Chen X, Wu Z, Qiu F. Hepatectomy for huge primary liver cancer: report of 171 patients. Zhonghua Wai Ke Za Zhi. 2000;38(1):6–9.
4. Wang Y, Chen H, Wu M, et al. Surgical treatment for the giant hepatic carcinomas occupying the central part of the liver. Chin J Surg. 2004;42(17):1025–8.
5. Zhang Z, Chen X. Technical points for hepatectomy of large hepatocellular carcinoma. J Hepatobiliary Surg. 2008;16(1):6–7.
6. Chen X, He S. Development and changes of surgical resection for giant hepatocellular carcinoma. Lingnan Mod Clin Surg. 2003;3(1):1–2.
7. Chen S, Rui J'a, Zhao H, et al. Clinical analysis of 583 cases with large primary liver cancer. Clin Med China. 2006;22(3):224–6.
8. Chen X, Zhang Z. Surgical treatment for recurrence after resection of large hepatocellular carcinoma. J Hepatobiliary Surg. 2009;17(1):3–4.
9. Chen X. Some opinions on hepatectomy for the treatment of giant hepatocellular carcinoma. J Clin Surg. 2001;9(1):1–2.
10. Wu Y, Zhang Z, Gao D, et al. A controlled study on the selection of comprehensive therapy in large hepatocellular carcinoma patients with portal vein tumor thrombosis. Chin J Pract Surg. 2014;34(8):757–61.
11. Chen XP, Qiu FZ, Wu ZD, et al. Effects of location and extension of portal vein tumor thrombus on long term outcomes of surgical treatment for hepatocellular carcinoma. Ann Surg Oncol. 2006;13(7):940–6.
12. Zhang G, Zhang Z, Xiang S, et al. Comparison of different hepatic inflow occlusion methods in hepatectomy for large liver cancer. Chin J General Surg. 2015;24(1):18–22.
13. Chen X, Qiu F, Wu Z. Hepatectomy for the treatment of huge primary liver cancer (PLC): a report of 65 cases. Chin J General Surg. 1998;13(6):332–4.
14. Chen X. Experience of liver resection for giant hepatocellular carcinoma. J Hepatobiliary Surg. 1994;2(4):193–4.
15. Cheng S, Wu M. Clinical study progress and outlook of liver cancer with portal vein tumor thrombosis. Chin J Minimally Invasive Neurosurg. 2007;7(1):6–7.

13 Surgical Treatments for Liver Cancer with Portal Vein Tumor Thrombus or Portal Hypertension

Xin Long and Xiaoping Chen

13.1 Surgical Treatment with Chinese Characteristics for Liver Cancer with Portal Vein Tumor Thrombosis

Liver cancer with portal vein tumor thrombosis (PVTT) is a significant adverse prognostic factor for patients with liver cancer. However, the incidence of PVTT is 12.5–39.7% in patients with liver cancer, up to 64.7% in autopsied patients with liver cancer, up to 90% in patients with advanced liver cancer, and 20–30% in patients with small liver cancer. The median survival time of patients with liver cancer complicated with PVTT in the natural course of the disease is 2.7–4.0 months, whereas that of patients with liver cancer without PVTT is 24.4 months. According to the Barcelona Clinic Liver Cancer (BCLC) staging system widely applied internationally, liver cancer with PVTT is classified as BCLC stage C. At present, there is no unified international standard for the treatment of liver cancer with PVTT, and the American Association for the Study of Liver Diseases (AASLD) and European Association for the Study of the Liver (EASL) recommend molecular targeted therapy (sorafenib/lenvatinib) as the only first-line treatment regimen, based on the BCLC staging system. The Hong Kong Liver Cancer Staging System recommends Trans-arterial chemoembolisation (TACE) as the first-line therapy for liver cancer with PVTT, but for tumors smaller than 5 cm in diameter with Child-Pugh class A liver function and intrahepatic vascular invasion, surgical resection is recommended. The Japan Society of Hepatology and the Asian Pacific Association for the Study of the Liver both recommend surgical resection as an option of the multiple treatment strategies for liver cancer with PVTT.

Ever since the beginning of the 1950s, scholars from China have explored the surgical treatment for liver cancer with PVTT and achieved a good prognosis. Since the 1990s, there have been growing reports on surgical treatment for liver cancer with PVTT, and the mechanism of PVTT formation was preliminarily explored. Entering the twenty-first century, as clinical experience accumulates and the study of PVTT deepens, standardized surgical treatment has been gradually established for liver cancer with PVTT. In the meantime, the prognosis of tumor thrombus in different sites of portal veins treated by surgical procedure was analyzed. In recent years, with the emergence of new evidence-based medical evidence, the treatment of liver cancer with PVTT in China tends to seek a comprehensive therapy with multiple treatment options, including surgical resection, TACE, radiotherapy, chemotherapy, molecular targeted therapy, immunotherapy, traditional Chinese medicine (TCM) treatment, liver transplantation (LT), and so on.

X. Long · X. Chen (✉)
Tongji Hospital Affiliated to Tongji Medical College, Huazhong University of Science & Technology, Wuhan, China

X. Chen (ed.), *Diagnosis and Treatment of Liver Cancer in China*,
https://doi.org/10.1007/978-981-97-7969-7_13

13.1.1 Mechanism of PVTT Formation

The PVTT formation is the pathological basis of intrahepatic spread and recurrence and metastasis of liver cancer. There are many studies on the mechanism of PVTT formation at home and abroad, but the specific mechanism is still unclear. Many factors cause the formation of PVTT, including pathological dissection of liver tumor, hemodynamic changes of portal veins, characteristics of tumor cells, changes in the tumor microenvironment, circulating tumor cells, immune escape, and others. The main anatomical basis of PVTT formation is that liver cancer is mainly nourished by the blood supply from hepatic arteries, but the portal vein branches, which are distributed around the tumor, do not supply blood to nourish the tumor, on the contrary, function as outflow vessels of the tumor like the hepatic veins. When tumor cells invade through the vessel wall into the vascular lumen, they sprout and extend in the lumen and protrude through the tumor envelope into portal veins, thus forming PVTT. In addition, the tumor thrombus attached to the vessel wall of portal veins is supplied with blood by the arteries like the primary tumor. With arterioles supplying the portal veins as the feeding arteries and portal veins as its outflow pathways, the PVTT can live and progress.

The vessel wall of hepatic veins is thin and easily compressed. As most liver cancer patients also have liver cirrhosis, the sclerotic nodules and fibrous connective tissue compress the hepatic veins, and the gradually growing tumor may also compress the hepatic veins to obstruct their blood outflow leading to regional portal hypertension. Compressed by large or multiple liver tumors, the normal lymphatic circulation in the liver is obstructed, and the liver micro-circulation is stagnated. Moreover, as there are a large number of arteriovenous fistulas in the tumor, arterial blood directly flows into portal veins and causes an even higher portal vein pressure, thereby leading to portal vein blood stasis and even varying degrees of reverse hepatic blood flow, which create conditions for PVTT formation and explain a higher probability of the co-occurrence of PVTT and hepatic vein tumor thrombosis. PVTT is closely associated with portal vein reflux, and the higher frequency and faster speed of venous reflux, the more chances for PVTT formation. Moreover, blood in portal venous reflux contains nutrients digested and absorbed and insulin, glucagon, and somatostatin secreted by the pancreas, which provide rich nutrients for tumor cell proliferation and are more conducive to PVTT formation.

Changes in tumor cells, including changes in gene expression profile, DNA methylation, post-transcriptional modification of histones, change of chromatin spatial structure and regulation of non-coding RNA, and changes in expression of adhesion molecules on the surface of liver cancer cells (cadherin, immunoglobulin superfamily, selectin, and integrin), enhance the self-renewal, migration, and invasion capacities of liver cancer cells, thereby promoting PVTT formation. The matrix metalloproteinases, chemokines, hypoxic conditions, Treg cells, vascular growth factors, thrombomodulin, and apolipoprotein in the tumor microenvironment provide indispensable conditions for PVTT formation. In addition, Treg cells in the microenvironment of portal veins and myeloid-derived suppressor cells inhibit the activity of immune cells. As a result, tumor cells can successfully escape the immunosurveillance and maintain sufficient proliferative activity after entering the portal vein system, forming PVTT.

The peripheral blood, portal vein system, and hepatic veins of patients with liver cancer all contain CTC, the number of which is positively related to the occurrence of PVTT and microvascular tumor thrombus after hepatectomy, indicating that CTC "homing" may cause PVTT formation.

In summary, the complex mechanism of PVTT formation involves multiple factors and requires further exploration.

13.1.2 Classification of PVTT

Although there are many staging systems for liver cancer, those independently classify PVTT according to PVTT extent or range at present include only the Vp Classification proposed by Japanese scholars in 2003 and Cheng's Classification proposed by Shanghai Eastern Hepatobiliary Surgery Hospital. The Japanese Vp Classification includes five types: Vp0 (no tumor thrombus); Vp1 (presence of a tumor thrombus in the tertiary branches of the portal vein and above); Vp2 (presence of a thrombus in the secondary branches); Vp3 (presence of a thrombus in the primary branches); and Vp4 (presence of a tumor thrombus in the main trunk of the portal vein or a contralateral portal vein branch). There is no statistical difference in the postoperative 5-year survival rate between Vp3 and Vp4 PVTT. Cheng's Classification divides PVTT into types I–IV according to the invasion sites, and the extent of the PVTT: type I refers to a tumor thrombus involving the secondary branches of the portal vein and above; type II refers to a tumor thrombus involving the primary branches of the portal vein; type III refers to a tumor thrombus involving the main trunk of the portal vein; and type IV refers to a tumor thrombus involving the superior mesenteric veins. The surgical outcomes of type I and type II PVTT are better than those of type III and type IV. These two classifications can classify PVTT relatively well and predict the prognosis, guiding liver cancer treatment with PVTT. However, the prognosis prediction capability of these classifications is only applicable to patients undergoing surgical resection without considering the liver function and tumor-related factors, and their clinical applications have certain limitations. It is necessary to classify PVTT since selecting the most appropriate treatment method based on different classifications can bring maximized benefits for patients, and the classification of PVTT still needs to be further improved.

13.1.3 Surgical Treatment of PVTT

The surgical treatment of PVTT is a surgery-based comprehensive therapy supplemented by preoperative downstaging therapies such as TACE, molecular targeted therapy, and radiotherapy to improve the surgical resection rate. Postoperative TACE, molecular targeted therapy, immunotherapy (Programmed death-1 (PD-1) or Programmed Cell Death-Ligand 1 (PD-L1) monoclonal antibody), and TCM treatment can also be supplemented to improve postoperative survival and quality of life.

13.1.3.1 Surgical Indications

In 2001, the Section of Hepatic Surgery, Branch of Surgery, Chinese Medical Association formulated the surgical indications of liver cancer with PVTT, which have been continuously improved with the accumulation of clinical experience and the emergence of new evidence-based medical evidence. The general condition of patients shall meet the following requirements for liver resection: The patient has a good general condition without organic lesions of vital organs, including the heart, lung, kidneys, and brain; liver function is normal or only slightly impaired, with a Child-Pugh class A score or class B score that can be restored to class A after significant improvements through short-term liver protection treatment; hepatic functional reserve (e.g., Indocyanine green retention rate at 15 min (ICGR15)) is basically within the normal range; there is no extrahepatic metastatic tumor which is unresectable. Local lesions shall meet the following requirements: (1) The tumor is resectable per the criteria for the indications of hepatectomy for liver cancer: a single liver cancer with a smooth surface, clearly-defined boundary or pseudo-envelope formation, and the liver tissue damaged by tumor is less than 30% (measurable by computed tomography (CT) or magnetic resonance imaging (MRI)); or although the liver tissue damaged by tumor is larger than 30%, there is an obvious compensatory enlargement of the uninvolved liver, accounting for more than 50% of total liver tissue; or multiple tumors restricted to one segment or lobe of the liver. (2) The main branch and/or main trunk is filled with tumor thrombus and is likely to endanger the patient's life if it further progresses. (3) The estimated formation time of tumor thrombus is short, and thrombus organization has not occurred yet. Patients with the above conditions are suitable for tumor thrombectomy via an incision of the main trunk of the portal vein synchronously with palliative hepatectomy (4). If hemihepatectomy is performed, the tumor thrombus may be removed by opening the portal vein stump instead of cutting the main trunk of the portal vein. (5) If the tumor thrombus is located in the small portal vein branches above the hepatic segment, the portal vein branches of this segment can be removed together when resecting the liver cancer. (6) If the lesion is found to be unresectable during the operation, intra-operative selective TACE or portal vein catheterization chemotherapy, radiofrequency therapy, microwave therapy, or cryotherapy can be performed after tumor thrombectomy via an incision of the main trunk of the portal vein.

13.1.3.2 Surgical Methods

A surgical resection is a treatment option for liver cancer with PVTT and mainly includes the following classes: (1) Hepatectomy removes the tumor thrombus with the tumor. Usually, the tumor thrombus is located in the primary branches of the portal vein and above. If the tumor occurs in the left liver and the tumor thrombus is located in the left branches of the portal vein or smaller branches, a left hemihepatectomy is performed; if the tumor occurs in the right liver and the tumor thrombus is located in the right branches of the portal vein or smaller branches, a right hemihepatectomy is performed; if the tumor occurs in the right posterior lobe and the tumor thrombus is located in the right posterior branches of the portal vein, right posterior lobectomy is performed; if the tumor occurs in the hepatic segment and the tumor thrombus is located in the corresponding segmental branches of the portal vein, liver segmentectomy, lobectomy, or hemihepatectomy is performed. (2) Hepatectomy+thrombectomy includes hepatectomy+thrombectomy via liver section access, hepatectomy+thrombectomy via an incision of the portal vein or portal vein endarterectomy after the removal of tumor thrombus, or portal vein reconstruction. This procedure is applicable to a tumor thrombus extending into the main trunk of the portal vein 1.0–2.0 cm beyond the liver resection line. After tumor resection, the blood flow of the portal vein's main trunk and contralateral portal veins is temporarily blocked. The tumor thrombus in the portal vein is removed through balloon catheter thrombectomy, biliary lithotomy forceps, or other instruments, aspirators, and other methods. If the tumor thrombus is challenging to remove or completely remove through the liver section, separate and expose the portal vein's main trunk or primary branches and longitudinally cut 1.5–2.0 cm from the anterior wall or right wall to remove the tumor thrombus directly. After removing the tumor thrombus, repeatedly flush it with normal saline and open the first hepatic hilum to allow tumor thrombus fragments to be flushed out by portal vein blood flow through the broken end of the portal vein. After confirming that there is no residual lesion with intra-operative ultrasound, close the broken end of the portal vein. After removing the tumor thrombus, portal vein endarterectomy can be performed. After the liver cancer and involved portal vein branches are resected, directly perform end-to-end venous anastomosis or venous bypass anastomosis using autologous blood vessels and artificial blood vessels. Studies confirmed that thrombectomy via the broken end of the liver, portal vein reconstruction after portal vein resection, and thrombectomy via portal vein section end with portal vein endarterectomy have no significant difference in prognosis, and the surgeons can make a selection among them according to the specific disease condition.

13.1.3.3 Surgical Effect

For patients undergoing tumor resection concurrently with portal vein thrombectomy, surgery can significantly improve their prognosis, which has been agreed upon by many scholars. In addition, portal hypertension resulting from PVTT has been relieved or alleviated to reduce gastroesophageal variceal hemorrhage and refractory ascites; meanwhile, gastrointestinal symptoms caused by PVTT, including fullness, anorexia, and diarrhea, can also be alleviated to varying degrees, the portal vein blood flow is restored, and the liver function is improved. Removing the tumor and tumor thrombus creates conditions and opportunities for subsequent further comprehensive treatment such as transarterial chemotherapy or portal vein chemotherapy, TACE, biotherapy, and so on. Xiaoping CHEN et al. summarized the data of 260 cases of liver cancer with PVTT, which were assigned to the tumor resection plus portal vein thrombectomy group, portal vein thrombectomy group, TACE group, and conservative treatment group. They found through analysis that the tumor resection plus portal vein thrombectomy group had a median survival time of 17.2 months and 1-, 3-, and 5-year overall survival (OS) rates of 67.7%, 40.3%, and 20.9%, respectively, which were significantly higher than those of the other three treatment groups. Many other retrospective studies in China showed that surgical treatment for liver cancer with PVTT is superior to TACE, hepatic artery ligation/hepatic artery infusion chemotherapy, systemic chemotherapy, and conservative treatment.

Table 13.1 summarizes the English literature published by Chinese scholars on the surgical treatment effect of liver cancer with PVTT. From the table, it can be seen that the postoperative survival of patients with PVTT varies greatly, with median survival time ranging from 5 to 22 months, 1-year OS rate ranging from 0% to 86.5%, 2-year OS rate ranging from 0% to 53.0%, 3-year OS rate ranging from 0% to 69.0%, 5-year OS rate ranging from 0% to 59%, 1-year TFS rate ranging from 0% to 50.7%, 2-year TFS rate ranging from 4.2% to 11.2%, 3-year TFS rate ranging from 0% to 17.8%, and 5-year TFS rate ranging from 0% to 10.1%. The above differences are also closely related to the site of PVTT except for factors such as tumor numbers, size, alpha-fetoprotein, intrahepatic recurrence, and metastasis. Altogether, if the tumor thrombus is located in the primary branches of the portal vein and above, surgical resection can provide a good survival benefit for patients; however, if the tumor thrombus is located in the main trunk of the portal vein and superior mesenteric vein, surgical resection cannot bring survival benefits for patients. Therefore, for resectable liver tumor patients, surgery is preferably considered if the tumor thrombus is in the primary branches of the portal vein and above; it is cautiously considered if the tumor thrombus is in the main trunk of the portal vein; it is not recommended if the tumor thrombus is in the superior mesenteric vein. For patients with tumor thrombus in the main trunk of the portal vein, surgery is suitable if the liver function is Child-Pugh class A. Xiaoping CHEN et al. showed that patients with organized tumor thrombus had a smaller postoperative survival benefit than those with proliferative, necrotic, and mixed tumor thrombus. Multivariate analysis found that the survival prognosis of patients with tumor thrombus attached to the vessel wall is poorer than that of patients with suspended tumor thrombus, and the prognosis of patients with the main trunk of portal vein filled with tumor thrombus is more dismal compared to those with the non-filled main trunk of the portal vein. Therefore, regarding whether surgery should be performed for patients with tumor thrombus in the portal vein main trunk, in addition to liver function, an important consideration indicator, the pathological type of tumor thrombus and whether the tumor thrombus is attached to the vessel wall and fills the portal vein main trunk should be considered.

13.1.3.4 Surgery-Based Comprehensive Treatment

In order to improve the surgical efficacy for patients with PVTT, reduce the risks of recurrence and metastasis, and prolong survival time, postoperative adjuvant therapy is usually required, including TACE, portal vein chemotherapy, hepatic artery infusion chemotherapy, molecular targeted therapy, TCM treatment, immunotherapy, and so on. For liver cancer patients with PVTT, postoperative adjuvant TACE, portal vein infusion chemotherapy, hepatic artery infusion chemotherapy, or combining multiple adjuvant therapies can improve their survival prognosis. However, most of the studies are single-center retrospective studies, and the effectiveness of adjuvant therapies requires further confirmation by large-sample, multicenter, prospective, randomized, and controlled studies.

Studies confirmed that Sorafenib, a postoperative molecular targeted drug, cannot prolong the survival time of liver cancer patients, nor can it

Table 13.1 Surgical treatment effect of liver cancer with PVTT

Author	Time/year	Number of subjects	Site of tumor thrombus	Median survival Time/month	Accumulated survival rate/%				TFS rate/%			
					1 year	2 years	3 years	5 years	1 year	2 years	3 years	5 years
Su Fet al.	2018	189	–	–	62.0	47.0	43.0	–	–	–	–	–
		75	Secondary branches of the portal vein and above	–	83.0	53.0	42.0	–	–	–	–	–
		77	Primary branches of the portal vein	–	55.0	42.0	25.0	–	–	–	–	–
		37	Main trunk of the portal vein	–	11.0	0.0	0.0	–	–	–	–	–
Liu S et al.	2018	232	–	–	–	–	–	–	–	–	–	–
		93	Secondary branches of the portal vein and above	32.0	–	–	–	–	–	–	–	–
		84	Primary branches of the portal vein	16.0	–	–	–	–	–	–	–	–
		55	Main trunk of the portal vein	14. 0	–	–	–	–	–	–	–	–
Zheng N et al.	2016	96	–	–	86. 5	–	60. 4	33. 3	–	–	–	–
		25	Secondary branches of the portal vein and above	–	–	–	–	–	–	–	–	–
		23	Primary branches of the portal vein	–	–	–	–	–	–	–	–	–
		23	Main trunk of the portal vein	–	–	–	–	–	–	–	–	–
		25	Superior mesenteric vein	–	–	–	–	–	–	–	–	–
Wang K et al.	2016	236	Secondary branches of the portal vein and above	15.9	–	–	–	–	–	–	–	–
		315	Primary branches of portal vein	12.5	–	–	–	–	–	–	–	–
		194	Main trunk of the portal vein	6.0	–	–	–	–	–	–	–	–
Xiao CZ et al.	2015	28	Secondary branches of the portal vein	–	53.6	–	25.0	25.0	28.6	–	10.7	10.7
		38	Primary branches of the portal vein	–	39.5	–	15.8	5.3	15.8	–	5.3	5.3
Zhang YF et al.	2016	208	–	–	48.3	–	18.7	13.9	–	–	–	–
		91	Secondary branches of the portal vein and above	–	41.3	–	10.7	10.7	–	–	–	–
		105	Primary branches of portal vein	–	11.1	–	0.0	0.0	–	–	–	–
		9	The main trunk of the portal vein	–	0.0	–	0.0	0.0	–	–	–	–

Xu JF et al.	2015	40	Primary branches of the portal vein	–	62.3	–	16.1	5.2	–	–	–	–
		16	Main trunk or left and right branches of the portal vein	–	31.5	–	0.0	0.0	–	–	–	–
JZ et al.	2014	90	–	8.2	28.0	20.0	15.0	–	–	–	–	–
		66	Primary branches of the portal vein	–	–	–	–	–	–	–	–	–
		24	Main trunk of the portal vein	–	–	–	–	–	–	–	–	–
Liu PH et al.	2014	108	–	–	84.0	–	69.0	59.0	–	–	–	
Tang QH et al.	2013	186	–	10.0	40.1	17.0	13.6	–	32.3	11.2	6. 1	–
		80	Secondary branches of the portal vein and above	–	43.1	–	–	–	–	–	–	–
		66	Primary branches of the portal vein	–	33.1	–	–	–	–	–	–	–
		40	Main trunk of the portal vein	–	22.4	–	–	–	–	–	–	–
Peng ZW et al.	2012	201	–	–	42.0	–	14.1	11.1	–	–	–	–
		27	Secondary branches of the portal vein and above	–	81.5	–	51.2	37.9	–	–	–	–
		68	Primary branches of the portal vein	–	46.3	–	17.2	17.2	–	–	–	–
		83	Main trunk of the portal vein	–	32.5	–	3.6	3.6	–	–	–	–
		23	Superior mesenteric vein	–	21.7	–	0.0	0.0	–	–	–	–
Chen JS et al.	2012	88	–	9. 0	31.1	18.3	15.2	–	–	–	–	–
		–	Primary branches of the portal vein and above	9.0	–	–	–	–	–	–	–	–
		–	Main trunk or left and right branches of the portal vein	5.0	–	–	–	–	–	–	–	–
Zhou Q et al.	2011	38	–	10.0	47.0	–	22.0	–	–	–	–	–
		13	Primary branches of the portal vein	–	–	–	–	–	–	–	–	–
		25	Main trunk of the portal vein	–	–	–	–	–	–	–	–	–

(continued)

Table 13.1 (continued)

Author	Time/year	Number of subjects	Site of tumor thrombus	Median survival Time/month	Accumulated survival rate/%				TFS rate/%			
					1 year	2 years	3 years	5 years	1 year	2 years	3 years	5 years
Shi J et al.	2011	441	–	–	38.6	23.8	16.1	–	14.3	6.6	4.2	–
		144	Secondary branches of the portal vein and above	–	54.8	33.9	26.7	–	–	–	–	–
		189	Primary branches of the portal vein	–	36.4	24.9	16.9	–	–	–	–	–
		86	Main trunk of the portal vein	–	25.9	12.9	3.7	–	–	–	–	–
		22	Superior mesenteric vein	–	11.1	0.0	0.0	–	–	–	–	–
Shi J et al.	2010	406	–	–	34.4	20.6	13.0	–	13.3	6.8	4.7	–
		139	Secondary branches of the portal vein and above	22.0	52.1	–	25.1	–	21.1	–	4.4	–
		169	Primary branches of the portal vein	15.0	38.2	–	1.7	–	13.6	–	6.4	
		78	Main trunk of the portal vein	10.0	24.7	–	3.6	–	3.0	–	0.0	–
		20	Superior mesenteric vein	8.0	18.3	–	0.0	–	0.0	–	0.0	–
Peng B et al.	2009	53	–	9.0	33.3	–	17.0	8.5	–	–	–	–
Liang LJ et al.	2008	53	–	6.2	23.4	5.8	5.8	–	8.4	4.2	4.2	–
		38	Primary branches of the portal vein	–	–	–	–	–	–	–	–	–
		15	Main trunk of the portal vein	–	–	–	–	–	–	–	–	–
Li Qet al.	2006	37	–	–	–	–	–	–	50.7	–	17.8	0.0
		16	Primary branches of the portal vein	–	–	–	–	–	–	–	–	–
		21	Main trunk of the portal vein	–	–	–	–	–	–	–	–	–
Peng B et al.	2006	63	–	7.8	18.0	–	14.8	1.6	–	–	–	–
Chen XP et al.	2006	438	–	–	–	–	–	–	–	–	–	–
		286	Primary branches of the portal vein and above	18.8	58.7	39.9	22.7	18.1	–	–	–	–
		152	Main trunk of the portal vein	10.1	39.5	20.4	5.7	0.0	–	–	–	–

Fan J et al.	2005	24	–	10.1	22.7	9.8	0.0	–	–	–	–	–
		16	Primary branches of the portal vein and above	–	–	–	–	–	–	–	–	–
		8	Main trunk or left and right branches of the portal vein	–	–	–	–	–	–	–	–	–
Xu X et al.	2004	29	–	–	22.2	14.8	–	–	–	–	–	–
Fan J et al.	2001	74	–	12.0	53.9	–	26.9	16.6	–	–	–	–
		58	Primary branches of the portal vein	13.0	59.7	–	27.4	8.8	–	–	–	–
		16	Main trunk of the portal vein	8.0	29.4	–	20.0	0.0	–	–	–	–

Note: "–" represents there is no such data or sites in the literature delay the recurrence of liver cancer; therefore, Sorafenib is not a reasonable option for postoperative treatment for patients with liver cancer combined with PVTT. Moreover, other targeted drugs such as lenvatinib, cabozantinib, apatinib, and immunotherapeutic drugs such as anti-PD-1 and PD-L1 monoclonal antibodies provide more options for postoperative adjuvant therapies for patients with liver cancer combined with PVTT. However, their effectiveness and safety still need to be further evaluated. Currently, there is no reliable evidence for postoperative adjuvant systemic intravenous chemotherapy or radiotherapy. Multi-center randomized clinical studies proved that the Chinese patent medicine Huaier Granule could significantly prolong the PFS of the disease after radical resection and reduce the risks of postoperative extrahepatic recurrence and metastasis, which opens up a new possibility of postoperative adjuvant therapy for liver cancer with PVTT.

While postoperative adjuvant therapy for patients with liver cancer combined with PVTT cannot be ignored, preoperative adjuvant therapy is also worthy of the same attention. Multiple preoperative low-dose radiotherapies for patients with liver cancer complicated with tumor thrombus in the main trunk of the portal vein can reduce the tumor thrombus, in some cases, even shrinking the thrombus back to the portal vein branches, improve the surgical resection rate, and reduce liver cancer-related mortality and recurrence risk. Preoperative TACE can necrotize and reduce the tumor by up to 50% for some patients and improve the patients' postoperative survival time. To date, few reports have been made at home and abroad on preoperative TACE for treating patients with liver cancer combined with PVTT.

13.1.3.5 LT

LT is the most effective option for liver cancer treatment, which removes not only the lesion but also the soil for the growth of liver cancer, that is, the diseased liver itself. However, the postoperative recurrence rate of LT can reach up to 60%. PVTT is an independent risk factor for postoperative liver cancer recurrence that affects long-term postoperative survival. The 2-year OS rate after LT for patients with liver cancer combined with PVTT is only 29.5%, the 3-year OS rate is only 23.6%, and the recurrence rate within 3 years is 100%. The median survival time after LT for patients with liver cancer combined with PVTT is 7 months, which is the same as TACE. The 1- and 3-year OS rates were lower than those of surgical resection. These clinical experiences demonstrated that after LT for patients with liver cancer combined with PVTT, the postoperative tumor recurrence rate was high, and the prognosis was poor, indicating that LT treatment is not suitable for patients with liver cancer combined with PVTT. So far, liver cancer with PVTT has been listed as a contraindication to LT internationally.

13.1.4 Summary

Different from European and American countries, surgical resection is preferred for resectable liver cancer with PVTT in China, which is supplemented by various forms of comprehensive postoperative therapies, including TACE, hepatic artery infusion chemotherapy, portal vein infusion chemotherapy, molecular targeted therapy, immunotherapy, and TCM treatment. In addition, preoperative comprehensive therapies such as radiotherapy, TACE, molecular targeted therapy, and immunotherapy are also being explored in the hope of eventually improving the quality of life and prolonging the survival time of patients. However, surgery-based comprehensive treatments with Chinese characteristics come from retrospective studies and have a low level of evidence; thus, large-sample, multi-center, prospective, randomized, and controlled studies are required to provide more reliable evidence.

13.2 Surgical Treatment with Chinese Characteristics for Liver Cancer with Portal Hypertension

There are many causes of liver cancer with portal hypertension, and those related to the tumor itself include PVTT, compression of portal veins by the tumor, and arteriovenous fistula in the tumor.

The concomitant diseases of liver cancer such as hepatitis B virus, hepatitis C virus, nonalcoholic steatohepatitis, and liver cirrhosis caused by aflatoxin and other reasons can lead to portal hypertension. In addition, portal vein or splenic vein embolization and portal vein cavernous transformation can cause prehepatic portal hypertension, and Budd-Chiari syndrome can cause post-hepatic portal hypertension. In case of tumor compression or arteriovenous fistula in the tumor, portal hypertension can be relieved after tumor resection. The surgical treatment of liver cancer with PVTT has been discussed in detail in the previous section. The following passage describes the surgical treatment with Chinese characteristics for liver cancer with portal hypertension.

Hepatitis B cirrhosis is a common disease in China, and liver cirrhosis is a common pathological basis of both liver cancer and portal hypertension. Liver cirrhosis develops liver cancer in one-third of the patients, and approximately 80% of patients with liver cancer have concomitant cirrhosis. Liver cirrhosis is also a common cause of portal hypertension, and in the meantime, 25–55% of patients with liver cancer combined with cirrhosis have concomitant portal hypertension. Therefore, diagnosing and treating liver cancer with portal hypertension is a problem that cannot be ignored in clinical practice.

13.2.1 Definition of Portal Hypertension

Portal hypertension is mainly characterized by a pathological increase in pressure gradient between the portal vein and inferior vena cava. The portal venous pressure is usually reflected by the hepatic venous pressure gradient (HVPG), that is, the difference between wedged hepatic venous pressure and free hepatic venous pressure. Normal HVPG is <5 mmHg, and an HVPG of ≥10 mmHg is considered clinically significant portal hypertension. The measuring of HVPG is an invasive and costly operation that brings intense discomfort to the patient and has a particular technical requirement for the operator, so HVPG cannot be widely applied in clinical practice. Clinically, portal hypertension is generally judged by its clinical manifestations, including gastroesophageal varices or an enlarged spleen with a platelet count of $<100 \times 10^9$/L.

13.2.2 Surgical Treatment for Liver Cancer with Portal Hypertension

LT is the optimal option for treating liver cancer with portal hypertension, which has been agreed upon at home and abroad. LT removes not only the lesion but also the cirrhotic liver, resolving the problem of portal hypertension. Currently, the standard criteria for LT include the Milian Criteria of Italy: a single tumor smaller than or equal to 5 cm in diameter or no more than three tumors, with the maximum diameter not exceeding 3 cm, and no vascular and lymph node invasion; and the University of California San Francisco Criteria: a single tumor smaller than or equal to 6.5 cm in diameter, or no more than three tumors, with the maximum diameter not exceeding 4.5 cm and the total tumor diameter not exceeding 8 cm, and no vascular and lymph node invasion. LT can be performed without a technical bottleneck and with a good prognosis. However, currently, there is a large base of liver cancer patients with portal hypertension and an acute shortage of liver donors, and the high cost of the procedure and long-term use of postoperative immunosuppressive agents make it unaffordable for average families. Therefore, for most patients, LT is often not the preferred regimen.

13.2.2.1 Hepatectomy

Surgical Indications

Hepatectomy for liver cancer with portal hypertension is controversial between Eastern and Western countries. Early retrospective studies indicated that patients with liver cancer complicated with portal hypertension who underwent hepatectomy had a high postoperative complication rate and poor long-term prognosis, and portal hypertension is a contraindication to hepatectomy. Based on these studies, both the 2001

EASL clinical guidelines and the 2005 AASLD clinical guidelines list portal hypertension as a surgical contraindication to hepatectomy for liver cancer. Even with the increase of clinical evidence and samples and the improvement of the level of evidence, so far, surgical treatment still has not been considered first-line therapy for liver cancer with portal hypertension by the EASL and AASLD clinical guidelines for liver cancer. However, in Asian countries, especially China, hepatectomy for liver cancer with portal hypertension is highly accepted. Back in 2001, the Section of Hepatic Surgery, Branch of Surgery, Chinese Medical Association formulated the surgical treatment methods and indications for primary liver cancer with cirrhosis and portal hypertension: (1) The patient has a good general condition without organic lesions of vital organs including heart, lung, kidney, and so on; liver function is normal or only slightly impaired, with a class A score or class B score that can be restored to class A after significant improvements through short-term liver protective treatment; the hepatic functional reserve is within the normal range; there is no extrahepatic metastatic tumor. (2) Local condition: For a resectable liver cancer with manifestations of a significantly enlarged spleen and hypersplenism (e.g., a white blood cell count of lower than 3×10^9/L and a platelet count of lower than 50×10^9/L), a splenectomy can be performed synchronously. For patients with significant gastroesophageal varices, especially those who had major bleeding due to rupture of gastroesophageal variceal veins, pericardial devascularization may be considered concurrently; for patients with severe gastric mucosal lesions, splenorenal shunt or other types of selective portocaval shunts shall be performed if the intra-operative condition of the patient permits. If the liver cancer is found unresectable intra-operatively with manifestations of a significantly enlarged spleen and hypersplenism (e.g., a white blood cell count of lower than 3×10^9/L and a platelet count of lower than 50×10^9/L) and there are no significant gastroesophageal varices, splenectomy is performed synchronously with intra-operative selective TACE, cryotherapy, or radiofrequency therapy; if there are significant gastroesophageal varices, especially if major bleeding had occurred due to rupture of gastroesophageal variceal veins, and there is no severe gastric mucosal lesion, splenectomy or splenic vein ligation plus coronary vein ligation may be performed; whether devascularization is performed depends on intra-operative findings of the patient. Then, intra-operative radiofrequency therapy or cryotherapy is performed; TACE is not suitable.

Safety Evaluation of Surgery

Strict evaluation should be performed preoperatively for patients with liver cancer complicated with portal hypertension, including the evaluation of tumor status, the patient's physical condition, and liver function, as well as the extent of portal hypertension. The evaluation of tumor resectability is the same as the surgical indications in the previous section. The patient has an The Eastern Cooperative Oncology Group (ECOG) score of 0–1 for performance status. Presently, liver function is mainly evaluated through the modified Child-Pugh score to obtain the classification of liver function, the ICGR15 to know the hepatic functional reserve, and the measurement of liver volume to assess the remnant liver volume. Class C liver function is contraindicated to surgery; if ICGR15 is >40%, there is a high risk for postoperative liver failure, and for patients with liver cirrhosis, the postoperative remnant liver volume is generally larger than 40%. In addition, the extent of liver cirrhosis shall also be evaluated, and the content of the preoperative scoring system for liver cirrhosis includes gastroesophageal varices, portal vein width, the thickness of spleen and platelet count, no or mild cirrhosis (0–1), moderate liver cirrhosis (2–3), and severe cirrhosis (≥4) (Table 13.2). Portal hypertension is clinically evaluated mainly through gastroscopy to understand the status of gastroesophageal varices, color Doppler ultrasound, routine blood tests, hemoglobin, and platelets to know the size of the spleen and hypersplenism status. Patients with liver cancer with portal hypertension have certain risks of biliary leakage, liver failure, and ascites after hepatectomy and risk of portal vein thrombosis forma-

Table 13.2 Preoperative scoring system for liver cirrhosis

	Score		
Clinical indicators	0	1	2
Gastroesophageal varices	None	Slight	Moderately to severely
Portal vein width/mm	<12	12–14	>14
Spleen thickness/cm	<4	4–5	>5
Platelet count/($\times 10^9$/L)	>100	70–100	<70

tion following splenectomy. However, the above complications are controllable through the selection of patients, strict preoperative evaluation, and fine perioperative management, and the patient is safe on the whole.

13.2.2.2 Surgical Methods

Treatment of Liver Cancer

The premise of liver resection for patients with portal hypertension is that ascites are absent or controllable with total serum bilirubin lower than 1.2 mg/dL. For resectable liver cancer, the extent of liver resection depends on serum total bilirubin, albumin, cholesterol, and prothrombin time. In case of a serum total bilirubin level of 0.7–1.2 mg/dL, albumin level of 35 g/L or lower, cholesterol level of 3.6 mmol/L or lower, and prothrombin time of 3–4 seconds, only minor liver resection (two liver segments and below) can be performed. In case of a serum total bilirubin level of <0.7 mg/dL, albumin level of >35 g/L, a cholesterol level of >3.6 mmol/L, and prolonged prothrombin time of <3 s, major liver resection (three liver segments and above) can be performed, but the remnant liver volume ratio should be >60%. Liver cancer patients with portal hypertension all have varying degrees of liver cirrhosis, and patients with mild or no cirrhosis are tolerable to segment 4 liver resection, but the incidence of liver failure is 9.1%; for patients with moderate liver cirrhosis, major liver resection has a significantly higher incidence of postoperative liver failure than minor liver resection (38.1% vs. 3%); for patients with severe liver cirrhosis who undergo liver resection of two liver segments and above, the incidence of postoperative liver failure is up to 63.2%. Therefore, with the aggravation of liver cirrhosis, minor liver resection shall be performed as far as possible under the condition of ensuring the incision margin. In addition, for a tumor smaller than 2 cm in diameter, microwave coagulation or RFA therapy can be selected to avoid postoperative liver failure caused by liver resection. For unresectable liver cancer found intra-operatively, only palliative treatment is performed.

13.2.2.3 Treatment of Portal Hypertension

Not Combining Resection with Splenectomy or Pericardial Devascularization

For patients with an enlarged spleen and mild hypersplenism (e.g., a white blood cell count of higher than 3×10^9/L and a platelet count of higher than 50×10^9/L and lower than 100×10^9/L), currently, there is no sufficient evidence proving the benefits of splenectomy for them, and therefore, portal hypertension may not be treated depending on the situation. In view of this situation, a multi-center, randomized, positive- and parallel-controlled clinical study of partial hepatectomy combined with splenectomy in patients with liver cancer combined with liver cirrhosis and hypersplenism is ongoing (Registration No: ChiCTR1900024695).

Splenectomy

In the case of an enlarged spleen, with a platelet count of <50×10^9/L, and insignificant gastroesophageal varices, resection can be combined with a splenectomy, and T cell subsets, and Th cell balance can be restored postoperatively, and white blood cell count and platelet count can return to normal. Moreover, the postoperative liver burden on metabolizing bilirubin can also be reduced to help recover liver function.

Pericardial Devascularization

For patients with severe gastroesophageal varices or with a red color sign as indicated by gastroscopy, and those who have had major bleeding due to rupture of gastroesophageal variceal veins, resection should be combined with pericardial devascularization. Pericardial devascularization has a high immediate hemostasis rate, low operative mortality, little impact on hepatic perfusion, and low incidence of postoperative hepatic encephalopathy, and is easy to operate and be popularized.

Shunt

For patients with severe gastric mucosal lesions, a splenorenal shunt or other types of selective portocaval shunts can be performed, but a large number of shunts reduce the blood flow of portal veins, further deteriorate postoperative liver function, and may increase the incidence of hepatic encephalopathy. At present, for patients with liver cancer combined with portal hypertension, hepatectomy is performed asynchronously with a shunt.

Surgical Effect

Surgical resection is safe and effective for patients with liver cancer combined with portal hypertension, whose OS rate and overall TFS rate are comparable to those of patients with liver cancer not combined with portal hypertension. Patients with liver cancer with portal hypertension who undergo hepatectomy or in combination with splenectomy or pericardial devascularization have a significantly superior survival prognosis than those treated by TACE or thermal ablation therapy and show no difference from patients with liver cancer not combined with portal hypertension. Chen XP et al. retrospectively analyzed 204 patients with liver cancer combined with portal hypertension and hypersplenism, 94 of whom received hepatectomy plus splenectomy, and 110 received hepatectomy only. There was no statistical difference between the two groups' extent of liver resection and postoperative complications. The two groups had no statistical differences in postoperative 5-year OS rate, but the 5-year overall TFS rate of the hepatectomy plus splenectomy group was superior to that of the hepatectomy alone group (37% vs. 27. 3%, P = 0.003) (Fig. 13.1). All patients in the hepatectomy plus splenectomy group received six cycles of postoperative chemotherapy, while only 15.5% in the hepatectomy group were tolerable to chemotherapy. This is because, after splenectomy, white blood cells and platelets in the body can return to normal, and the

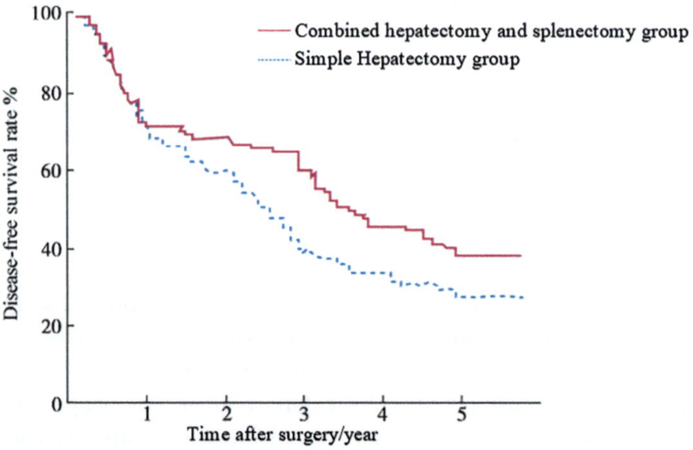

Number of patients in danger/case						
Combined hepatectomy and splenectomy group	94	67	64	56	43	35
Simple Hepatectomy group	110	77	65	43	36	30

Fig. 13.1 Patients in the hepatectomy plus splenectomy group have a significantly higher TFS than those in the hepatectomy alone group

liver metabolism can be affected by splenectomy to alleviate the progression of liver cirrhosis and improve liver function and immunity of the body, thereby enabling patients to receive subsequent therapies and improving their survival prognosis. Moreover, splenectomy or combined pericardial devascularization can reduce portal vein blood flow and the risk of gastroesophageal variceal hemorrhage, which is beneficial to the patient's long-term survival. This study indicated that hepatectomy combined with splenectomy is an effective option for treating liver cancer with liver cirrhosis and hypersplenism. Therefore, portal hypertension is not a surgical contraindication to hepatectomy for liver cancer; instead, an extended surgical method is required for hypersplenism and gastroesophageal varices resulting from portal hypertension, which is more conducive to improving the patient's survival prognosis.

Therefore, hepatectomy is a first-line treatment measure for liver cancer with portal hypertension in China, and an extended surgical method with concurrent splenectomy is required for patients with a significantly enlarged spleen and hypersplenism. For patients with significant gastroesophageal varices, especially those who had major bleeding due to rupture of gastroesophageal variceal veins, concurrent pericardial devascularization is required.

13.3 Non-surgical Treatment

With regard to patients with unresectable liver cancer combined with cirrhosis and portal hypertension (unresectable due to the presence of multiple, giant tumors, extensive tumor thrombus in portal veins, etc.), interventional procedure or radiotherapy, targeted therapy, immunotherapy, TCM treatment, and other options can be selected if the liver function and physical condition of the patient permits. In the case of an enlarged spleen with severe hypersplenism, splenic artery embolization may be selected. In the case of gastroesophageal variceal hemorrhage, endoscopic treatment is preferred.

13.4 Summary

For the treatment of liver cancer with portal hypertension, LT is preferred if the condition permits, but hepatectomy combined with splenectomy or pericardial devascularization is still the mainstream treatment option.

Suggested Reading

1. Poon RT, Fan ST, Tsang FH, et al. Locoregional therapies for hepatocellular carcinoma: a critical review from the surgeon's perspective. Ann Surg. 2002;235(4):466–86.
2. Minagawa M, Makuuchi M. Treatment of hepatocellular carcinoma accompanied by portal vein tumor thrombus. World J Gastroenterol. 2006;12(47):7561–7.
3. Kumar S, Gao L, Yeagy B, et al. Virus combinations and chemotherapy for the treatment of human cancers. Curr Opin Mol Ther. 2008;10(4):371–9.
4. Wu Y, Zhiwei Z. Surgical treatment of liver cancer with portal vein tumor thrombosi. J Hepatopancreatobiliary Surg. 2015;27(2):171–4.
5. Llovet JM, Bustamante J, Castells A, et al. Natural history of untreated nonsurgical hepatocellular carcinoma: rationale for the design and evaluation of therapeutic trials. Hepatology. 1999;29(1):62–7.
6. Bruix J, Sherman M. Management of hepatocellular carcinoma: an update. Hepatology. 2011;53(3):1020–2.
7. Tsochatzis E, Meyer T, O'Beirne J, et al. Transarterialchemoembolisation is not superior to embolisation alone: the recent European Association for the Study of the liver (EASL) European Organisation for Research and Treatment of Cancer (EORTC) guidelines. Eur J Cancer. 2013;49(6):1509–10.
8. Bruix J, Llovet JM. Prognostic prediction and treatment strategy in hepatocellular carcinoma. Hepatology. 2002;35(3):519–24.
9. Yau T, Tang VY, Yao TJ, et al. Development of Hong Kong liver cancer staging system with treatment stratification for patients with hepatocellular carcinoma. Gastroenterology. 2014;146(7):1691–700.
10. Omata M, Cheng AL, Kokudo N, et al. Asia Pacific clinical practice guidelines on the management of hepatocellular carcinoma: a 2017 update. Hepatol Int. 2017;11(4):317–70.
11. Kudo M, Matsui O, Izumi N, et al. JSH consensus based clinical practice guidelines for the management of hepatocellular carcinoma: 2014 update by the liver cancer study group of Japan. Liver Cancer. 2014;3(3–4):458–68.

12. Zhou Xinda Y, Yeqin LZ, et al. Clinical analysis of 19 primary liver cancer cases survived over 10 years after resection. Tumor. 1989;9(3):115–7.
13. Xiaoping C, Shuai X, Zhiyong H. Investigation of extent of liver resection for liver cancer combined with liver cirrhosis. Chinese Journal of Digestive Surgery. 2019;18(4):303–6.
14. Xiao H, Zhang B, Mei B, et al. Hepatic resection for hepatocellular carcinoma in patients with portal hypertension: a long term benefit compared with transarterial chemoembolization and thermal ablation. Medicine (Baltimore). 2015;94(7):e495.
15. Yu Yeqin X, Dongbo ZY, et al. Hepatectomy combined with portal vein thrombectomy for the treatment of liver cancer (a report of 25 cases). Chinese J Pract Surg. 1994;14(1):18–9.
16. Ting Z. Analysis of clinical diagnosis and treatment of 38 moderate or advanced primary liver cancer combined with portal vein tumor thrombosis cases. J Pract Oncol. 1996;11(4):166–8.
17. Zheng Yaxin Y, Yeqin LK, et al. Correlations between portal vein tumor thrombogenesis and expression of P53 and PCNA in hepatocellular carcinoma. Chinese J Digest. 1996;16(2):75–8.
18. AnYiming CS, Guoying H. Effect of Hemorheological change on cancer embolism in portal vein of primary liver cancer. Chinese J Microcirculation. 1996;6(4):42–3.
19. Anzhong L. Diagnosis and differential diagnosis of portal vein tumor thrombosis. J Hepatobiliary Surg. 2000;8(5):397–8.
20. Xiaoping C, Bixiang Z, Guangwan Z, et al. Basis and clinical study of hepatocellular carcinoma with portal vein tumor thrombosis. J Abdom Surg. 2003;16(6):343–6.
21. Zhefu L, Xiaoping C. Clinical progress in primary liver cancer with portal vein tumor thrombosis. Med J Qilu. 2008;23(2):182–3.
22. Minghui M, Jinghong Y, Wei D. Surgical treatment for hepatocellular carcinoma with portal vein tumor thrombosis. J Surg Concept Pract. 2000;5(4):231–4.
23. Rongping G, Xiaojun L, Yunfei Y, et al. Significance of removing portal vein tumor thrombus and TACE in improving outcome of resection for primary liver cancer with portal vein tumor thrombus. Chin J Hepatobiliary Surg. 2000;6(5):54–6.
24. Jia F, Jian Z, Zhaoyou T, et al. Hepatocellular carcinoma with tumor thrombi in the portal vein. A comparison of therapeutic effects by different treatments. Chinese J Oncol. 2000;22(3):71–3.
25. Hepatobiliary Surgery Group, Chinese Society of Surgery, Chinese Medical Association. Selection of surgical treatments for primary liver cancer. J Abdom Surg. 2001;14(1):60–1.
26. Hepatobiliary Surgery Group, Chinese Society of Surgery, Chinese Medical Association. 2004 guidelines for surgical treatment of primary hepatocellular carcinoma. Chinese J Hepatol. 2005;13(5):329–30.
27. Shuqun C, Jianqiang C, Minshan C, et al. Chinese expert consensus on multidisciplinary diagnosis and treatment of hepatocellular carcinoma with portal vein tumor thrombus (2018). J Clin Hepatol. 2019;35(4):737–43.
28. Shuqun C, Han C, Jiahe Y, et al. Significance of typing of tumor thrombi in determination of treatment and assessment of prognosis of hepatocellular carcinoma with tumor thrombi in the portal vein. Nat Med J China. 2004;84(1):7–9.
29. Chen XP, Qiu FZ, Wu ZD, et al. Effects of location and extension of portal vein tumor thrombus on long term outcomes of surgical treatment for hepatocellular carcinoma. Ann Surg Oncol. 2006;13(7):940 946.
30. Jiazhou Y, Yuequn L. Progress in surgical treatment of liver cancer with portal vein tumor thrombosis: Barcelona clinic liver cancer prognosis and treatment strategy. Chinese J Bases Clin Gen Surg. 2019;26(5):532–7.
31. Ying T, Jiamei Y. Formation and treatment of portal vein tumor thrombosis for primary liver cancer. Chinese J Pract Surg. 2003;23(6):56–8.
32. Toyosaka A, Okamoto E, Mitsunobu M, et al. Pathologic and radiographic studies of intrahepatic metastasis in hepatocellular carcinoma; the role of efferent vessels. HPB Surg. 1996;10(2):97–103.
33. Zhiquan W, QiuShuangjian SZ, et al. Relationship of portal vein tumor thrombosis formation with the characteristics of liver blood supply. World Chinese J Digestol. 2004;12(1):249–50.
34. Lei D, Xinmin L. Study on the causes of portal vein tumor thrombosis formation for liver cancer. Chinese J Ultrasound Med. 1999;15(6):25–6.
35. Chenhe Y, Xin Y, Xiangyu W, et al. Research progress in the molecular mechanism of portal vein tumor thrombus (PVTT) in hepatocellular carcinoma (HCC). Fudan Univ J Medical Sci. 2019;46(2):261–6.
36. Ou H, Huang Y, Xiang L, et al. Circulating tumor cell phenotype indicates poor survival and recurrence after surgery for hepatocellular carcinoma. Dig Dis Sci. 2018;63(9):2373–80.
37. Ikai I, Yamamoto Y, Yamamoto N, et al. Results of hepatic resection for hepatocellular carcinoma invading major portal and/or hepatic veins. Surg Oncol Clin N Am. 2003;12(1):65–75.
38. Shuqun C, Mengchao W, Han C, et al. Tumor thrombus types influence the prognosis of hepatocellular carcinoma with the tumor thrombi in the portal vein. Hepato-Gastroenterology. 2007;54(74):499–502.
39. Shi J, Lai EC, Li N, et al. A new classification for hepatocellular carcinoma with portal vein tumor thrombus. J Hepatobiliary Pancreat Sci. 2011;18(1):74–80.
40. Xiaoping C, Zhiwei Z. Norms and clinical interpretation guidelines from the hepatology branch of the Chinese Medical Association. J Clin Hepatol. 2013;29(1):25–7.
41. Weidong J, Wenbin L. Surgical treatment of hepatocellular carcinoma with portal vein tumor thrombus. J Clin Hepat. 2015;31(6):859–62.
42. Shi J, Lai EC, Li N, et al. Surgical treatment of hepatocellular carcinoma with portal vein tumor thrombus. Ann Surg Oncol. 2010;17(8):2073–80.

43. Fan J, Wu ZQ, Tang ZY, et al. Multimodality treatment in hepatocellular carcinoma patients with tumor thrombi in portal vein. World J Gastroenterol. 2001;7(1):28–32.
44. Fan J, Zhou J, Wu ZQ, et al. Efficacy of different treatment strategies for hepatocellular carcinoma with portal vein tumor thrombosis. World J Gastroenterol. 2005;11(8):1215–9.
45. Peng ZW, Guo RP, Zhang YJ, et al. Hepatic resection versus transcatheter arterial chemoembolization for the treatment of hepatocellular carcinoma with portal vein tumor thrombus. Cancer. 2012;118(19):4725–36.
46. Liu PH, Lee YH, Hsia CY, et al. Surgical resection versus transarterial chemoembolization for hepatocellular carcinoma with portal vein tumor thrombosis: a propensity score analysis. Ann Surg Oncol. 2014;21(6):1825–33.
47. Zheng N, Wei X, Zhang D, et al. Hepatic resection or transarterial chemoembolization for hepatocellular carcinoma with portal vein tumor thrombus. Medicine (Baltimore). 2016;95(26):e3959.
48. Ye JZ, Zhang YQ, Ye H, et al. Appropriate treatment strategies improve survival of hepatocellular carcinoma patients with portal vein tumor thrombus. World J Gastroenterol. 2014;20(45):17141–7.
49. Wang K, Guo WX, Chen MS, et al. Multimodality treatment for hepatocellular carcinoma with portal vein tumor thrombus: a large scale, multicenter, propensity mathching score analysis. Medicine (Baltimore). 2016;95(11):e3015.
50. Liang L, Chen TH, Li C, et al. A systematic review comparing outcomes of surgical resection and non surgical treatments for patients with hepatocellular carcinoma and portal vein tumor thrombus. HPB(Oxford). 2018;20(12):1119–29.
51. Su F, Chen KH, Liang ZG, et al. Comparison of three dimensional conformal radiotherapy and hepatic resection in hepatocellular carcinoma with portal vein tumor thrombus. Cancer Med. 2018;7(9):4387–95.
52. Liu S, Guo L, Li H, et al. Postoperative adjuvant trans arterial chemoembolization for patients with hepatocellular carcinoma and portal vein tumor thrombus. Ann Surg Oncol. 2018;25(7):2098–104.
53. Xiao CZ, Wei W, Guo ZX, et al. A prognosis model for patients with hepatocellular carcinoma and portal vein tumor thrombus following hepatic resection. Oncol Lett. 2015;10(5):2787–94.
54. Zhang YF, Guo RP, Zou RH, et al. Efficacy and safety of preoperative chemoembolization for resectable hepatocellular carcinoma with portal vein invasion: a prospective comparative study. Eur Radiol. 2016;26(7):2078–88.
55. Xu JF, Liu XY, Wang S, et al. Surgical treatment for hepatocellular carcinoma with portal vein tumor thrombus: a novel classification. World J Surg Oncol. 2015;13:86.
56. Tang QH, Li AJ, Yang GM, et al. Surgical resection versus conformal radiotherapy combined with TACE for resectable hepatocellular carcinoma with portal vein tumor thrombus: a comparative study. World J Surg. 2013;37(6):1362–70.
57. Chen JS, Wang Q, Chen XL, et al. Clinicopathologic characteristics and surgical outcomes of hepatocellular carcinoma with portal vein tumor thrombosis. J Surg Res. 2012;175(2):243–50.
58. Zhou Q, Wang Y, Zhou X, et al. Prognostic analysis for treatment modalities in hepatocellular carcinomas with portal vein tumor thrombi. Asian Pac J Cancer Prev. 2011;12(11):2847–50.
59. Peng BG, He Q, Li JP, et al. Adjuvant transcatheter arterial chemoembolization improves efficacy of hepatectomy for patients with hepatocellular carcinoma and portal vein tumor thrombus. Am J Surg. 2009;198(3):313–8.
60. Liang LJ, Hu WJ, Yin XY, et al. Adjuvant intraportal venous chemotherapy for patients with hepatocellular carcinoma and portal vein tumor thrombi following hepatectomy plus portal thrombectomy. World J Surg. 2008;32(4):627–31.
61. Li Q, Wang J, Sun Y, et al. Efficacy of postoperative transarterial chemoembolization and portal vein chemotherapy for patients with hepatocellular carcinoma complicated by portal vein tumor thrombosis a randomized study. World J Surg. 2006;30(11):2004–11.
62. Peng B, Liang L, He Q, et al. Surgical treatment for hepatocellular carcinoma with portal vein tumor thrombus. Hepato-Gastroenterology. 2006;53(69):415–9.
63. Xu X, Zheng S, Liang TB, et al. Orthotopic liver transplantation for patients with hepatocellular carcinoma complicated by portal vein tumor thrombi. Hepatobiliary Pancreat Dis Int. 2004;3(3):341–4.
64. Bruix J, Takayama T, Mazzaferro V, et al. Adjuvant sorafenib for hepatocellular carcinoma after resection or ablation(STORM): a phase 3, randomised, double blind, placebo controlled trial. Lancet Oncol. 2015;16(13):1344–54.
65. Chen Q, Shu C, Laurence AD, et al. Effect of Huaier granule on recurrence after curative resection of HCC: a multicentre, randomised clinical trial. Gut. 2018;67(11):2006–16.
66. Li N, Feng S, Xue J, et al. Hepatocellular carcinoma with main portal vein tumor thrombus: a comparative study comparing hepatectomy with or without neoadjuvant radiotherapy. HPB (Oxford). 2016;18(6):549–56.
67. Yoshidome H, Takeuchi D, Kimura F, et al. Treatment strategy for hepatocellular carcinoma with major portal vein or inferior vena cava invasion: a single institution experience. J Am Coll Surg. 2011;212(5):796–803.
68. Wang ZX, Song SH, Teng F, et al. A single center retrospective analysis of liver transplantation on 255 patients with hepatocellular carcinoma. Clin Transpl. 2010;24(6):752–7.
69. Llovet JM, Bruix J. Novel advancements in the management of hepatocellular carcinoma in 2008. J Hepatol. 2008;48(Suppl 1):20–37.

70. European Association for the Study of the Liver. EASL clinical practice guidelines: management of hepatocellular carcinoma. J Hepatol. 2018;69(1):182–236.
71. Sanyal AJ, Bosch J, Blei A, et al. Portal hypertension and its complications. Gastroenterology. 2008;134(6):1715–28.
72. Zhong JH, Li H, Xiao N, et al. Hepatic resection is safe and effective for patients with hepatocellular carcinoma and portal hypertension. PLoS One. 2014;9(9):e108755.
73. Zhou SJ, Zhang EL, Liang BY, et al. Morphologic severity of cirrhosis determines the extent of liver resection in patients with hepatocellular carcinoma and child Pugh grade a cirrhosis. J Surg Res. 2016;200(2):444–51.
74. Xiaoping C. Surgical treatment status for portal hypertension. J Abdom Surg. 2007;20(2):70–1.
75. Xiaoping C. Emphasis should be laid on the selection of surgical methods for portal hypertension. J Clin Surg. 2007;15(3):150–1.
76. Llovet JM, Fuster J, Bruix J. Intention to treat analysis of surgical treatment for early hepatocellular carcinoma: resection versus transplantation. Hepatology. 1999;30(6):1434–40.
77. Bruix J, Castells A, Bosch J, et al. Surgical resection of hepatocellular carcinoma in cirrhotic patients: prognostic value of preoperative portal pressure. Gastroenterology. 1996;111(4):1018–22.
78. Cucchetti A, Ercolani G, Vivarelli M, et al. Is portal hypertension a contraindication to hepatic resection. Ann Surg. 2009;250(6):922–8.
79. Jang CW, Kwon HJ, Kong H, et al. Impact of clinically significant portal hypertension on surgical outcomes for hepatocellular carcinoma in patients with compensated liver cirrhosis: a propensity score matching analysis. Ann Hepatobil Pancreat Surg. 2016;20(4):159–66.
80. Ohkubo T, Midorikawa Y, Nakayama H, et al. Liver resection of hepatocellular carcinoma in patients with portal hypertension and multiple tumors. Hepatol Res. 2018;48(6):433–41.
81. Xiaoping C, Zhixin C. Surgical treatment for hepatocellular carcinoma with portal hypertension and hypersplenism. Chinese J Pract Surg. 2004;24(12):716–8.
82. Zhiyong H, ErLei Z, Xiaoping C. Staging the severity of liver cirrhosis and decision of surgical treatment for hepatocellular carcinoma: Tongji experience. Chinese J Surg. 2019;57(6):408–11.
83. Zhang EL, Zhang ZY, Wang SP, et al. Predicting the severity of liver cirrhosis through clinical parameters. J Surg Res. 2016;204(2):274–81.
84. Chen XP, Zhang ZW, Zhang BX, et al. Modified technique of hepatic vascular exclusion: effect on blood loss during complex mesohepatectomy in hepatocellular carcinoma patients with cirrhosis. Langenbeck's Arch Surg. 2006;391(3):209–15.
85. Chen XP, Wu ZD, Huang ZY, et al. Use of hepatectomy and splenectomy to treat hepatocellular carcinoma with cirrhotic hypersplenism. Br J Surg. 2005;92(3):334–9.
86. Dong KS, Liang BY, Zhang ZY, et al. Histologic severity of liver cirrhosis: a key factor affecting surgical outcomes of hepatocellular carcinoma in patients with portal hypertension. Asian J Surg. 2019;42(12):981–9.
87. Guangshun Y, Ning Y. Surgical treatment for liver cancer with portal hypertension. Chinese J Pract Surg. 2002;22(9):552–3.
88. He W, Zeng Q, Zheng Y, et al. The role of clinically significant portal hypertension in hepatic resection for hepatocellular carcinoma patients: a propensity score matching analysis. BMC Cancer. 2015;15:263.

Part IV

Interventional Therapy for Liver Cancer

14 Overview of Interventional Therapy for Liver Cancer

Hai-Dong Zhu and Gao-Jun Teng

Interventional therapy is one of the main treatments methods for intermediate-stage and advanced liver cancer. Interventional therapy of primary liver cancer began in the 1970s. After more than 40 years of innovation and development, endovascular interventional therapy, represented by transcatheter arterial chemoembolization (TACE), has become the most widely used treatment for intermediate-stage and advanced liver cancer that cannot be surgically resected. Endovascular interventional therapy for liver cancer mainly includes transcatheter arterial infusion, transcatheter arterial embolization (TAE), and TACE. In particular, TACE can be further divided into conventional TACE, drug-eluting bead TACE, and transcatheter arterial radioembolization, which is also known as selective internal radiation therapy.

In 1953, Seldinger invented the arteriographic method via percutaneous femoral artery puncture and guidewire-guided cannulation using trocar needles, guidewires, and catheters, pioneering the technique of transcatheter endovascular therapy. In 1963, Carroll first proposed the theory of blood supply for liver cancer, which laid the theoretical foundation for endovascular therapy of liver cancer. Subsequently, Carroll performed a series of studies on the anatomical characteristics of the blood supply of liver cancer, providing the anatomical basis for the transarterial treatments for liver cancer. In 1970, Watkins *et al.* first reported hepatic arterial infusion chemotherapy (HAIC) for primary liver cancer. In 1974, Doyon *et al.* first reported TAE for liver tumors. The same year, Takashima *et al.* studied the value of hepatic arteriography in the diagnosis of liver cancer. In 1976, Goldstein *et al.* also investigated the use of TAE in treating liver cancer. In 1979, Nakakuma *et al.* discovered that lipiodol injected through the hepatic artery could be selectively retained in liver tumors and be used for embolization of the feeding arteries of liver cancer, ushering in a new era of interventional treatment for liver cancer. The same year, Gui LIN *et al.* explored the diagnosis of primary liver cancer by selective angiography. In 1981, Zijiang LIU *et al.* reported the femoral artery cannulation technique. The same year, Dushan RONG, Gui LIN, Nengshu HE, and Enhui WU published articles to promote interventional radiology across the nation, and Zijiang LIU launched interventional radiology workshops to popularize the Seldinger technique nationwide, which greatly boosted the popularity of TACE in China. In 1983, Zhiying LIN *et al.* reported 13 cases of primary liver cancer treated with TAE using gelatin sponge particles. The same year, Nakakuma K *et al.* conducted an animal study on the mechanism of TACE for primary liver cancer. In 1984, Gui LIN reported the preliminary clinical results of TAE in 13

H.-D. Zhu · G.-J. Teng (✉)
Zhongda Hospital, Southeast University, Nanjing, China
e-mail: gjteng@seu.edu.cn

X. Chen (ed.), *Diagnosis and Treatment of Liver Cancer in China*,
https://doi.org/10.1007/978-981-97-7969-7_14

cases of primary liver cancer. In addition, his cadaver study on the blood supply and microvascular manifestations of metastatic liver cancer was published. He also investigated the changes in blood circulation before and after interventional therapy for liver cancer. Since iodized oil can be selectively retained in the tumor for a long time, Xuehao WANG *et al.* innovated radioactive iodized oil by labeling, mixed with doxorubicin or mitomycin C, and prepared a ^{125}I-iodized oil anticancer emulsion in 1986. The emulsion was then injected through the hepatic artery to treat unresectable primary liver cancer. In 1987, Junyuan GUO *et al.* reported the clinical results of TACE using lipiodol mixed with an anticancer drug for liver cancer and published a review article on TACE for liver cancer in the same year. In 1991, Yuchen JIA compared the efficacy of hepatic arterial infusion with chemoembolization for liver cancer. The same year, Jianming TIAN *et al.* investigated the effect of the inferior phrenic artery on the treatment outcomes for liver cancer. In 1993, Zhi WANG *et al.* studied the postoperative pharmacokinetics of lipiodol and cisplatin after TACE. In 1993, Chihua FANG *et al.* reported the use of a hepatic artery infusion pump to treat primary liver cancer, and in 1994, Qiyong GUO *et al.* reported the direct injection of boiling saline for treating liver tumors, providing more options and new ideas for liver cancer treatments. In 1996, Yonghua DONG *et al.* explored the prognostic factors associated with liver cancer after interventional therapy.

At the same time, materials for interventional therapy kept evolving. In 1981 and 1983, Konno *et al.* and Yamada *et al.* applied lipiodol-based drugs and gelatin sponges, respectively, to treat liver cancer. In 1985, Gansheng FENG *et al.* conducted animal experiments and clinical studies to test the traditional Chinese medicine Bletilla as an embolic agent. In 1989, Yinghua ZOU *et al.* investigated the use of domestic polyvinyl alcohol microspheres in hepatic artery embolization in animal experiments and preliminary clinical studies. In 1991, Li YANG *et al.* published experimental and preliminary clinical results of hepatic artery embolization with Dextran MMC microspheres. The same year, Zhiping YAN *et al.* reported a preliminary clinical study on brachytherapy using yttrium-90 (^{90}Y) glass microspheres for primary liver cancer. Then, in 1992, they published a review article on detailed descriptions of the types and dosages of radioactive microspheres and their applications in treating liver cancer. In 1994, Baowei DONG *et al.* reported the results of ultrasound-guided direct intratumoral injection of ^{90}Y glass microspheres for treating liver cancer. In 1999, Gao-Jun TENG *et al.* reported that hepatic arterial embolization using phosphorus-32 (^{32}P) glass microspheres caused damage to the liver tissue, proving the safety and efficacy of this treatment. By 2001, ^{32}P glass microspheres had been used for liver cancer and become an effective treatment for intermediate-stage and advanced liver cancer.

Since the 21st century, many studies on endovascular treatments for liver cancer have been conducted in China based on previous endovascular techniques. Considering the dual blood supply from the hepatic artery and portal vein, Jingjian SUN *et al.* used TACE combined with portal vein chemotherapy or chemoembolization to treat liver cancer in 2002. Preliminary results showed that this approach more adequately blocked the blood supply to the tumor and tumor thrombus, increased the concentration of drugs in the lesions, and effectively led to necrosis of the tumors, satellite lesions, and intrahepatic metastases. In 2004, Ke XU *et al.* analyzed the important interventional techniques and protocols for patients with liver cancer at different stages and various comorbidities. The same year, in Gang ZHANG *et al.*'s investigation on the association between post-TACE iodized oil deposition and blood supply to primary liver cancer, it was found that the characteristics of blood supply were closely related to iodized oil deposition after TACE. In 2016, Ming CHAO *et al.*'s examination on the combination therapy of TACE and bicarbonate for large tumors demonstrated significantly improved antitumor efficacy of TACE. In 2017, based on portal vein stenting for portal vein tumor thrombosis (PVTT), Gao-Jun TENG *et al.* innovated a portal vein irradiation stent and demonstrated its safety and efficacy for PVTT in a single-center study. In 2018, Ming ZHAO *et al.*'s study on HAIC using oxaliplatin in combination with fluorouracil and calcium folinate demonstrated safety and efficacy profiles.

At present, the approaches to endovascular therapy for liver cancer are diverse, and the techniques are continuously developing in clinical settings in China. The *Guidelines for Diagnosis and Treatment of Primary Liver Cancer in China (2011, 2017, 2019, and 2022 Editions)* enabled the continuous standardization and generalizability of endovascular therapy for liver cancer in China, thus ensuring the efficacy of this treatment option.

Suggested Reading

1. Seldinger SI. The seldinger technique. AJR Am J Roentgenol. 1984;142:5–7.
2. Carroll R. Infarction of the human liver. J Clin Pathol. 1963;16(2):133.
3. Rogers W, Edlich RF, Lewis DV, et al. Tumor blood flow: I. Blood flow in transplantable tumors during growth. Surg Clin North Am. 1967;47(6):1473–82.
4. Nilsson LAV, Zettergren L. Effect of hepatic artery ligation on induced primary liver carcinoma in rats. APMIS. 2010;71(2):187–93.
5. Ackerman NB. Experimental studies on the circulatory dynamics of intrahepatic tumor blood supply. Cancer. 1972;31(3):211.
6. Choichiko K. Hepatic angiography of experimental transplantable tumor. Investig Radiol. 1970;5(5):341–7.
7. Watkins E, Khazei AMJ, Nahra KS. Surgical basis for arterial infusion chemotherapy of disseminated carcinoma of the liver. Surg Gynecol Obstet. 1970;130(4):581–605.
8. Doyon D, Mouzon A, Jourde AM, et al. Hepatic, arterial embolization in patients with malignant liver tumours (author's transl). Ann Radiol (Paris). 1974;17(6):593–603.
9. Tsutomu T. A new angiographic technique in the diagnosis of so-called "Hypovascular" tumor SS-hepatic arteriography. Nippon Shokakibyo Gakkai Zasshi. 1974;71(10):1042–9.
10. Harvey M. Transcatheter occlusion of abdominal tumors. Radiology. 1976;120(3):539–45.
11. Lin G. The role of selective angiography in diagnosing primary liver cancer. Chinese J Surg. 1982;20(2):71–3.
12. Liu ZJ, Wu RQ. Selective cerebral angiography with femoral artery cannulation. Chinese J Radiol. 1981;15(4):244–7.
13. Rong DS, Kong QD, Lin G, et al. Overview of surgical radiology. Chinese J Radiol. 1981;15(4):304–7.
14. Liu YQ. Interventional radiology: review, prospects, and measures. Chinese J Radiol. 2002;36(12):5–6.
15. Lin ZY, Lu JZ, Cao YZ, et al. Hepatic arterial embolization therapy for primary liver cancer. Chinese J Oncol. 1983;5(3):197–201.
16. Lin G. Blood supply and microvascular manifestations of metastatic liver tumors. Tumor. 1984;4(4):152–4.
17. Lin G, Hagerstrand I, Lunderquist A. Portal blood supply of liver metastases. AJR Am J Roentgenol. 1984a;143(1):53–5.
18. Lin G, Lunderquist A, Gerstrand IH, et al. Postmortem examination of the blood supply and vascular pattern of small liver metastases in man. Surgery. 1984b;96(3):517–26.
19. Ekelund L, Lin G, Jeppsson B. Blood supply of experimental liver tumors after intraarterial embolization with gelfoam powder and absolute ethanol. Cardiovasc Intervent Radiol. 1984;7(5):234–9.
20. Wang XH, Du JH, Li LS. Analysis of 12 cases of liver cancer diagnosed by hepatic arteriography with oil-based contrast. Acta Univ Med Nanjing. 1986;6(3):39–40.
21. Guo JY, Huang ZC, Run D, et al. Intra-arterial chemoembolization of liver cancer with lipiodol anticancer drug mixture. J Clin Radiol. 1987;6(6):281–3.
22. Xie QK, Guo JY. Hepatic arterial embolization for hepatic malignancies. J Clin Radiol. 1987;6(1):46–50.
23. Cn JY, Wang ZT. Comparative study of the efficacy of intra-arterial drug infusion and chemoembolization in liver cancer. Chinese J Radiol. 1991;25(4):197–9.
24. Tian JM, Wang ZT. Diagnostic value of selective inferior phrenic arteriography for liver cancer. Chinese J Radiol. 1991;25(5):300–2.
25. Wang Z, Guo YJ. Pharmacokinetic study in liver cancer patients after chemoembolization with lipiodol cisplatin. Chinese J Radiol. 1993;27(12):863–4.
26. Fang CH, He ZP. Hepatic arterial infusion pump for treating primary liver cancer. Qinghai Med J. 1993;23(3):21–2.
27. Guo QY, Chen LY, Honda N, et al. A new treatment method for hepatocellular carcinoma—percutaneous transhepatic boiling saline injection. Chinese J Med Imaging. 1994;2(1):16–20.
28. Dong YH, Lin G. Cox regression model analysis of prognostic factors of patients after interventional treatment for liver cancer. Chinese J Radiol. 1996;30(12):833–6.
29. Konno T. Use of a lipid lymphographic agent, lipiodol, as a carrier of high molecular weight antitumor agent, smancs, for hepatocellular carcinoma. Gan Kagaku Ryoho Cancer Chemoth. 1982;9(11):2005–15.
30. Yamada R, Sato M, Kawabata M, et al. Hepatic artery embolization in 120 patients with unresectable hepatoma. Radiology. 1983;148(2):397–401.
31. Feng GS, Yan XQ, Wang LY. Experimental study of a new embolic material, the Chinese herb Bletilla. Cancer Res Prev Treat. 1985;12(1):33–5.
32. Feng GS. Animal experimental study and clinical application of the Chinese herb Bletilla as a vascular embolic agent. Natl Med J China. 1985;19(4):193–6.

33. Zou YH, Chen ML. Experimental study of hepatic arterial embolization with domestic PVA microspheres. Chinese J Radiol. 1989;23(6):330–2.
34. Yan ZP, Lin G, Zhao HY. Preliminary clinical application of 90 yttrium glass microsphere internal beam radiation therapy for primary liver cancer. Chinese J Radiol. 1994;28(1):55–7.
35. Dong BW, Liang P, Jin XH, et al. Ultrasound-guided intratumoral injection of 90 yttrium glass microspheres for the comprehensive treatment of liver cancer. Natl Med J China. 1994;74(8):471–3.
36. Guo JH, Teng GJ. Experimental evaluation of liver tissue injury by ^{32}P glass microsphere hepatic arterial embolization. Chinese J Radiol. 1999;33(10):667.
37. Liu L, Teng GJ, Jiang Z, et al. Experimental and clinical studies of regional delivery of ^{32}P glass microspheres for the treatment of liver cancer. Bull Med Res. 2001;30(10):22–3.
38. Sun J, Yang JM. Progress of TACE combined with PCV/E for liver cancer. Chinese J Pract Surg. 2002;22(5):307–8.
39. Dai X, Han MJ, Su HY, et al. Staging study of recurrent metastasis after hepatic arterial chemoembolization for primary liver cancer. J China Clin Med Imaging. 2004;15(11):613–5.
40. Zhang G, Zhou XP, Guan YS. Study on the correlation between post-operative iodinated oil deposition and blood supply after TACE for primary liver cancer. J Med Imaging. 2004;14(9):718–21.
41. Lu J, Guo JH, Zhu HD, et al. Safety and efficacy of irradiation stent placement for malignant portal vein thrombus combined with transarterial chemoembolization for hepatocellular carcinoma:a single-center experience. J Vasc Interv Radiol. 2017;28(6):786–94.
42. Lyu N, Kong Y, Pan T, et al. Hepatic arterial infusion of oxaliplatin, fluorouracil, and leucovorin in hepatocellular cancer with extrahepatic spread. J Vasc Interv Radiol. 2019;30(3):349–57.
43. Ministry of Health of the People's Republic of China. Guidelines for diagnosis and treatment of primary liver cancer (2011 edition). J Clin Hepatol. 2011;27(11):1141.
44. Bureau of Medical Administration. Health and Family Planning Commission of the People's Republic of China. Guidelines for Diagnosis and Treatment of Primary Liver Cancer (2017 Edition). Chinese J Hepatol. 2017;25(12):886–95.
45. Bureau of Medical Administration, National Health Commission of the People's Republic of China. Guidelines for diagnosis and treatment of primary liver cancer (2019 Edition). J Multidiscip Cancer Manag. 2020;6(2):55–85.
46. Forner A, Gilabert M, Bruix J, et al. Treatment of intermediate-stage hepatocellular carcinoma. Nat Rev Clin Oncol. 2014;11(9):525–35.

15 Transvascular Interventional Therapy for Liver Cancer

Hai-Dong Zhu and Gao-Jun Teng

While the hepatic artery provides more than 90% of the blood supply to liver cancer, the portal vein only supplies a small amount of blood to the peripheral and capsule of the tumor. In contrast, 70–75% of the blood supply to normal liver tissue comes from the portal vein, while only 25–30% originates from the hepatic artery, which provides the anatomical and theoretical basis for transcatheter arterial chemoembolization (TACE). As blood flow to the tumor is blocked to induce tumor necrosis, TACE deposits chemotherapy drugs in and around the tumor, thus promoting local chemotherapy to the tumor. The global BRIDGE study demonstrated that TACE is the most widely used treatment in patients with primary liver cancer across different stages and plays an important role in managing primary liver cancer. In 2002, a randomized controlled study by Llovet *et al.* confirmed that, compared to the best supportive care, TACE can prolong survival of patients with unresectable liver cancer and is the recommended first-line treatment for intermediate-stage liver cancer by the Barcelona Clinic Liver Cancer (BCLC) staging system. According to the *Guidelines for Diagnosis and Treatment of Primary Liver Cancer in* China *(2017 Edition)*, TACE is indicated for liver cancer of stages Ib–IIIb. Meanwhile, TACE can be used to downstage liver cancer to make subsequent radical treatment possible. Based on Xin JIN and Jiahong DONG *et al.*'s analysis of 58 cases of large liver cancer receiving TACE for downstaging in 2011, some large liver cancers can be successfully treated by radical resection and liver transplantation following TACE downstaging with satisfactory long-term prognosis. In addition, TACE can also be used as an adjuvant therapy after radical resection of liver cancer. In 2005, Tao XI and Feng SHEN performed prophylactic TACE after liver resection, showing the ability of prophylactic TACE to significantly reduce the postoperative recurrence rate within 2 years. Later, in 2008, Tianhao WANG and Jia FAN *et al.* analyzed the efficacy of postoperative adjuvant TACE on survival after radical resection of massive primary liver cancer. They found that postoperative adjuvant TACE prolonged long-term survival, and this effect was more prominent in high-risk patients with residual tumors.

Among the side effects after TACE, post-embolization syndrome, characterized by fever, pain, nausea, and vomiting, is most common. Fever and pain are mainly caused by local tissue ischemia and necrosis after embolizing the hepatic artery, while nausea and vomiting are mainly associated with chemotherapy drugs. Other common side effects include bleeding at the puncture site, decreased white blood cell count, transient abnormal liver function, impaired renal function, and

H.-D. Zhu · G.-J. Teng (✉)
Zhongda Hospital, Southeast University, Nanjing, China
e-mail: gjteng@seu.edu.cn

X. Chen (ed.), *Diagnosis and Treatment of Liver Cancer in China*,
https://doi.org/10.1007/978-981-97-7969-7_15

dysuria. In 1993, Jianxin WU *et al.* summarized the diagnosis and management of five complications after TACE in 208 patients with liver cancer. In 2008, Guangsheng ZHAO and Ke XU *et al.* analyzed the causes and prevention of severe postoperative complications in 573 patients with primary liver cancer. They found that severe complications after TACE were often associated with poor preoperative liver function, portal hypertension, a large volume of chemoembolic drugs, drug reflux, or embolic material migration. Therefore, severe complications may be avoided or alleviated if appropriate timing and standardization of TACE are adopted. On the contrary, given the palliative feature of TACE, poor control of the lesions may become a problem after multiple sessions of TACE. As a result, the concept of "TACE resistance/failure" has been proposed, and many scholars believe that TACE should be discontinued and replaced by other treatment regimens after TACE resistance occurs.

Indications for endovascular interventions are generally based on Eastern Cooperative Oncology Group performance status (PS) and liver function. The main indications for conventional TACE (cTACE) for liver cancer at all stages include the following:

1. Early stage: (a) Tumor can be surgically resected, but the patient cannot or does not intend to undergo surgery for other reasons (e.g., advanced age, severe cirrhosis, etc.) or local ablation is not feasible due to the location of the tumor; (b) downstaging treatment prior to surgical resection or liver transplantation, especially when the expected waiting time for liver transplantation exceeds 6 months.
2. Intermediate stage: Large tumor or multiple lesions but without tumor-related symptoms, macrovascular invasion, or extrahepatic metastasis.
3. Advanced stage: The portal vein is not completely obstructed or completely obstructed but with good collateral compensation between the hepatic artery and portal vein.
4. Others: Bleeding from a ruptured liver tumor or from portal hypertension caused by hepatic arterioportal shunt, management of bleeding, and embolization of arteriovenous fistula. The indications for transcatheter arterial embolization (TAE) and drug-eluting bead (DEB)-TACE are similar to cTACE. Transcatheter arterial radioembolization (TARE) can act as an alternative to cTACE in patients with intermediate-stage liver cancer where cTACE is not suitable or in patients with massive liver cancer invading the portal vein or presenting with cTACE resistance.

15.1 cTACE

Infusing iodized oil emulsions via a catheter, cTACE is the most widely used non-surgical treatment for liver cancer. The most common monotherapy agent is doxorubicin or epidoxorubicin, and the most common combination drug is cisplatin, doxorubicin, and mitomycin C. The dosage of chemotherapy drugs is generally based on the patient's liver function and body weight, but it can be empirical sometimes. The BRIDGE study showed that TACE is the most common first-line treatment for liver cancer in China, accounting for up to 51%. Even if TACE is not performed as the first-line treatment, 48–72% of the patients will receive TACE as the subsequent treatment. TACE can effectively shrink the tumor and prolong the patient's survival. Even if a slight impairment to liver function occurs, it can be recovered in the short term without affecting the patient's prognosis. Furthermore, TACE can be used alone or in combination in patients with liver cancer having portal vein tumor thrombus (PVTT) and/or distant metastases. A meta-analysis by Silva *et al.* demonstrated that only 1% of patients with liver cancer having PVTT developed liver failure after TACE, with a median survival of 11 months for patients with thrombosis in the branches and 5 months for those in the main trunk. Another meta-analysis suggested that in patients with relatively good liver function, TACE remains safe and can prolong the overall survival of patients despite distant metastases. Based on the growing clinical evidence, increasingly more scholars have advocated for expanding the indications for TACE in the BCLC staging system.

15.2 TAE

TAE mainly uses embolic agent(s) without chemotherapy drug(s) to embolize the blood vessels supplying the tumor. Currently, the most commonly used embolic materials include iodized oil followed by particles, gelatin sponge particles, microspheres, and polyvinyl alcohol (PVA) particles. The dosage of iodized oil is typically 5–20 mL, which can be adjusted according to the tumor load but generally does not exceed 30 mL. Although TACE has become the dominant transcatheter treatment, the efficacy advantage of TACE over TAE has not yet been confirmed. Both TAE and TACE can effectively treat primary liver cancer with comparable efficacy. However, compared with TACE, TAE can avoid damage to the liver induced by chemotherapy drugs. It has been suggested that tumor necrosis after TACE is mainly induced by the embolic effect. TAE can achieve good local control of the tumor without impairing liver function by chemotherapy drugs if the tumor-feeding arteries can be super-selectively embolized, which is particularly important for patients with a history of hepatitis B cirrhosis.

15.3 DEB-TACE

Compared with cTACE, DEB-TACE enables sustained drug release, achieving embolization and local high-concentration chemotherapy simultaneously. However, current clinical evidence cannot support its superiority over cTACE on the benefit of survival. According to the PRECISION V study in 2010 that compared the safety and efficacy of the two treatments for liver cancer, DEB-TACE outperformed cTACE in local tumor control (63% vs. 52%), but the difference was not statistically significant ($P = 0.11$). However, for patients in critical condition (i.e., Child-Pugh B liver function, PS of 1, bilobar lesions, or tumor recurrence), the DEB-TACE group showed higher rates of complete response (27% vs. 22%, $P = 0.091$), objective response (52% vs. 44%, $P = 0.038$), and disease control (63% vs. 52%, $P = 0.026$). At the same time, DEB-TACE was significantly safer than cTACE and effectively lowered the postoperative complication rate. In 2014, the PRECISION study comparing DEB-TACE and cTACE planned to enroll 214 patients, but the study was suspended after recruiting 177 because the treatment outcomes failed to meet the expectations. A meta-analysis that included four randomized controlled trials and eight retrospective studies showed that compared with cTACE, DEB-TACE could not prolong the patient's survival (Table 15.1).

Table 15.1 Summary of comparative studies on DEB-TACE versus cTACE

Study	Patient number	Efficacy criteria	OR rate (%)	Median/mean survival (mon)	Survival rate (%)
Lammer, 2010	93 vs. 108	EASL	51.6 vs. 43.5	N/A	N/A
Dhanase Karan, 2010	45 vs. 26	N/A	N/A	20.3/– vs. 13.4/–	N/A
Ferrer Puchol, 2011	47 vs. 25	RECIST	36.1 vs. 15.3	22.4/25.5 vs. 23.6/22.9	N/A
Song, 2012	60 vs. 69	mRECIST	81.6 vs. 49.4	–/32.2 vs.–/24.7	1 year, 88 vs. 67
Kloeckner, 2015	76 vs. 174	N/A	N/A	12.3/– vs. 13.6/–	N/A
Kucukay, 2015	53 vs. 73	N/A	N/A	–/37.4 vs.–/39	1 year, 95.9 vs. 84.9 2 years, 92.3 vs. 74.6

(continued)

Table 15.1 (continued)

Study	Patient number	Efficacy criteria	OR rate (%)	Median/mean survival (mon)	Survival rate (%)
Arabi, 2015	35 vs. 25	mRECIST	35 vs. 36	N/A	2 years, 58 vs. 60
MegíasVericat, 2015	30 vs. 30	N/A	N/A	N/A	5 years, 20 vs. 30
Rahman, 2016	45 vs. 34	mRECIST	39 vs. 29	8.3/– vs. 4.9/–	N/A
Baur, 2016	14 vs. 18	N/A	N/A	9.2/– vs. 10.8/–	N/A
Massani, 2017	28 vs. 54	N/A	N/A	22.7/29.4 vs. 21.8/27	N/A
Lee, 2017	106 vs. 144	mRECIST	86.8 vs. 78.3	46.6/– vs. 44.9/–	N/A

Note: *DEB-TACE* drug-eluting bead transcatheter arterial chemoembolization, *cTACE* conventional transcatheter arterial chemoembolization, *OR* objective response, *EASL* European Association for the Study of Liver Disease, *RECIST* Response Evaluation Criteria in Solid Tumors, *mRECIST* modified Response Evaluation Criteria in Solid Tumors, *N/A* non-applicable

15.4 TARE

TARE refers to the injection of radioactive microspheres into the tumor-feeding arteries. At present, the two main types of ^{90}Y microspheres are resin microspheres and glass microspheres, which were first used in patients with liver cancer accompanying PVTT. Biederman *et al.*'s retrospective study comparing the safety and efficacy of resin and glass microspheres demonstrated a median survival of 3.7 and 9.4 months ($P < 0.001$), respectively, and that glass microspheres were associated with fewer complications. In 2014, Muxing LI *et al.*'s meta-analysis on the efficacy of TARE using ^{90}Y microspheres for unresectable primary liver cancer showed that compared with TACE, TARE significantly improved the tumor response rate and long-term survival rate. In 2018, Bin CHEN *et al.* noted in a systematic review and meta-analysis of TARE using ^{90}Y microspheres vs. cTACE for unresectable primary liver cancer that compared with TACE, TARE could significantly improve the 3-year survival rate. In addition, patients receiving TARE had a lower incidence of serious complications than those receiving cTACE, though the difference was not statistically significant. In 2017, the SARAH trial compared the efficacy and safety of TARE to sorafenib in treating liver cancer with PVTT, demonstrating a median survival of 8.0 and 9.9 months ($P = 0.18$), respectively. Similarly, in 2018, the SIRveNIB trial generated a median survival of 8.8 months in the TARE group, vs. 10.0 months in the sorafenib group ($P = 0.36$) without statistical difference. Given its better safety profile, TARE has been increasingly used, especially in patients with PVTT, and serves as a downstaging treatment prior to liver transplantation in the United States. Fortunately, except for Taiwan, Hong Kong, and some hospitals in Hainan, TARE is gradually approved for treating liver cancer in China (Table 15.2).

Table 15.2 Summary of comparative studies on TARE versus TACE

Study	Number of patients	Efficacy	Safety
Moreno-Luna, 2013	61 vs. 55	Median survival, 15 vs. 14.4 (mon) 2-year survival rate, 30% vs. 24%	Fever, 7% vs. 21% Asthenia, 46% vs. 20%
El Fouly, 2015	44 vs. 42	Overall survival, 16.4 vs. 18 (mon) TTP, 13.3 vs. 6.8 (mon)	Pain, 5% vs. 83% Asthenia, 40% vs. 73% Vomiting, 0 vs. 38%
Kolligs, 2015	13 vs. 15	Best overall response rate, 30.8% vs. 13.3% Disease control rate, 76.9% vs. 73.3%	Adverse events, 33.3% vs. 23.1%
Kooby, 2010	27 vs. 44	Median survival, 6 vs. 6 (mon)	Serious adverse events, 18% vs. 24%
Carr, 2010	99 vs. 691	Median survival, 11.5 vs. 8.5 (mon)	N/A
Salem, 2011	123 vs. 122	Median survival, 20.5 vs. 17.4 (mon) TTP, 13.3 vs. 8.4 (mon)	Pain, 15% vs. 38% Liver injury, 11% vs. 29%

Note: *TARE* transcatheter arterial radioembolization, *TACE* transcatheter arterial chemoembolization, *TTP* time to progression

15.5 Summary

Endovascular interventions play an important role in the treatment of primary liver cancer. They can be used to prolong survival for patients with unresectable intermediate-stage and advanced liver cancer. Also, endovascular interventions can be applied as downstaging treatments prior to subsequent radical resection or liver transplantation. Endovascular interventions can be performed in a variety of ways. The therapeutic agents used can be a combination of multiple chemotherapy drugs. The drug delivery materials can be iodized oil emulsions or microspheres. The embolic agents can be gelatin sponge particles, PVA particles, microspheres, and so on. To date, whether some treatment regimens are superior to others still remain controversial. Repeated TACE may cause impaired liver function and even TACE resistance, and post-TACE recurrence and metastasis may also be problematic. Therefore, combination therapy of TACE and other treatments, no doubt, is a future research direction.

Suggested Reading

1. Lencioni R, Baere TD, Soulen MC, et al. Lipiodol transarterial chemoembolization for hepatocellular carcinoma: a systematic review of efficacy and safety data. Hepatology. 2016;64(1):106–16.
2. Cheung A, Amarapurkar D, Chao Y, et al. Re-evaluating transarterial chemoembolization for the treatment of hepatocellular carcinoma: consensus recommendations and review by an international expert panel. Liver Int. 2014;34(2):174–83.
3. Park JW, Chen M, Colombo M, et al. Global patterns of hepatocellular carcinoma management from diagnosis to death: the BRIDGE study. Liver Int. 2015;35(9):2155–66.
4. Llovet JM, Real MI, Monta AX, et al. Arterial embolisation or chemoembolisation versus symptomatic treatment in patients with unresectable hepatocellular carcinoma: a randomised controlled trial. Lancet. 2002;359(9319):1734–9.
5. Lo CM, Ngan H, Tso WK, et al. Randomized controlled trial of transarterial lipiodol chemoembolization for unresectable hepatocellular carcinoma. Hepatology. 2002;35(5):1164–71.
6. Jian Z, Sun H, Wang Z, et al. Guidelines for Diagnosis and Treatment of Primary Liver Cancer in China (2017 Edition). Liver Cancer. 2018;7(3):235–60.
7. Galle PR, Forner A, Llovet JM, et al. EASL clinical practice guidelines: management of hepatocellular carcinoma. J Hepatol. 2018;69(1):182–236.

8. Jin X. Experience of transhepatic arterial cannulation chemoembolization for downstaging treatment in 58 patients with large liver cancer. Natl Med J China. 2011;91(14):950–5.
9. Xi T, Shen F, Wu MC. The significance of prophylactic hepatic arterial chemoembolization for delaying recurrence after liver cancer surgery. China Cancer. 2005;14(3):161–3.
10. Wang TH, Ren ZG, Ye QH, et al. Effect of postoperative adjuvant hepatic arterial chemoembolization on survival after radical resection of giant liver cancer. Tumor. 2008;28(11):994–6.
11. Wu JX, Yu ZJ. Diagnosis and treatment of five complications after arterial chemoembolization of primary liver cancer (with analysis of 208 cases). Jiangsu Med J. 1993;19(8):422–4.
12. Zhao GS, Xu K, Liang SN, et al. Causes and prevention of serious complications after TACE for primary liver cancer. J Intervent Radiol. 2008;17(11):773–5.
13. Yu CX, Teng GJ. Progress of research on transcatheter arterial chemoembolization resistance. J Intervent Radiol. 2017;26(12):1063–7.
14. Group K L C S. 2014 Korean Liver Cancer Study Group-National Cancer Center Korea practice guideline for the management of hepatocellular carcinoma. Korean J Radiol. 2015;16(3):465–522.
15. Graziadei IW, Sandmueller H, Waldenberger P, et al. Chemoembolization followed by liver transplantation for hepatocellular carcinoma impedes tumor progression while on the waiting list and leads to excellent outcome. Liver Transplant. 2003;9(6):557–63.
16. Chow PKH, Pin CS, Ng DCE, et al. National Cancer Centre Singapore Consensus Guidelines for hepatocellular carcinoma. Liver Cancer. 2016;5(2):97–106.
17. Chen TJ, Li HW. Observation of the effect of arterial chemoembolization on survival and postoperative liver function in patients with primary liver cancer. Heilongjiang Med J. 2018;42(12):27–9.
18. Silvaj P, Berger NG, Tsai S, et al. Transarterial chemoembolization in hepatocellular carcinoma with portal vein tumor thrombosis: a systematic review and meta-analysis. HPB. 2017;19(8):659–66.
19. Zhao Y, Cai G, Zhou L, et al. Transarterial chemoembolization in hepatocellular carcinoma with vascular invasion or extrahepatic metastasis: a systematic review. Asia Pac J Clin Oncol. 2013;9(4):357–64.
20. Gaba RC, Lokken RP, Hickey RM, et al. Quality improvement guidelines for transarterial chemoembolization and embolization of hepatic malignancy. J Vasc Interv Radiol. 2017;28(9):1210–23.
21. Mauri G, Varano GM, Orsi F. TAE for HCC: when the old way is better than the new ones. Cardiovasc Intervent Radiol. 2016;39(6):799–800.
22. Li CY, Sun LJ. Effectiveness of TAE and TACE in the treatment of primary liver cancer and the effect on liver function classification. Lab Med Clin. 2019;16(18):2634–6.
23. Giovanni MG. TAE for HCC: when the old way is better than the new ones. Cardiovasc Intervent Radiol. 2016;39(6):799–800.
24. Llovet JM, Real MI, Monta AX, et al. Arterialembolisation or chemoembolisation versus symptomatic treatment in patients with unresectable hepatocellular carcinoma: a randomised controlled trial. Lancet. 2002;359(9319):1734–9.
25. Hall B, Gonzalez MV, Willis SL, et al. Pharmacokinetic and safety study of doxorubicin-eluting beads in a porcine model of hepatic arterial embolization. J Vasc Interv Radiol. 2006;17(8):1335–43.
26. Lammer J, Malagari K, Vogl T, et al. Prospective randomized study of doxorubicin-eluting-bead embolization in the treatment of hepatocellular carcinoma: results of the PRECISION V study. Cardiovasc Intervent Radiol. 2010;33(1):41–52.
27. Chen Y, Wei XY, Cao K, et al. Efficacy of drug-eluting bead hepatic arterial chemoembolization for the treatment of intermediate to advanced primary liver cancer. Chinese J Clin Oncol Rehab. 2017;24(6):77–80.
28. Golfieri R, Giampalma E, Renzulli M, et al. Randomised controlled trial of doxorubicin-eluting beads vs conventional chemoembolisation for hepatocellular carcinoma. Br J Cancer. 2014;111(2):255–64.
29. Facciorusso A, Maso MD, Muscatiello N. Drug-eluting beads versus conventional chemoembolization for the treatment of unresectable hepatocellular carcinoma: a meta-analysis. Dig Liver Dis. 2016;48(6):571–7.
30. Dhanasekaran R, Kooby DA, Staley CA, et al. Prognostic factors for survival in patients with unresectable hepatocellular carcinoma undergoing chemoembolization with doxorubicin drug-eluting beads: a preliminary study. HPB. 2010;12(3):174–80.
31. Puchol F, Parra CL, Esteban E, et al. Comparison of doxorubicin-eluting bead transarterial chemoembolization(DEB-TACE)with conventional transarterial chemoembolization(TACE)for the treatment of hepatocellular carcinoma. Radiologia. 2011;53(3):246–53.
32. Song MJ, Chun HJ, Song DS, et al. Comparative study between doxorubicin-eluting beads and conventional transarterial chemoembolization for treatment of hepatocellular carcinoma. J Hepatol. 2012;57(6):1244–50.
33. Kloeckner R, Weinmann A, Prinz F, et al. Conventional transarterial chemoembolization versus drug-eluting bead transarterial chemoembolization for the treatment of hepatocellular carcinoma. BMC Cancer. 2015;15:465.
34. Kucukay F, Badem S, Karan A, et al. A single-center retrospective comparison of doxorubicin-loaded hepasphere transarterial chemoembolization with conventional transarterial chemoembolization for patients with unresectable hepatocellular carcinoma. J Vasc Interv Radiol. 2015;26(11):1622–9.
35. Arabi M, Benmousa A, Bzeizi K, et al. Doxorubicin-loaded drug-eluting beads versus conventional transarterial chemoembolization for nonresectable hepatocellular carcinoma. Saudi J Gastroenterol. 2015;21(3):175–80.

36. Meg AS, Vericat JE, Marcos GAR, Briz LEP, et al. Trans-arterial chemoembolization with doxorubicin-eluting particles versus conventional trans-arterial chemoembolization in unresectable hepatocellular carcinoma: a study of effectiveness, safety and costs. Radiologia. 2015;57(6):496–504.
37. Rahman FA, Naidu J, Ngiu CS, et al. Conventional versus doxorubicin-eluting beads transarterial chemoembolization for unresectable hepatocellular carcinoma: a tertiary medical Centre experience in Malaysia. Asian Pac J Cancer Prev. 2014;17(8):4037.
38. Johannes B, Christian R, Christoph-Thomas G, et al. Transarterial chemoembolization with drug-eluting beads versus conventional transarterial chemoembolization in locally advanced hepatocellular carcinoma. Hepat Med. 2016;8:69–74.
39. Massani M, Stecca T, Ruffolo C, et al. Should we routinely use DEBTACE for unresectable HCC? cTACE versus DEBTACE: a single-center survival analysis. Updat Surg. 2017;69(1):1–7.
40. Lee YK, Jung KS, Kim DY, et al. Conventional versus drug-eluting beads chemoembolization for hepatocellular carcinoma: emphasis on the impact of tumor size. J Gastroenterol Hepatol. 2017;32(2):487–96.
41. Kennedy A, Nag S, Salem R, et al. Recommendations for radioembolization of hepatic malignancies using yttrium-90 microsphere brachytherapy: a consensus panel report from the radioembolization brachytherapy oncology consortium. Int J Radiat Oncol Biol Phys. 2007;68(1):13–23.
42. Biederman DM, Titano J, Tabori NE. Outcomes of Radioembolization in the treatment of hepatocellular carcinoma with portal vein invasion: resin versus glass microspheres. J Vasc Interv Radiol. 2016;27(6):812–21.
43. Li MX, Zhang XF, Cheng JW, et al. Meta-analysis of the efficacy of transarterial radioembolization with yttrium 90 microspheres for unresectable primary liver cancer. Chinese J Hepat Surg. 2014;3(6):26–30.
44. Chen B, Jia Z, Xie SS, et al. Systematic evaluation and meta-analysis of yttrium 90 microsphere radioembolization versus conventional transhepatic arterial infusion chemoembolization for surgically unresectable hepatocellular carcinoma-a review series on yttrium 90 microsphere radioembolization (VI). J Intervent Radiol. 2018;27(9):102–8.
45. Val Rie V, Helena P, Eric A, et al. Efficacy and safety of selective internal radiotherapy with yttrium-90 resin microspheres compared with sorafenib in locally advanced and inoperable hepatocellular carcinoma(SARAH): an open-label randomised controlled phase 3 trial. Lancet Oncol. 2017;18(12):1624–36.
46. Salem R, Lewandowski RJ, Mulcahy MF, et al. Radioembolization for hepatocellular carcinoma using Yttrium-90 microspheres: a comprehensive report of long-term outcomes. Gastroenterology. 2010;138(1):52–64.
47. Kim MD, Park SI, Won JY, et al. Conventional versus drug-eluting beads chemoembolization for hepatocellular carcinoma: emphasis on the impact of tumor size. J Gastroenterol Hepatol. 2017;32(2):487–96.
48. El Fouly A, Ertle J, El Dorry A, et al. In intermediate stage hepatocellular carcinoma: radioembolization with yttrium 90 or chemoembolization? Liver Int. 2015;35(2):627–35.
49. Kolligs FT, Bilbao JI, Jakobs T, et al. Pilot randomized trial of selective internal radiation therapy vs. chemoembolization in unresectable hepatocellular carcinoma. Liver Int. 2015;35(6):1715–21.
50. Kooby DA, Egnatashvili V, Srinivasan S, et al. Comparison of Yttrium-90 Radioembolization and Transcatheter arterial chemoembolization for the treatment of Unresectable hepatocellular carcinoma. J Vasc Interv Radiol. 2010;21(2):224–30.
51. Carr BI, Kondragunta V, Buch SC, et al. Therapeutic equivalence in survival for hepatic arterial chemoembolization and yttrium 90 microsphere treatments in unresectable hepatocellular carcinoma: a two-cohort study. Cancer. 2010;116(5):1305–14.
52. Salem R, Lewandowski RJ, Kulik L, et al. Radioembolization results in longer time-to-progression and reduced toxicity compared with chemoembolization in patients with hepatocellular carcinoma. Gastroenterology. 2011;140(2):497–507.

16 Other Local Treatment Options in Interventional Therapy for Liver Cancer

Hai-Dong Zhu and Gao-Jun Teng

16.1 Non-Vascular Interventional Therapy

16.1.1 Percutaneous Ethanol Injection (PEI)

PEI can dehydrate tumor cells and nearby vascular endothelial cells, coagulate and denature proteins, and eventually cause necrosis and fibrosis formation in tumor tissues. In 1983, Sugiura reported the treatment of liver cancer by percutaneous hepatic puncture and intratumoral injection of absolute ethanol under ultrasound guidance, which gained wide attention and application because of its ideal route of drug delivery, simple and safe operation, and minimally invasive characteristics. Many scholars also carried out extensive research related to ethanol injection for liver cancer in the 1980s. Xiaoguang ZHANG and Lanxi GENG *et al.* investigated the role of direct ethanol injection *ex vivo* and in patients with intermediate-stage to advanced liver cancer. In 1990, Chung *et al.* reported the results of ethanol injection in controlling tumor rupture bleeding. For tumors < 3 cm in diameter, direct percutaneous injection into the tumor is quite effective. With the continuous development of other treatment options, multi-point coverage or combination with transcatheter arterial chemoembolization transcatheter arterial chemoembolization (TACE) is now being adopted to improve treatment effects for single or multiple tumor(s) 3–5 cm in diameter.

16.1.2 Radiofrequency Ablation (RFA)

RFA induces coagulative necrosis of the tumor by cauterizing it at high temperatures. Meanwhile, the vascular tissue around the tumor coagulates to form a reaction zone, which can block the blood supply to the tumor and prevent its metastasis.

Research on RFA for liver cancer first began in the 1990s. In 1993, Rossi *et al.* systematically reported the successful treatment of small liver cancer using RFA. In 1999, Qingjiu MA and Jinsheng WU *et al.* reported the progress of RFA for liver cancer. For liver tumors < 5 cm in diameter, both the tumor volume and alpha-fetoprotein (AFP) values were significantly decreased. In the early 21st century, research on RFA emerged continually. In the beginning, single-electrode ablation was adopted in RFA. With the steady advances in technology, a variety of RFA methods gradually appeared in the clinic, including monopolar, multipolar, HittRFA, Cool-tip RFA, etc. In the meantime, there is ongoing research on RFA combined with other treatments. Studies have demonstrated that RFA can enhance the immunity of the body,

H.-D. Zhu · G.-J. Teng (✉)
Zhongda Hospital, Southeast University,
Nanjing, China
e-mail: gjteng@seu.edu.cn

X. Chen (ed.), *Diagnosis and Treatment of Liver Cancer in China*,
https://doi.org/10.1007/978-981-97-7969-7_16

stimulate macrophage activity, and bolster the cytotoxic effect of natural killer cells. At present, RFA has been widely proven a safe and effective first-line ablation technique, as well as the one that is most commonly used. Compared with PEI, disease control and efficacy of RFA are improved. The European Association for the Study of the Liver (EASL) guidelines suggest that RFA combined with TACE can significantly prolong patients' overall survival.

16.1.3 Microwave Ablation (MWA)

MWA mainly treats liver tumors of 3–5 cm in diameter as well as those near the blood vessels and gallbladder by percutaneously puncturing a specialized electrode into the tumor and heating it to induce tumor necrosis by thermal coagulation. MWA was used to treat liver cancer in 1990; however, compared to RFA, early microwave regimens showed no significant difference in prolonging overall survival. Chinese scholars also gradually began conducting research on MWA for liver cancer in the 1990s. Xinda ZHOU and Wenxin HU *et al.* first performed microwave hepatectomy in China. They also investigated MWA for unresectable liver tumors. After 6–7 years of development, with the continuous improvement of the equipment and the accumulation of treatment experience, MWA has achieved satisfactory clinical efficacy. A variety of MWA devices are emerging on the market. The shape and volume of ablation produced by different devices are completely different, which makes individualized treatment regimens for tumors with different shapes possible. However, compared with RFA, MWA is not significantly superior in treating liver tumors of 3–5 cm in diameter, and there is also controversy in the incidence of complications between the two.

16.1.4 High-Intensity Focused Ultrasound (HIFU)

HIFU uses a special focusing device to focus ultrasound from outside the body into a selected treatment area within the body, forming a high-energy density zone at its focal point, which instantly generates high temperature and causes irreversible coagulative necrosis, denaturation, and apoptosis of tissues in the treatment area. HIFU also has the effects of destroying tumor-feeding arteries and stimulating the body's immunity and the benefits of being non-invasive and reproducible with extensive indications and demonstrates synergistic effects with various treatment methods. In 1942, Lynn *et al.* reported the effects of focused ultrasound on paraffin blocks and performed experiments on damage to the liver of cattle and the nervous system of cats and dogs. In 1993, Vallancien first reported the use of ultrasound for human liver metastases. Meanwhile, scholars conducted a large number of animal experiments, which confirmed the ablative effect of HIFU on liver tissues and implantation tumors, laying a foundation for the clinical application of liver cancer with HIFU. The JC-type HIFU tumor treatment system developed by the Institute of Medical Ultrasound Engineering of Chongqing Medical University has been used in clinical practice and achieved wide recognition. In China, Feng WU *et al.* also pioneered extensive clinical studies using this system and confirmed that HIFU is safe and effective in treating liver cancer.

16.1.5 Irreversible Electroporation (IRE)

IRE is a novel technique for tumor treatment using high voltage and short pulses to act on the target cell membranes to cause irreversible formation of nano-scale pores in the phospholipid bilayer of the cell membrane, resulting in cell death. It does not destroy the extracellular matrix, which protects the blood vessels, bile ducts, and other structures from damage and is safer than thermal ablation when treating lesions near large blood vessels, bile ducts, or gallbladder.

As early as 1754, Nollet systematically recorded erythema on the skin of animals and humans that had been exposed to electric sparks. However, it was not until 1982 that Neumann used electric field pulses to temporarily penetrate the cell membrane to allow entry of exogenous DNA into the cell, forming a stable transformed strain, which marked the beginning of electroporation application in modern medicine. In 2005, Davalos *et al.* proposed that IRE, as a novel ablation method, avoided some of the side effects of thermal ablation, making its application in the field of tumor ablation possible. In 2011, the U.S. Food and Drug Administration approved the IRE nanoknife device for clinical use, and in 2015, the China Food and Drug Administration (CFDA) (now National Medical Products Administration NMPA) approved IRE for the treatment of pancreatic tumors and liver tumors. A series of clinical studies on IRE for primary liver cancer demonstrated that IRE is a safe and effective local ablation method.

16.1.6 Cryotherapy

Cryotherapy uses high-pressure argon and helium as cold and heat media to freeze and rewarm local tumor tissues and destroy tumor cell structure, resulting in cell shrinkage, rupture, and death, and can cause occlusion of microvessels, leading to ischemic necrosis of the tumor. With the advantages of reducing the tumor load, activating the immune function of the body, and being less invasive, rapid recovery, and cost-efficiency, it has become one of the important approaches to treating for liver cancer.

As early as the 1840s, the British physician Arnott had reported cryogenic treatment of malignant tumors of the breast and uterus. However, it was not until 1961, when Cooper and Lee developed a continuous cryosurgical device with probes utilizing liquid nitrogen, that cryotherapy entered a phase of rapid development. However, due to the limitations of conditions, there were still many complications with poor treatment outcomes. In 1998, Endocare successfully developed a new argon-helium superconducting surgical system, Argon Helium Knife, providing a new option for the local treatment of liver cancer. In the following year, the Cancer Center of Zhujiang Hospital of Southern Medical University first introduced this technique into China. Subsequent studies confirmed that argon-helium knife for liver cancer can achieve a complete response rate of 82.8–97.2%, with 3- and 5-year survival rates of 65.5% and 59.5%, respectively. Meanwhile, other research findings also suggested that an argon-helium knife combined with TACE or PEI has better efficacy.

A summary of non-vascular interventional therapy for liver cancer is shown in Table 16.1.

Table 16.1 Non-vascular interventional therapy for liver cancer

Type	Benefits	Weakness
PEI	Easy to operate, safe, minimally invasive and inexpensive	Poor overall efficacy, and currently not often used alone
RFA	Most widely used clinically and well-documented	Poor efficacy for tumors adjacent to the liver capsule, blood vessels, gallbladder, diaphragm, or > 3 cm
MWA	Good anti-heat sink effect; shorter operation time than RFA; effective for tumors ≤ 5 cm	Poor efficacy for tumors > 5 cm; greatly varied efficacy among different devices
HIFU	Non-invasive, highly reproducible, broad indications	Susceptible to rib condition; limited clinical evidence
IRE	No heat sink effect; can be used for ablation of paravascular tumors	High incidence of needle tract seeding; requires multiple needle punctures; limited evidence; requires general anesthesia
Cryotherapy	Less invasive, fast recovery, cost efficiency	Limited clinical evidence

Note: *PEI* percutaneous ethanol injection, *RFA* radiofrequency ablation, *MWA* microwave ablation, *HIFU* high-intensity focused ultrasound, *IRE* irreversible electroporation

16.2 Radiotherapy

The high radiosensitivity of the liver has led to the limitation of conventional external beam radiotherapy in liver cancer by the poor tolerance of the liver. Since the efficacy of whole liver radiotherapy is unsatisfactory, it is rarely used in clinical practice. In recent years, with advanced modern radiotherapy technology, different measures, such as conformality of projection and modulation of dose, have improved the precision of and expanded the indications for liver cancer radiotherapy. The main means of radiotherapy for liver cancer include internal (brachytherapy) and external beam radiotherapy. Among them, the treatment modes of external beam radiotherapy mainly include the following.

16.2.1 Conventional Radiotherapy

The routine radiation fields for liver cancer mainly include the whole liver field, strip field, and local field. The whole liver field is mainly used in patients with diffuse intrahepatic metastases cautiously, with a recommended dose of 1–1.5 Gy. The strip field mainly divides the liver into several strip areas, each about 2.5 cm wide, which are radiated sequentially. With the development of three-dimensional (3D) conformal and other precision radiotherapy techniques, conventional radiotherapy (CRT) has been basically eliminated.

16.2.2 Three-Dimensional CRT

Based on computerized virtual reconstruction technology, 3D CRT designs radiation field parameters with the help of the radiation treatment planning system (TPS), calculates radiation dose based on the radiation tolerance dose model of normal liver tissue, and accurately captures the patient's liver radiation treatment location, while also enabling the monitoring of the radiotherapy effect according to the specified radiation treatment plan. Compared with conventional (2D) radiation methods, 3D CRT offers at least two important advantages: (1) it allows higher doses and minimizes the dose to uninvolved liver regions and surrounding critical organs; and (2) it enables a better quantitative understanding of the relationship between treatment dose, volume and risk of complications, and the acquisition of the tissue and surrounding counterparts. In terms of short-term results, 3D CRT can significantly improve the control rate of primary liver cancer, while significantly reducing the side effects of radiotherapy.

16.2.3 Intensity-Modulated Radiotherapy (IMRT)

IMRT is an advanced form of CRT that better facilitates the delivery of radiation dose compared to 3D CRT. Using computer-aided automatic optimization, called inverse processing planning, the intensity of each beam is adjusted to obtain the desired target coverage while minimizing the dose to normal tissue. This type of therapy includes volume-modulated arc therapy (VMAT) and helical tomotherapy (HT). VMAT provides an intensity-modulated beam as the gantry rotates. HT delivers the radiation dose in slices through a rotating gantry, similar to that of a spiral CT scanner. In addition, it is possible to deliver different doses to different targets simultaneously, known as simultaneous-integrated boost IMRT, which can deliver higher doses to the tumor while delivering lower doses to subcritical disease areas. A comparative study on 3D CRT, fixed-angle IMRT, and VMAT in radiotherapy for small to large liver cancer by Chen *et al.* suggested that, compared to 3D CRT or IMRT, VMAT is associated with the lowest risk of radiation-induced liver injury for tumors in the right lobe (lowest V20 and V30).

16.2.4 Stereotactic Body Radiotherapy (SBRT)

SBRT integrates stereotactic technology with 3D conformal multifield radiation technology. In the main body positioning framework, with the aid of body frame fixation and image guidance technology, this technique uses less fractionated high-dose radiation and provides better dose distribution and treatment effects. It is mainly applied to patients with liver cancer < 6 cm in diameter and Child-Pugh A/B liver function, with 1- and 2-year local control rates of 72–100% and 62–100%, respectively, and 1- and 2-year survival rates of 72.7–100% and 45.3–87.9%, respectively. For patients with Child-Pugh A cirrhosis or tumor < 3 cm in diameter, ≥ 10 Gy per dose/3–5 fractions are mostly used. The 2019 edition National Comprehensive Cancer Network guideline (NCCN) recommends a total SBRT dose of 30–50 Gy with 3–5 fractions for liver cancer. With the benefits of good local control and adequate tolerability, it is recognized as one of the alternatives for small liver cancers that are not suitable for surgery.

16.2.5 Proton Beam Radiotherapy

Protons are positively charged particles. After proton beams generated by modern accelerators enter the human body, molecular ionization and molecular excitation are induced by proton–electron collisions. The ionized and excited molecules have large internal energy, which has a destructive effect on biological macromolecules (such as DNA) that play a key role in cellular life activity. Upon entering the human body, the proton beam forms a sharp Bragg peak, and the energy after the peak drops off without further damagings other tissues. Therefore, by adjusting different energies and controlling the width of the Bragg peak, the high-energy region can be placed exactly at tumors with different depths and sizes. Previously, it was thought that the liver could only receive a maximum dose of 30 Gy over a 3-week period, but proton radiotherapy can surpass this limit due to the Bragg peak effect of protons, which allows most of the dose in the target area. Although respiratory gating technology is available, respiratory motion still affects the positioning of proton radiotherapy in the liver, making it still difficult to achieve precise tracking of liver cancer in real time. Furthermore, the device of the proton radiotherapy system is extremely complex, bulky in size, and expensive to build.

Suggested Reading

1. Sugiura N. Percutaneous intratumoral injection of ethanol under ultrasound imaging for treatment of small hepatocellular carcinoma. Acta Hepatol Jpn. 1983;24:920–3.
2. Jia YC. Recent progress in the interventional treatment of liver cancer. J Intervent Radiol. 1995;4(2): 112–5.
3. Castells J, Bruix C, Bru J, et al. Treatment of small hepatocellular carcinoma in cirrhotic patients: a cohort study comparing surgical resection and percutaneous ethanol injection. Hepatology. 2010;18(5):1121–6.
4. Geng LX, Xu WD. B ultrasound-guided percutaneous ethanol injection for the treatment of intermediate and advanced liver cancer. J Clin Hepatol. 1988;3(3):45.
5. Zhang XG, Tian YC. PEIT for treating small hepatocellular carcinoma. Shaanxi Med J. 1989;18(4):40–1.
6. Chung SC, Lee TW, Kwok SP, et al. Injection of alcohol to control bleeding from ruptured hepatomas. BMJ. 1990;301(6749):421.
7. Xie F, Xu L, Huang YQ, et al. Proton beam radiotherapy for liver cancer. J Hepatobiliary Surg. 2007;15(4):314–6.
8. Okad A, Shuich I. Local ablation therapy for hepatocellular carcinoma. Semin Liver Dis. 1999;19(3): 323–8.
9. Forner A, Reig M, Bruix J. Hepatocellular carcinoma. Lancet. 2018;391(10127):1301–14.
10. Galle PR, Forner A, Llovet JM, et al. EASL clinical practice guidelines: management of hepatocellular carcinoma. J Hepatol. 2018;69(1):182–236.
11. Rossi S. Percutaneous ultrasound-guided radiofrequency electrocautery for the treatment of small hepatocellular carcinoma. J Interv Radiol. 1993;8:97–103.
12. Ma QJ, Zhao BS. Percutaneous puncture radiofrequency treatment with cluster electrodes for liver cancer: a report of 35 cases. Chinese J Pract Surg. 1999;19(10):595–6.
13. Jiang AN, Yang W. Research progress of radiofrequency ablation electrode needle for liver tumor. J Intervent Radiol. 2017;26(5):466–70.
14. Galanakis N, Kehagias E, Matthaiou N, et al. Transcatheter arterial chemoembolization com-

bined with radiofrequency or microwave ablation for hepatocellular carcinoma: a review. Hep Oncologia. 2018;5(2):7.
15. Haen SP, Pereira PL, Salih HR, et al. More than just tumor destruction: immunomodulation by thermal ablation of cancer. Clin Dev Immunol. 2011;2011:1–19.
16. Zhou Y, Zhao Y, Li B, et al. Meta-analysis of radiofrequency ablation versus hepatic resection for small hepatocellular carcinoma. BMC Gastroenterol. 2010;10(1):1–7.
17. Kenji ON. Comparison of therapeutic effects between radiofrequency ablation and percutaneous microwave coagulation therapy for small hepatocellular carcinomas. J Gastroenterol Hepatol. 2009;24(2):223–7.
18. Shibata T, Iimuro Y, Yamamoto Y, et al. Small hepatocellular carcinoma: comparison of radio-frequency ablation and percutaneous microwave coagulation therapy. Radiology. 2002;223(2):331–7.
19. Zhou XD. Microwave surgery in the treatment of liver cancer. Chinese J Surg. 1993;31(3):153–5.
20. Hu WX, Yu SH. Clinical study of microwave therapy for hepatobiliary tumors. Chin J Clin Oncol. 1994;5:374–5.
21. Solbiati L, Goldberg SN, Ierace T, et al. Radiofrequency ablation of hepatic metastases: post-procedural assessment with a US microbubble contrast agent-early experience. Radiology. 1999;211(3):643–9.
22. Hoffman N, Dige R, Rempp H, et al. Comparison of four microwave ablation devices: an experimental study in ex vivo bovine liver. Radiology. 2013;268(1):89–97.
23. Poulou LS. Percutaneous microwave ablation vs radiofrequency ablation in the treatment of hepatocellular carcinoma. World J Hepatol. 2015;7(8):1054–63.
24. Facciorusso A, Maso MD, Muscatiello N. Microwave ablation versus radiofrequency ablation for the treatment of hepatocellular carcinoma: a systematic review and meta-analysis. Int J Hyperth. 2016;32(3):339–44.
25. Guan LM, Wang ZB, Wu F, et al. Pathological observation on the damage of human breast cancer cells and their feeding vessels by high-intensity focused ultrasound. Chinese J Clin Med. 2006;13(4):675.
26. Zhang Y, Deng J, Feng J, et al. Enhancement of antitumor vaccine in ablated hepatocellular carcinoma by high-intensity focused ultrasound. World J Gastroenterol. 2010;16(28):3584–91.
27. Jin CB, Ran LF, Yang W, et al. Preliminary clinical observation of HIFU combined with stereotactic body radiotherapy for the treatment of liver malignancies. Chinese J Ultrasound Med. 2011;27(7):659.
28. Li Z, Mi DH, Yang KH, et al. Meta-analysis of TACE combined with HIFU for the treatment of primary liver cancer. J Evid Based Med. 2013;13(5):292–9.
29. Lynn JG. A new method for the generation and use of focused ultrasound in experimental biology. J Gen Physiol. 1942;26(2):179–93.
30. Vallancien G, Chartier-Kastler E, Harouni M, et al. Focused extracorporeal pyrotherapy: experimental study and feasibility in man. Semin Urol. 1993;11(1):7–9.
31. Chen L, Rivens I, Haar G, et al. Histological changes in rat liver tumours treated with high-intensity focused ultrasound. Ultrasound Med Biol. 1993;19(1):67–74.
32. Prat F, Centarti M, Sibille A, et al. Extracorporeal high-intensity focused ultrasound for VX2 liver tumors in the rabbit. Hepatology. 1995;21(3):832–6.
33. Rowland IJ, Rivens I, Chen L, et al. MRI study of hepatic tumours following high intensity focused ultrasound surgery. Br J Radiol. 1997;70(830):144–53.
34. Sibille A, Prat F, Chapelon JY, et al. Extracorporeal ablation of liver tissue by highintensity focused ultrasound. Oncology. 1993;50(5):375–9.
35. Yang R. High-intensity focused ultrasound in the treatment of experimental liver cancer. Arch Surg. 1991;126(8):1002–9.
36. Wu F, Wang ZB, Chen WZ, et al. Extracorporeal high intensity focused ultrasound ablation in the treatment of 1038 patients with solid carcinomas in China: an overview. Ultrason Sonochem. 2004;11(3–4):149–54.
37. Wu F, Wang ZB, Chen WZ, et al. Extracorporeal high intensity focused ultrasound ablation in the treatment of patients with large hepatocellular carcinoma. Ann Surg Oncol. 2004;11(12):1061–9.
38. Wu F, Wang Z, Chen W. Advanced hepatocellular carcinoma: treatment with high-intensity focused ultrasound ablation combined with transcatheter arterial embolization. Radiology. 2005;235(2):659–67.
39. Wu F, Wang ZB, Chen WZ, et al. Extracorporeal focused ultrasound surgery for treatment of human solid carcinomas: early Chinese clinical experience. Ultrasound Med Biol. 2004;30(2):245–60.
40. Beebe SJ, Fox PM, Rec LJ, et al. Nanosecond, high-intensity pulsed electric fields induce apoptosis in human cells. FASEB J. 2003;17(11):1493–5.
41. Lee EW, Thai S, Kee ST. Irreversible electroporation: a novel image-guided cancer therapy. Gut Liver. 2010;4(Suppl 1):S99–S104.
42. Charpentier KP, Wolf F, Noble L, et al. Irreversible electroporation of the liver and liver hilum in swine. HPB (Oxford). 2015;13(3):168–73.
43. Phillips MA, Narayan R, Padath T, et al. Irreversible electroporation on the small intestine. Br J Cancer. 2012;106(3):490–5.
44. Ivorra A, Rubinsky B. Historical review of irreversible electroporation in medicine. Irrevers Electrop. 2010;1:21.
45. Neumann EM, Schaefer-Ridder M, Wang Y, et al. Gene transfer into mouse lyoma cells by electroporation in high electric fields. EMBO J. 1982;1(7):841–5.
46. Davalos RV, Mir LM, Rubinsky B. Tissue ablation with irreversible electroporation. Ann Biomed Eng. 2005;33(2):223–31.
47. Cannon R, Ellis S, Hayes D, et al. Safety and early efficacy of irreversible electroporation for hepatic tumors in proximity to vital structures. J Surg Oncol. 2013;107(5):544–9.
48. Kimura T, Aikata H, Takahashi S, et al. Stereotactic body radiotherapy for patients with small hepatocel-

lular carcinoma ineligible for resection or ablation therapies. Hepatol Res. 2015;45(4):378–86.
49. Niu LZ, Li ZH, Li R, et al. Safety and short-term efficacy of irreversible electroporation ablation for hepatic malignancies. Chinese J Radiol. 2016;50(7):526–30.
50. Gage A, Baust J. Mechanisms of tissue injury in cryosurgery. Cryobiology. 1998;37(3):171–86.
51. Hoffmann NE, Bischof JC. The cryobiology of cryosurgical injury. Urology. 2002;60(2 Suppl 1):40–9.
52. Min YS, Young-Suk L, Jin PM, et al. Stereotactic body radiation therapy as an alternative treatment for small hepatocellular carcinoma. PLoS One. 2013;8(11):e79854.
53. Cooper IS, Lee AS. Cryostatic congelation: a system for producing a limited, controlled region of cooling or freezing of biologic tissues. J Nerv Ment Dis. 1961;133(3):259–63.
54. Zhang JR. Argon helium knife cryoablation of tumors. China Cancer. 2007;16(5):335–7.
55. Chen Y, Gao SG, Chen JM, el al. Risk factors for the long-term efficacy, recurrence, and metastasis in small hepatocellular carcinomas. Cell Biochem Biophys. 2015;72(2):627–31.
56. Rong G, Bai W, Dong Z, et al. Long-term outcomes of percutaneous cryoablation for patients with hepatocellular carcinoma within Milan criteria. PLoS One. 2015;10(4):e0123065.
57. Pan F, Jiang Y, Zhang XJ, et al. Argon helium knife cryotherapy in 145 cases of small liver cancer. Military Med J Southeast China. 2012;5:419–21.
58. Li Z, Mi DH, Yang KH, et al. Systematic evaluation of the efficacy and safety of hepatic arterial chemoembolization combined with argon helium knife for the treatment of liver cancer. Chin J Evid Based Med. 2013;13(1):31–8.
59. Gu XY, Jiang Z. Observation on the efficacy of combined argon helium knife cryotherapy and absolute alcohol injection for the treatment of liver cancer. Modern Med J. 2003;6:23–4.
60. Zhong JH, Ma L, Li LQ. Postoperative therapy options for hepatocellular carcinoma. Scand J Gastroenterol. 2014;49(6):649–61.
61. Lee JH, Kim DH, Ki YK, et al. Three-dimensional conformal radiotherapy for portal vein tumor thrombosis alone in advanced hepatocellular carcinoma. R Radiat Oncol J. 2014;32(3):170–8.
62. Kennedy AS. Radiation oncology approaches in liver malignancies[J]. Am Soc Clin Oncol Educ Book. 2014;34:e150–5.
63. Schaub SK, Hartvigson PE, Lock MI, et al. Stereotactic body radiation therapy for hepatocellular carcinoma: current trends and controversies. Technol Cancer Res Treat. 2018;17:153303381879021.
64. Lazarev S, Hardy-Abeloos C, Factor O, et al. Stereotactic body radiation therapy for centrally located hepatocellular carcinoma: outcomes and toxicities. J Cancer Res Clin Oncol. 2018;144(10):2077–83.
65. Rdenes CHR, Price TR, Perkins SM, et al. Phase I feasibility trial of stereotactic body radiation therapy for primary hepatocellular carcinoma. Clin Transl Oncol. 2010;12(3):218–25.
66. Kwon JH, Bae SH, Kim JY, et al. Long-term effect of stereotactic body radiation therapy for primary hepatocellular carcinoma ineligible for local ablation therapy or surgical resection. Stereotactic radiotherapy for liver cancer. BMC Cancer. 2010;10(1):475.
67. Park SH, Kim JC, Kang MK. Technical advances in external radiotherapy for hepatocellular carcinoma. World J Gastroenterol. 2016;22(32):7311–21.

Part V

Molecular Targeted Drugs for Liver Cancer

The occurrence, development, and metastasis of hepatocellular carcinoma (HCC) are closely related to gene mutation, cellular signal transduction pathway, and tumor microenvironment. The basis of molecular targeted therapy for HCC is to block the pivotal driving signals in tumor progression. The systemic treatment for HCC includes conventional systemic chemotherapy, molecular targeted therapy, and the new emerging immunotherapy. The recent 10 years have witnessed the rapid development of systemic therapy drugs in HCC. Accordingly, the clinical practice of advanced HCC has changed dramatically, and the prognosis of HCC patients has also been improved greatly. At present, systemic treatment has been extended to adjuvant therapy for early and intermediate HCC. The whole-course management of systemic treatment, as well as the combination of local regional therapy with systemic treatment, has also been emphasized in the management of intermediate and advanced HCC.

17 Developments and Current Status of Molecular Targeted Therapy for Liver Cancer

Xin Yin, Zhenggang Ren, and Shukui Qin

The data on the prevalence of malignant tumors in China released by the National Cancer Center in January 2019 showed that there were 370,000 new cases of primary liver cancer in China, accounting for about 44% of global cases, and 326,000 deaths, accounting for about 42% of global deaths. Among them, HCC accounts for 85–90% of all liver cancers. Judging from the latest data on the incidence and mortality of liver cancer, China still ranks first among high-risk HCC regions in the world. Only 15–20% of the patients with HCC are diagnosed at an early stage and suitable for surgical resection, whereas approximately 80% of the HCC patients are diagnosed at intermediate or advanced stage, losing the chance to receive surgical resection. Therefore, the improvement of systemic therapy for intermediate or advanced HCC has become the key to improving the prognosis of patients with HCC.

In 2007, the first molecular-targeted drug sorafenib ushered in a new era of molecular-targeted therapy for HCC. The SHARP and ORIENTAL clinical studies established the therapeutic status of sorafenib as the standard first-line therapy for advanced HCC. The SHARP clinical study conducted in Europe and America confirmed that sorafenib could improve the prognosis of patients with advanced HCC with a median survival of 10.7 months. The ORIENTAL clinical study conducted in the Asia-Pacific region showed that sorafenib was also effective in hepatitis B virus-related HCC, and the median overall survival (mOS) of patients treated with sorafenib was 6.5 months, which was superior to that of the patients in the placebo group. Nevertheless, the efficacy of sorafenib for patients in the Asia-Pacific region was not as good as that for patients in Europe and America. Obviously, the difference in efficacy of sorafenib between the East and West is attributed to different etiology of liver disease. A meta-analysis published in the *Journal of Clinical Oncology* in 2017 investigated the efficacy of sorafenib in HCC patients infected with different hepatitis viruses. Patients enrolled in the ORIENTAL clinical study in the Asia-Pacific region were mainly HBV-infected patients, while patients enrolled in the SHARP clinical study in Europe and America were mainly infected by hepatitis C virus (HCV). The results showed that the survival benefit of sorafenib in HCV-positive HCC patients was higher than that in hepatitis B virus (HBV)-positive HCC patients.

In the decade following the emergence of sorafenib, many first-line and second-line molecular targeted drugs have been evaluated in different clinical trials but failed to obtain positive results in the end, including sunitinib, brivanib,

X. Yin · Z. Ren
ZhongShan Hospital Fudan University,
Shanghai, China

S. Qin (✉)
Nanjing Jinling Hospital, Nanjing, China
e-mail: qinsk@csco.org.cn

X. Chen (ed.), *Diagnosis and Treatment of Liver Cancer in China*,
https://doi.org/10.1007/978-981-97-7969-7_17

linifanib, and lapatinib, whose efficacy was no better than that of sorafenib. After 2017, successive approval of new molecular targeted drugs such as lenvatinib, regorafenib, cabozantinib, and ramucirumab, and the application of immune checkpoint inhibitors (ICIs) has led to a diversified therapeutic pattern and significantly improved the efficacy of systemic treatment in advanced HCC. In 2019, the positive results of a phase III IMbrave150 trial demonstrated superior survival results for atezolizumab plus bevacizumab versus sorafenib in advanced HCC, which heralded a new era of molecular targeted therapy combined with immunotherapy and set a new benchmark for survival benefits. This combination and others reported in phase II trials (e.g., lenvatinib plus pembrolizumab, camrelizumab combined with apatinib or nivolumab plus ipilimumab) increase objective responses in advanced HCC to 30–40%, encouraging the exploration of their effects on the management of intermediate or even early-stage HCC.

17.1 Development of Systemic Chemotherapy for HCC

Chemotherapy has been used in the systemic treatment for HCC since the 1950s. As a common digestive system tumor in clinical practice, most chemotherapy drugs in HCC are not effective, and the efficacy of chemotherapy alone is less than 20%. 5-Fluorouracil (5-FU), adriamycin, cisplatin, and mitomycin have been used in chemotherapy for HCC. However, several large randomized controlled trials evaluating systemic chemotherapy for HCC failed to demonstrate survival benefits for patients with advanced HCC.

In 2011, a phase II clinical trial of arsenic trioxide (arsenic acid injection) for the treatment of intermediate and advanced HCC presided by Professor Yan SUN showed an objective response rate of 6.9% and a disease control rate (DCR) of 76.5%. Thus, arsenic acid injection has also been approved by the National Medical Products Administration for the treatment of HCC. However, due to its limited efficacy, arsenic acid treatment has not been widely recognized in Western countries.

In 2010, a multicenter clinical study in the Asia-Pacific region (EACH) led by Professor Shukui QIN investigated the efficacy and safety of the oxaliplatin-based FOLFOX4 regimen versus adriamycin monotherapy in advanced HCC. The results showed that, compared to doxorubicin monotherapy, FOLFOX4 chemotherapy could improve the tumor objective response rate and DCR and prolong the progression-free survival (PFS) and overall survival of patients. The clinical study results of EACH are widely recognized in HCC treatment worldwide and have been listed as the first-line treatment strategy for advanced HCC by the U.S. National Comprehensive Cancer Network (NCCN) Guidelines, the Chinese *Guidelines for the Diagnosis and Treatment of Primary Liver Cancer* (2019 Edition), and the guidelines for liver cancer in Japan, South Korea, and other countries.

17.2 Evidence Review of Molecular Targeted Drugs for HCC

Sorafenib was approved as a first-line therapy for advanced HCC in 2007, and several phase III clinical studies (including first-line, second-line, adjuvant therapy, etc.) were subsequently conducted (Table 17.1). Various systemic therapy drugs for advanced HCC have been studied from 2007 to 2017, but most clinical trials failed to obtain the desired positive results. The new drugs in several clinical studies were all aborted in phase III due to high toxicity or poor efficacy. For example, sunitinib failed due to severe side effects; brivanib (BRISK-FL study) failed to demonstrate superior efficacy in the endpoint, although the time to progression (TTP) and overall survival were not significantly different from sorafenib; and linifanib also failed to reach the primary endpoint due to greater toxicity, although the overall survival was not significantly different from sorafenib and the TTP was prolonged. The failure of several large clinical studies was mainly due to the complex etiologies of HCC, such as HBV, HCV, and alcoholic and non-alcoholic liver disease. The prognosis of HCC with different background liver disease

Table 17.1 Phase III clinical trials of molecular targeted drugs for hepatocellular carcinoma completed in recent years

Drug name	Registration No.	Study populations	Study design	Results
Sorafenib	NCT00105443	Patients with advanced HCC who received first-line therapy	Sorafenib vs. placebo	Positive result
	NCT00692770	HCC patients who received postoperative adjuvant therapy	Sorafenib vs. placebo	Negative result
	NCT00855218	Patients with BCLC stage B HCC	Sorafenib combined with TACE vs. TACE	Negative result
	NCT00990860	Patients with BCLC stage B HCC(Asian-Pacific region)	Sorafenib combined with TACE vs. TACE	Negative result
	NCT01217034	Patients with BCLC stage BHCC	Sorafenib combined with TACE vs. TACE	Positive result(PFS only)
Sunitinib	NCT00699374	Patients with advanced HCC who received first-line therapy	Sunitinib vs. sorafenib	Discontinuation in phase III
Brivanib	NCT00858871	Patients with advanced HCC who received first-line therapy	Brivanib vs. sorafenib	Discontinuation in phase III
Linifanib	NCT01009593	Patients with advanced HCC who received first-line therapy	Linifanib vs. sorafenib	Discontinuation in phase III
Lenvatinib	NCT01761266	Patients with advanced HCC who received first-line therapy	Lenvatinib vs. sorafenib	Positive result (non-inferiority)
Everolimus	NCT01035229	Patients with HCC who received second-line therapy after failure of sorafenib treatment	Everolimus vs. placebo	Discontinuation in phase III
Regorafenib	NCT01774344	Patients with HCC who received second-line therapy after failure of sorafenib treatment	Regorafenib vs. placebo	Positive result
Cabozantinib	NCT01908426	Patients with HCC who received second-line therapy after failure of sorafenib treatment	Cabozantinib vs. placebo	Positive result
Ramucirumab	NCT02435433	Patients with HCC who received second-line therapy after failure of sorafenib treatment (AFP $\geq$400 ng/mL)	Ramucirumab vs. placebo	Positive result
Nivolumab	NCT02576509	Patients with unresectable HCC who received first-line therapy	Nivolumab vs. Sorafenib	Negative result

(continued)

Table 17.1 (continued)

Drug name	Registration No.	Study populations	Study design	Results
Pembrolizumab	NCT02702401	Patients with unresectable HCC who received second-line therapy after failure of sorafenib treatment	Pembrolizumab vs. placebo	Negative result
Atezolizumab + Bevacizumab	NCT03434379	Patients with unresectable HCC who received first-line therapy	Atezolizumab + bevacizumab vs. sorafenib	Positive result
Sintilimab + bevacizumab biosimilar	NCT03794440	Patients with unresectable HCC who received first-line therapy	Sintilimab + bevacizumab biosimilar vs. sorafenib	Positive result
Donafenib	NCT0264598	Patients with unresectable HCC who received first-line therapy	Donafenib vs. sorafenib	Positive result
Apatinib	NCT02329860	Patients with unresectable HCC who received second-line therapy after failure of sorafenib treatment	Apatinib vs. placebo	Positive result
Tremelimumab +durvalumab	NCT03298451	Patients with unresectable HCC who received first-line therapy	Tremelimumab +durvalumab vs. sorafenib	Positive result

showed significant heterogeneity in response to molecular targeted drugs.

In 2018, the international multicenter clinical study REFLECT, in which Professor Shukui QIN was the leading principal investigator in China, obtained non-inferiority results. Lenvatinib became the second first-line drug approved for the treatment of HCC after sorafenib. The REFLECT study showed that the mOS of patients was 13.6 months in the lenvatinib group and 12.3 months in the sorafenib group, reaching its non-inferiority endpoint. All secondary endpoints including the PFS, TTP, and overall response rate (ORR) were better in the lenvatinib group than those in the sorafenib group, as assessed by the modified Response Evaluation Criteria in Solid Tumors. The data from the subgroup of HBV-related HCC patients treated with lenvatinib showed superiority over the sorafenib group, with an mOS of 15.0 months, a PFS of 9.2 months, a TTP of 11.0 months, and an ORR of 21.5%.

For patients with HCC who had disease progression following first-line targeted therapy and then received second-line therapy, especially for patients with advanced HCC who had disease progression on sorafenib, new molecular targeted drugs for second-line therapy, such as regorafenib, cabozantinib, ramucirumab, nivolumab, and pembrolizumab (ICI) showed encouraging results and have been successively approved by the U.S. Food and Drug Administration (FDA) and recommended by the NCCN Guidelines. For example, the CheckMate-040 study investigated the efficacy of the immunotherapy drug nivolumab in advanced HCC, which enrolled 262 patients previously treated with sorafenib and took safety, tolerance, and tumor objective response rate as the primary study endpoints. The results showed that nivolumab had clinically significant efficacy in second-line therapy for advanced HCC. A separate analysis of the Asian population revealed similar results compared to the total population. In addition, the efficacy of nivolumab in HCC patients with different etiologies (infected or uninfected with HBV/HCV) was similar to that in the total population. Based on the results of this study, nivolumab was approved by the U. S. FDA in 2017 for the treatment of HCC patients previously treated with sorafenib. Another immunotherapy clinical study, Keynote-224, a non-randomized, multicenter, open-label phase II clinical trial, enrolled 104 Child-Pugh A patients with advanced HCC who had failed to respond to sorafenib therapy. The study results showed that patients treated with pembrolizumab had an mPFS of 4.9 (3.4–7.2) months, an mOS of 12.9 (9.7–15.5) months, an ORR of 17%, and a DCR of 62%. 15% of patients experienced Grade 3 side effects or above, including elevated aspartate aminotransferase and alanine aminotransferase, and diarrhea. In view of the efficacy and safety of pembrolizumab in HCC, the U.S. FDA granted accelerated approval to pembrolizumab as second-line therapy for patients with HCC who had failed to respond to sorafenib therapy in November 2018.

The incorporation of nivolumab and pembrolizumab into the American Association for the Study of Liver Diseases (AASLD) guideline on HCC as second-line systemic therapy was made in advance of the phase III trial results. Unfortunately, the subsequent phase III trial results (CheckMate459 (NCT02576509) 459 and KEYNOTE-240 (NCT02702401) both did not meet their primary endpoints of overall survival and PFS in patients with advanced HCC. These results, although disappointing, would appear to be consistent with the opinion that ICIs may well be most efficacious as combination therapy.

Thus, a number of ICI combinations have entered into phase III clinical trials comparing them with sorafenib in HCC patients naive to systemic therapy. The much-awaited open-label phase III IMbrave150 (NCT03434379) trial evaluated the efficacy of atezolizumab plus bevacizumab compared with sorafenib therapy as a first-line treatment in 501 patients with HCC. Patients treated with atezolizumab plus bevacizumab had significantly improved 12-month OS rate versus patients treated with sorafenib (67.2% vs. 54.6%, respectively). Additionally, the median PFS was 6.8 months in the combination group versus 4.3 months in the sorafenib group (HR for disease progression or death 0.59; 95% CI, 0.47–0.76; $p < 0.001$). Based on IMbrave150 study, the combination of atezolizumab and bevacizumab is recommended as a first-line preferable treatment in advanced HCC by NCCN, AASLD, and European Society for Medical Oncology (ESMO) guidelines. In addition to atezolizumab and bevacizumab combination, other two phase III clinical trials (ORIENT-32 (NCT03794440) and HIMALAYA (NCT03298451)) successfully achieved their primary endpoint in comparison with sorafenib as first-line treatment for unresectable HCC. Recently, the combinations of sintilimab+bevacizumab biosimilar and tremelimumab +durvalumab are also recommended by the 2022 NCCN guidelines or Chinese Guidelines for the Diagnosis and Treatment of Primary Liver Cancer (2022 edition).

Suggested Reading

1. Bray F, Ferlay J, Soerjomataram I, et al. Global cancer statistics 2018: GLOBOCAN estimates of incidence and mortality worldwide for 36 cancers in 185 countries. CA Cancer J Clin. 2018;68:394–424.
2. Rongshou Z, Kexin S, Siwei Z, et al. Report of cancer epidemiology in China, 2015. Chinese J Oncol. 2019;41(1):19–28.
3. Zhou J, Sun HC, Wang Z, et al. Guidelines for diagnosis and treatment of primary liver cancer in China (2017 Edition). Liver Cancer. 2018;7:235–60.
4. Villanueva A. Hepatocellular Carcinoma. N Engl J Med. 2019;380:1450–62.
5. Llovet JM, Ricci S, Mazzaferro V, et al. Sorafenib in advanced hepatocellular carcinoma. N Engl J Med. 2008;359:378–90.
6. Jackson R, Psarelli E, Berhane S, et al. Impact of viral status on survival in patients receiving sorafenib for advanced hepatocellular cancer: a meta-analysis of randomized phase III trials. J Clin Oncol. 2017;35:622.
7. Finn RS, Qin S, Ikeda M, et al. Atezolizumab plus Bevacizumab in Unresectable Hepatocellular Carcinoma. N Engl J Med. 2020;382(20):1894–905.
8. Feng-lian QU, Xue-zhi HAO, Shu-kui QIN, et al. Multicenter phase II clinical trial of arsenic trioxide injection in the treatment of primary hepatocarcinoma. Chinese J Oncol. 2011;33(9):697–701.
9. Qin S, Bai Y, Lim HY, et al. Randomized, multicenter, open-label study of oxaliplatin plus fluorouracil/leucovorin versus doxorubicin as palliative chemotherapy in patients with advanced hepatocellular carcinoma from Asia. J Clin Oncol. 2013;31:3501–8.
10. Kudo M, Finn RS, Qin S, et al. Lenvatinib versus sorafenib in first line treatment of patients with unresectable hepatocellular carcinoma: a randomised phase 3 non-inferiority trial. Lancet. 2018;391(10126):1163–73.
11. El-Khoueiry AB, Sangro B, Yau T, et al. Nivolumab in patients with advanced hepatocellular carcinoma (CheckMate 040): an open-label, non-comparative, phase 1/2 dose escalation and expansion trial. Lancet. 2017;389(10088):2492–502.
12. Zhu AX, Finn RS, Edeline J, et al. Pembrolizumab in patients with advanced hepatocellular carcinoma previously treated with sorafenib (KEYNOTE-224): a non-randomised, open-label phase 2 trial. Lancet Oncol. 2018;19(7):940–52.
13. Ren Z, Xu J, Bai Y, et al. ORIENT-32 study group. Sintilimab plus a bevacizumab biosimilar (IBI305) versus sorafenib in unresectable hepatocellular carcinoma (ORIENT-32): a randomised open-label, phase 2-3 study. Lancet Oncol. 2021;22(7):977–90.
14. Kelley RK, Sangro B, Harris W, et al. Safety, efficacy, and pharmacodynamics of Tremelimumab plus Durvalumab for patients with unresectable hepatocellular carcinoma: randomized expansion of a phase I/II study. J Clin Oncol. 2021;39(27):2991–3001.

18 Application of Efficacy Evaluation Criteria for Molecular Targeted Therapy for Liver Cancer

Xin Yin, Zhenggang Ren, and Shukui Qin

It is difficult to completely cure cancers. The prolonging of overall survival (OS) has long been the gold standard for evaluating the efficacy of targeted therapy and drug approval in clinical practice. OS has the advantages of objective evaluation and less influence from investigators' observation bias, but it also has the disadvantage of long observation time and being easily affected by later-line therapies. The U.S. Food and Drug Administration (FDA) determined the improvement of OS as the main evaluation index in the standard drug approval process in 2017. However, if a drug is intended to treat a serious life-threatening disease and can provide significant improvement in the disease or fill the treatment gap, it can enter the accelerated approval pathway under certain conditions and adopt surrogate endpoints to support drug approval. The surrogate endpoints recommended by the U.S. FDA in clinical trials of new drugs include progression-free survival (PFS), time to progression, event-free survival, objective response rate (ORR), complete response (CR), disease-free survival, and time to treatment failure. Among these recommended outcome indexes, the surrogate endpoint of PFS is more relevant to OS. PFS as a trial endpoint has the advantage of short observation time and small sample size required for the study. The disadvantage of PFS is derived from its subjectivity, which is prone to cause evaluation bias, and difficult to determine the direct impact on patient survival. Considering the lack of objectivity of the surrogate endpoints, the National Medical Products Administration has established relatively strict approval criteria for new drugs. The *Guidelines on General Considerations for Clinical Trials of Drugs* issued by the National Medical Products Administration in 2017 pointed out that the primary endpoint of a clinical trial should reflect the primary clinical effects of the drug and should be selected based on the primary purpose of the study. Surrogate endpoints are indexes related to primary endpoints but are not direct evidence of clinical benefits themselves. A surrogate endpoint can be used as a primary index only when it is highly likely or known to be reasonably predictive of the primary endpoint. Therefore, survival benefit is still the main supporting basis for molecular targeted drugs approval by the National Medical Products Administration.

OS is the main efficacy evaluation criterion for anti-tumor therapies. In addition, the objective evaluation criteria to judge tumor treatment response include post-treatment tumor ORR, disease control rate, and PFS, which are also related to ORR. At present, the treatment efficacy evaluation criteria in HCC include World Health

X. Yin · Z. Ren
ZhongShan Hospital Fudan University, Shanghai, China

S. Qin (✉)
Nanjing Jinling Hospital, Nanjing, China
e-mail: qinsk@csco.org.cn

X. Chen (ed.), *Diagnosis and Treatment of Liver Cancer in China*,
https://doi.org/10.1007/978-981-97-7969-7_18

Organization (WHO) criteria, Response Evaluation Criteria in Solid Tumors (RECIST), RECIST 1.1, modified RECIST (mRECIST), and immune RECIST (iRECIST) for efficacy evaluation of immunotherapy.

18.1 WHO Criteria

In 1981, WHO published the efficacy evaluation criteria for anti-tumor therapy for the first time, that is, WHO criteria, which specify the relevant terms and measurement criteria for the efficacy evaluation of solid tumors. According to the WHO criteria, the treatment effect is evaluated by measuring the tumor in two diameters, calculating its product, and then classifying the treatment response as CR, partial response (PR), stable disease (SD), and progressive disease (PD). CR + PR is defined as the presence of a response to tumor treatment, and PD is defined as no response to treatment. The WHO criteria have been used for efficacy evaluation in solid tumors since they were proposed. However, there are some deficiencies in efficacy evaluation in HCC, for instance, the presence of different types of tumor lesions, including measurable lesions, evaluable lesions, and evaluable but unmeasurable lesions. WHO criteria do not evaluate tumor lesions based on different tumor types nor clearly specify the minimum number of lesions to be measured.

18.2 RECIST

In 1999, the European Organization for Research and Treatment of Cancer, the National Cancer Institute of America, and the National Cancer Institute of Canada put forward RECIST based on WHO criteria. RECIST follow the efficacy description of CR, PR, SD, and PD in WHO criteria and change the lesion measurement method from two-dimensional measurement to one-dimensional measurement. RECIST are mainly applicable to the efficacy evaluation of conventional cytotoxic drugs that induce tumor cell apoptosis or directly kill tumor cells, thus resulting in tumor volume reduction.

18.3 RECIST 1.1

RECIST 1.1, issued in 2009, include the imaging manifestations of lymph nodes during tumor treatment as evaluation indexes based on RECIST. According to RECIST 1.1, CR is defined as the disappearance of all tumors, PR and PD are defined as ≥30% reduction and ≥ 20% increase in the sum of the longest diameter of tumors, respectively, and those failing to meet the requirements of PR and PD are classified as SD. Compared with RECIST, RECIST 1.1 redefine the number of measurable target lesions, append the evaluation guide for pathological lymph nodes, clearly specify the percentage and absolute value for evaluating disease progression, and further refine the progression of non-target lesions. RECIST 1.1 have played an important role in clinical practice since they were proposed and now have become the most widely used efficacy evaluation criteria in solid tumors in international multicenter clinical trials.

18.4 mRECIST

Since RECIST 1.1 mainly evaluate the change in tumor size following anti-tumor treatment, it cannot evaluate the treatment-induced tumor necrosis, which may underestimate the efficacy of local regional therapy. In 2010, the American Association for the Study of Liver Diseases—Journal of the National Cancer Institute guidelines proposed amendments to the efficacy evaluation criteria revised based on RECIST, known as mRECIST, aiming at supplementing the concept of viable (enhancing) tumor region from previous studies to RECIST. Studies have generally found that the new mRECIST are more scientific for evaluating the efficacy of TACE, and the observation of long-term outcomes also suggests that mRECIST can better predict the prognosis. However, mRECIST also have certain limitations, especially in patients receiving TACE. When CT is used for measurement, there are sparse punctate or diffuse lipiodol deposits, and it is difficult to accurately identify the enhancing part of the tumors due to the interference of lipiodol after enhancement. The impact of lipiodol deposition can be overcome by MRI evaluation.

18.5 Immune-Related Response Criteria

Immunotherapy, as an emerging treatment, has been applied to solid tumors including malignant melanoma, lung cancer, liver cancer, colorectal cancer, and so on. The tumor response pattern of immunotherapy differs from chemotherapy and targeted therapy, due to its special anti-tumor mechanism. Immunotherapy can maintain a durable response after treatment discontinuation, challenging the previous concept of continuous treatment for advanced tumors until progression. Initially, the efficacy evaluation criteria in solid tumors (RECIST 1.1) are clinically used to evaluate the efficacy of immunotherapy drugs. However, the evaluation based on RECIST 1.1 is generally carried out at week 8 after treatment, and immunotherapy has such problems as slow response and tumor pseudoprogression. The traditional evaluation criteria for solid tumors cannot accurately reflect the efficacy of immunotherapy. Immune-related response criteria (irRC) are the first criteria developed based on evolved WHO criteria, which are adapted for the assessment of response to immunotherapy. The irRC were formulated based on data from clinical trials of ipilimumab in patients with advanced melanoma, showing delayed but durable treatment responses in a subset of patients. There are two major points in the formulation of irRC: (1) allowing for the continuation of immunotherapy at first progression, but requiring the confirmation of progression at least 4 weeks after initial assessment with a repeat imaging and (2) allowing for the appearance of new lesions, which are no longer considered as PD but incorporated into the total tumor burden. At baseline tumor assessment, the sum of the largest perpendicular diameters of all target lesions (5 lesions per organ and up to 15 in total) is calculated, and at each subsequent tumor assessment, baseline lesions and new measurable lesions (≥5. 0 mm × 5. 0 mm) are incorporated into the total tumor burden. The irRC could avoid early discontinuation of treatment in a subset of patients with advanced disease who respond to immunotherapy. However, there are also some problems with irRC. The irRC are based on bi-dimensional measurements of tumor lesions, as WHO criteria are, which may exaggerate the actual extent of tumor change, especially when the lesion changes slightly. The irRC increase variability in assessments in comparison to RECIST, which are based on one-dimensional measurements. The majority of initial clinical studies of immunotherapy were assessed according to RECIST, rendering comparisons difficult between findings of clinical studies.

18.6 Immune Therapy Related RECIST (irRECIST)

The irRECIST were proposed based on irRC at the 2014 Congress of the European Society for Medical Oncology. The most significant change from irRC is the re-adoption of one-dimensional measurement in irRECIST. In irRECIST, the measurable lesion is defined as non-lymph nodal metastases >10 mm in the long axis and lymph nodal lesions >15 mm in the short axis. Disappearance of all target lesions and lymph nodal lesions <10 mm in short axis with no appearance of new lesions is defined as CR.A ≥ 30% decrease in the tumor burden compared with the baseline, and no unequivocal progression in the nontarget lesions with no appearance of new lesions is defined as PR. ≥5 mm increase in the sum of longest diameters of measurable target lesions and ≥ 20% increase in tumor burden, progression of nontarget lesions, or the appearance of a new lesion is defined as irPD. An important aspect of irRECIST is that the irPD must also be reassessed at least 4 weeks later, and if the repeat assessment shows a new unequivocal progression from the prior imaging assessments, or the appearance of another new lesion, a confirmed disease progression is defined.

18.7 iRECIST

In early 2017, to harmonize the interpretation of data between different trials assessing immunotherapy drugs, the RECIST working group along with immunotherapy subcommittees created a modified version of RECIST1.1 for immunotherapy, the iRECIST. The principles and imaging techniques for evaluating tumor response are basically consistent with RECIST 1.1, except that the abbreviations of response types are preceded by an "i," such as iCR, iPR, and iSD. The most prominent change in iRECIST is the introduction of two new concepts, namely, the immunity unconfirmed progressive disease (iUPD) and the immunity confirmed progressive disease (iCPD). Other changes include the evaluation of new lesions, the response evaluation after iUPD evaluation, and how iUPD is confirmed. According to iRECIST, the reevaluation time is generally 4–6 weeks, but no more than 8 weeks. However, for certain tumor immunotherapy with a high incidence of pseudoprogression (such as treatment of melanoma with ipilimumab) or in cases where no remedial therapy is available, the evaluation time can be appropriately extended. For patients assessed as iCPD, ongoing follow-up evaluation is recommended as long as conditions allow, regardless of whether the patient continues to receive the treatment or not. In addition, the difference between the evaluation results based on RECIST 1.1 and iRECIST can also provide a reference for a future revision of iRECIST. Due to the short time following the proposal of iRECIST, RECIST 1.1 remain the primary evaluation criteria and iRECIST are used as secondary or investigational evaluation criteria in most clinical trials.

Suggested Reading

1. Hodi FS, Hwu WJ, Kefford R, et al. Evaluation of immune-related response criteria and RECIST v1. 1 in patients with advanced melanoma treated with pembrolizumab. J Clin Oncol. 2016;34:1510–7.
2. Seymour L, Bogaerts J, Perrone A, et al. iRECIST: guidelines for response criteria for use in trials testing immunotherapeutics. Lancet Oncol. 2017;18:e143–52.
3. Miller AB, Hoogstraten B, Staquet M, et al. Reporting results of cancer treatment. Cancer. 1981;47:207–14.
4. Therasse P, Arbuck SG, Eisenhauer EA, et al. New guidelines to evaluate the response to treatment in solid tumors. European organization for search and treatment of cancer, National Cancer Institute of the United States, National Cancer Institute of Canada. J Natl Cancer Inst. 2000;92:205–16.
5. Eisenhauer EA, Therasse P, Bogaerts J, et al. New response evaluation criteria in solid tumours: revised RECIST guideline (version 1.1). Eur J Cancer. 2009;45:228–7.
6. Lencioni R, Llovet JM. Modified RECIST(mRECIST assessment)for hepatocellular carcinoma. Semin Liver Dis. 2010;30:52–60.
7. Gavanier M, Ayav A, Sellal C, et al. CT imaging findings in patients with advanced hepatocellular carcinoma treated with sorafenib: alternative response criteria(Choi, European Association for the Study of the liver, and modified response evaluation criteria in solid tumor(mRECIST))versus RECIST 1. 1. Eur J Radiol. 2016;85:103–12.
8. Wolchok JD, Hoos A, O'Day S, et al. Guidelines for the evaluation of immune therapy activity in solid tumors: immune-related response criteria. Clin Cancer Res. 2009;15:7412–20.

Molecular Targeted Drugs for Liver Cancer

19

Xin Yin, Zhenggang Ren, and Shukui Qin

Sorafenib is the first molecular targeted drug approved by the U.S. Food and Drug Administration (FDA) in advanced hepatocellular carcinoma (HCC). As an oral tyrosine kinase inhibitor, sorafenib inhibits tumor proliferation and angiogenesis by blocking the RAF/MEK/ERK signaling pathway and inhibiting vascular endothelial growth factor (VEGF) and PDGFR. Two international multicenter clinical studies, SHARP and ORIENTAL, confirmed the efficacy and safety of sorafenib in advanced HCC, initiating an era of molecular targeted therapy for HCC. The SHARP clinical study mainly enrolled HCC patients with hepatitis C virus infection in Europe and America, showing a median overall survival (mOS) of 10.7 and 7.9 months, a disease control rate (DCR) of 43% and 33%, and an imaging-based median time to progression (TTP) of 5.5 and 2.8 months in the sorafenib and placebo groups, respectively, with overall survival (OS) prolonged by 44% and TTP prolonged by 73%. The ORIENTAL trial, conducted in the Asia-Pacific region in hepatitis B virus-infected patients with advanced HCC, showed an mOS of 6.5 and 4.2 months, a DCR of 35% and 16%, and an imaging-based median TTP of 2.8 and 1.4 months in the sorafenib and placebo groups, respectively, with OS prolonged by 47% and TTP prolonged by 74%.

Following the approval of sorafenib as the first-line drug for advanced HCC in 2007, many large-scale international phase III clinical trials of anti-vascular molecular targeted drugs, such as brivanib, sunitinib, and linifanib, have been successively carried out. However, none of these drugs surpassed sorafenib in efficacy for HCC, and all the trials ended in failure. Therefore, during the 10 years after the approval of sorafenib, there has been no new progress in first-line molecular targeted therapy for HCC.

Lenvatinib (E7080) is a novel tyrosine kinase inhibitor. In 2018, an open-label, multicenter, phase III non-inferiority study (REFLECT) demonstrated that lenvatinib was noninferior to sorafenib in OS (13.6 months vs. 12.3 months) and showed advantages in the secondary endpoints of progression-free survival (PFS) (7.4 vs. 3.7 months), TTP (8.9 vs. 3.7 months), objective response rate (ORR) (24.1% vs. 9.2% as per RECIST), and DCR (75.5% vs. 60.8%). Based on the REFLECT study, lenvatinib was approved by the U.S. FDA and China National Medical Products Administration as the first-line treatment of advanced HCC in September and November 2018, respectively.

At the 2020 ASCO annual meeting, a new TKI drug designed by a Chinese company reported its positive phase III results. In a first-line treatment

X. Yin · Z. Ren
ZhongShan Hospital Fudan University, Shanghai, China

S. Qin (✉)
Nanjing Jinling Hospital, Nanjing, China
e-mail: qinsk@csco.org.cn

X. Chen (ed.), *Diagnosis and Treatment of Liver Cancer in China*,
https://doi.org/10.1007/978-981-97-7969-7_19

setting, donafenib (ZGDH3, NCT02645981) had a longer OS than sorafenib: the mOS was 12.1 vs.10.3 months (HR = 0.831, P = 0.0363). Additionally, donafenib exhibited favorable safety and tolerability compared to sorafenib: drug-related AEs of grade ≥ 3 occurred in 37.5% of patients in the donafenib group versus 49.7% in the sorafenib group (P = 0.0018), and the incidence of treatment interruptions due to drug-related AEs was 30.3% in the donafenib group, compared to 42.5% in the sorafenib group (P = 0.0013). Based on the ZGDH3 study, donafenib has also been approved for the marketing application in China as the first-line treatment of advanced HCC by the China National Medical Products Administration (NMPA).

In recent years, immunotherapy-based combination therapies have become new anti-tumor strategies and have made remarkable progress. A number of clinical studies on different regimens of immunotherapy-based combination therapy for HCC are underway, and data on immunotherapy combined with chemotherapy, radiation therapy, and anti-angiogenic therapy are constantly updated, changing the pattern of comprehensive treatment of HCC. Basic research has found that molecular targeted drugs with anti-VEGF receptor effects can alleviate the immunosuppressive tumor microenvironment mediated by VEGF and promote T-lymphocyte infiltration in the tumor microenvironment, thus enhancing the efficacy of anti-PD-1/PD-L1 antibodies. In November 2019, the European Society for Medical Oncology (ESMO) Asia Congress announced the results of the IMBrave150 phase III clinical trial, in which atezolizumab combined with bevacizumab achieved an ORR of 36% and significant improvements in OS and PFS over sorafenib for unresectable HCC. This combination regimen has achieved the longest OS of 19.2 months ever seen in first-line phase III studies. Based on the IMBrave150 data, the U.S. FDA has granted the combination regimen of atezolizumab + bevacizumab as the first-line therapy in advanced or metastatic HCC.

ORIENT-32 is a randomized, open-label, multicenter phase 2/3 clinical trial evaluating the efficacy and safety of Sintilimab (PD-1 inhibitor) combined with bevacizumab bioanalog IBI305 in the first-line treatment of unresectable hepatitis B-associated HCC. The results showed the median PFS for Sintilimab with IBI305 was 4.6 and 2.8 months for sorafenib monotherapy (HR = 0.56, P < 0.001). The median OS for Sintilimab with IBI305 was not reached and 10.4 months for sorafenib monotherapy (HR = 0.57, P < 0.001). Based on the results of the ORIENT-32 study, NMPA approved the marketing application of Sintilimab combined with bevacizumab for first-line treatment in HCC in 2021.

Tremelimumab is a fully human IgG2 monoclonal antibody (mAb) that binds to CTLA-4 and results in inhibition of B7-CTLA-4-mediated downregulation of T-cell activation. Tremelimumab has previously been demonstrated to induce a significant tumor response in patients with metastatic colorectal cancer and melanoma. AstraZeneca recently released positive results from the phase 3 HIMALAYA trial. Data show that durvalumab (D, PD-L1inhibitor) combined with tremelimumab (T) significantly improved the prognosis of unresectable HCC patients versus sorafenib. In terms of the main study endpoints, STRIDE therapy (T300 + D1500 mg 1 dose followed by D Q4 weekly) significantly prolonged the median OS (16.4 vs. 13.8 months) and reduced the risk of death by 22% (HR = 0.78, P = 0.0035). The 3-year OS rates in the STRIDE group and sorafenib group were 30.7% and 20.2%, respectively. Based on the HIMALAYA trial, the STIRDE therapy will become the first first-line immunotherapy as a new treatment choice in the management of advanced HCC.

For a long time, it has been very difficult to explore the second-line therapy after sorafenib treatment failure, and many international large-scale phase III clinical studies ended in failure, including the anti-angiogenic small molecule targeted drug brivanib, the mTOR inhibitors everolimus and tivantinib (ARQ 197), and the mAb ramucirumab (REACH study). Regorafenib, a newly developed TKI drug with a molecular structure similar to sorafenib, can inhibit a variety of kinases in the tumor microenvironment and have the effects of anti-angiogenesis and anti-tumor cell proliferation. In 2016, the RESORCE clinical study of regorafenib as a second-line therapy for advanced HCC achieved positive results. A total of 567 patients with advanced HCC who have progressed on sorafenib treatment were included in the study and randomized to receive either regorafenib or placebo. The results showed that regorafenib prolonged patients' median survival (10.6 vs. 7.8 months, $P < 0.0001$) and median PFS (3.1 vs. 1. 5 months, $P < 0.0001$) compared to placebo. Based on the RESORCE study, regorafenib was successively approved in America and China in patients with advanced HCC who develop tumor progression after sorafenib treatment.

Cabozantinib is a new multi-targeted anti-tumor drug, which was initially used in the treatment of advanced medullary thyroid cancer and renal cancer. The results of the CELESTIAL clinical study in 707 patients with advanced HCC who had failed in first-line molecular targeted therapy showed an mOS of 10.2 and 8.0 months (HR = 0.76, $P = 0.005$), an mPFS of 5.2 and 1.9 months (HR = 0.44, $P < 0.001$), a tumor ORR of 4% and less than 1% ($P = 0.009$), and a DCR of 64% and 33% in the cabozantinib and placebo groups, respectively. CELESTIAL is another successful phase III clinical study of second-line treatment for advanced HCC after regorafenib, providing a new option for second-line therapy of HCC.

Patients with advanced HCC with elevated alpha-fetoprotein (AFP) have a poor prognosis. About half of HCC patients have an AFP level ≥ 400 ng/mL after sorafenib treatment failure, and effective therapeutic drugs are needed for these patients. Ramucirumab is a human IgG1 mAb, which can inhibit the activation of VEGFR2 ligands. In the previous randomized, controlled phase III clinical study (REACH), ramucirumab as a second-line therapy for patients with advanced HCC who progressed on sorafenib failed to significantly improve OS in the entire group, while a prolonged OS was observed in a subgroup with baseline AFP ≥400 ng/mL, indicated by the subgroup analysis in REACH study. The REACH-2 clinical study further evaluated the efficacy and safety of ramucirumab in patients with advanced HCC with AFP ≥400 ng/mL. The results showed that the mOS of patients treated with ramucirumab was longer than that of placebo (8.5 vs. 7.3 months, HR = 0.710, $P = 0.0199$). The mPFS was also better in the ramucirumab-treated group than in the placebo group (2.8 vs. 1.6 months, HR = 0.452, $P < 0.001$). REACH-2 is the first phase III clinical study with positive results in patients with HCC screened by tumor marker, bringing new options for second-line therapy of patients with elevated baseline AFP.

Apatinib, a VEGFR-2 inhibitor, has been investigated as second-line therapy in Chinese advanced HCC patients through a phase III study AHELP, which showed significantly longer OS and PFS compared to placebo and exhibited a tolerable safety profile. The mOS was 8.7 versus 6.8 months (HR = 0.785, $P = 0.0476$), the mPFS was 4.5 versus 1.9 months (HR = 0.471, $P < 0.001$), the ORR was 10.7% versus 1.5% per RECIST v1.1, and no new safety signals were noted. According to the AHELP study, Apatinib was approved for the marketing application in the treatment of advanced HCC as a second-line molecular targeted drug by NMPA.

Suggested Reading

1. Lovet JM, Ricci S, Mazzaferro V, et al. Sorafenib in advanced hepatocellular carcinoma. N Engl J Med. 2008;359:378–90.
2. Cheng AL, Kang YK, Chen Z, et al. Efficacy and safety of Sorafenib in patients in the Asia-Pacific region with advanced hepatocellular carcinoma:a phase III randomised, double-blind, placebo-controlled trial. Lancet Oncol. 2009;10:25–34.
3. Kudo M, Finn RS, Qin S, et al. Lenvatinib versus sorafenib in first line treatment of patients with unresectable hepatocellular carcinoma: a randomised phase 3 non-inferiority trial. Lancet. 2018;391:1163–73.
4. Qin S, Bi F, Gu S, et al. Donafenib versus Sorafenib in first-line treatment of Unresectable or metastatic hepatocellular carcinoma: a randomized, open-label, parallel-controlled phase II-III trial. J Clin Oncol. 2021;39(27):3002–11.
5. Finn RS, Qin S, Ikeda M, et al. Atezolizumab plus bevacizumab in unresectable hepatocellular carcinoma. N Engl J Med. 2020;382(20):1894–905.

6. Ren Z, Xu J, Bai Y, et al. ORIENT-32 study group. Sintilimab plus a bevacizumab biosimilar (IBI305) versus sorafenib in unresectable hepatocellular carcinoma (ORIENT-32): a randomised, open-label, phase 2-3 study. Lancet Oncol. 2021;22(7):977–90.
7. Chambers CA, Kuhns MS, Egen JG, Allison JP. CTLA-4-mediated inhibition in regulation of T cell responses: mechanismsand manipulation in tumor immunotherapy. Annu Rev Immunol. 2001;19:565–94.
8. Song X, Kelley RK, Khan A, et al. Exposure-response (E-R) efficacy and safety (E-S) analyses of tremelimumab as monotherapy or in combination with durvalumab in patients (pts) with unresectable hepatocellular carcinoma (uHCC). J Clin Oncol. 2021;39:abstr 313.
9. Zhu AX, Park JO, Ryoo BY, et al. Ramucimmab versus placebo as second line treatment in patients with advanced hepatocellular carcinoma following first-line therapy with sorafenib(REACH): a randomised, double-blind, multicentre, phase 3 trial. Lancet Oncol. 2015;16:859–70.
10. Bruix J, Qin S, Merle P, et al. Regorafenib for patients with hepatocellular carcinoma who progressed on sorafenib treatment(RESORCE): a randomised, double-blind, placebocontrolled, phase 3 trial. Lancet. 2017;389:56–66.
11. Abou-Alfa GK, Meyer T, Cheng AL, et al. Cabozantinib in patients with advanced and progressing hepatocellular carcinoma. N Engl J Med. 2018;379:54–63.
12. Zhu AX, Kang YK, Yen CJ, et al. Ramucirumab after sorafenib in patients with advanced hepatocellular carcinoma and increased α-fetoprotein concentrations(REACH-2): a randomised,double-blind,placebo-controlled,phase 3 trial. Lancet Oncol. 2019;20:282–96.
13. Qin S, Li Q, Gu S, et al. Apatinib as second-line or later therapy in patients with advanced hepatocellular carcinoma (AHELP): amulticentre, double-blind, randomised, placebo-controlled, phase 3 trial. Lancet Gastroenterol Hepatol. 2021;6(7):559–68.

Sequential Therapy and Whole-Course Management of Molecular Targeted Therapy for Liver Cancer

20

Xin Yin, Zhenggang Ren, and Shukui Qin

According to the current international authoritative guidelines for hepatocellular carcinoma (HCC), the approved first-line therapy drugs include atezolizumab plus bevacizumab, sorafenib, and lenvatinib, while there are more options for second-line molecular targeted drugs, including regorafenib, cabozantinib, and ramucirumab. In the sequential therapy of advanced HCC with first-line and second-line drugs, the timing of treatment switch is very important. Generally, switching to a second-line targeted therapy drug is required for patients with progression on first-line drug therapy. However, the specific causes and patterns of disease progression should also be analyzed specifically. If the patient has disease progression due to insufficient dose caused by side effects of the first-line drug, dose recovery should be considered after the side effects are alleviated or tolerated, rather than therapy switching. Similarly, the pattern of progression on first-line therapy also influences the choice of subsequent therapy. If rapid disease progression occurs while the patient is receiving an adequate dose of first-line therapy drug, it should be switched to second-line drugs as soon as possible. However, if the tumor progresses slowly, it can be considered that the first-line drug is still partially effective and may be used in combination with an immune checkpoint inhibitor to improve the overall efficacy.

To date, multiple second-line molecular targeted drugs after progression on sorafenib have been approved. The median overall survival (mOS) of patients with advanced, unresectable HCC who received sequential treatment with sorafenib followed by regorafenib reached 26 months. Second-line therapy with cabozantinib in advanced HCC after progression on sorafenib could improve OS by 2.2 months (CELESTIAL study). Sequential treatment with second-line ramucirumab following sorafenib could improve the OS of HCC patients with alpha-fetoprotein (AFP) ≥400 ng/mL by 1.2 months (REACH-2 study). Sequential treatment with second-line apatinib after sorafenib failure can obtain 4.5 months of progression-free survival (PFS) and 8.7 months of OS (AHELP study). In second-line immunotherapy, the disease control rate (DCR) was over 50% and the mOS was up to 15.6 months (CheckMate-040) in patients treated with nivolumab after progression on sorafenib, with no difference between the Asian population and the global population. Pembrolizumab showed a DCR of 62% and an OS of 12.9 months in patients who had previously failed to respond to sorafenib therapy

X. Yin · Z. Ren
ZhongShan Hospital Fudan University, Shanghai, China

S. Qin (✉)
Nanjing Jinling Hospital, Nanjing, China
e-mail: qinsk@csco.org.cn

X. Chen (ed.), *Diagnosis and Treatment of Liver Cancer in China*,
https://doi.org/10.1007/978-981-97-7969-7_20

(Keynote 224 study). At the 2019 American Society of Clinical Oncology Annual Meeting, Taiwanese scholars reported a single-center study suggesting that second-line treatment with lenvatinib was also effective in HCC patients who progressed on sorafenib. This study included 70 patients with HCC admitted from 2017 to 2018, 65.7% of whom had received sorafenib followed by oral lenvatinib (10 mg/day) as second-line treatment after progression on sorafenib, the results of which showed a median PFS of 5.3 months and an OS of 8.5 months in patients. In 2019, a Japanese multicenter study retrospectively analyzed the results of 131 cases with unresectable advanced HCC treated with lenvatinib from 15 centers. The study found that the tumor objective response rate of lenvatinib was 40% in first-line therapy and 41% in second-line therapy, while the DCR was basically the same in first- and second-line therapies. The actual study data showed that the patients could also benefit from lenvatinib whether it is used as first- or second-line therapy.

Since there is no standard third-line targeted therapy drug for HCC, treatment options for patients failing second-line therapy have become a challenge in the systemic treatment of HCC. In clinical practice, multiple strategies can be chosen based on patients' performance status and liver function reserve, for instance, the combined use of vascular targeted therapy with immunotherapy, immunotherapy combined with chemotherapy, combined use of immune checkpoint inhibitors, and so on. According to the tumor progression during systemic therapy, corresponding local regional therapy also can be given, such as molecular targeted therapy combined with Trans-arterial Chemo-Embolization (TACE) or hepatic arterial infusion chemotherapy, immunotherapy combined with local ablation therapy, or radiation therapy. Actually, the treatment modality of advanced HCC differs from other late-stage solid tumors. Patients with HCC who have developed distant metastasis can be treated by local regional therapies for liver lesions on the basis of systemic therapy. If there is no progression of extrahepatic lesions but only progression of intrahepatic lesions, intrahepatic local treatments should be carried out first. The implementation of local regional therapy should be adjusted if extensive intrahepatic progression occurs.

Management of side effects of molecular targeted therapy is an important part of the whole-course management for advanced HCC. Molecular targeted therapy often causes fatigue, diarrhea, hypertension, rash, hand-foot syndrome, and so on. It is quite important to control the side effects to the maximum extent and achieve optimal clinical treatment effects to improve the prognosis of patients. Although side effects of molecular targeted therapies vary in the type, frequency, and severity of reactions, they usually occur at the early stage of medication and do not worsen with the continuation of treatment. Most patients have mild side effects (Grade 1/2), which can be effectively controlled by conventional methods without interruption of treatment. The side effects associated with molecular targeted drugs can be relieved by actively communicating with patients about possible side effects and taking preventive measures in advance.

With the emergence of molecular targeted therapy and immunotherapy, systemic therapy for HCC has entered a diversified and multimodality era, and the survival of patients with advanced HCC has been prolonged significantly. The treatment modality of advanced HCC should also involve chronic liver disease management. Only by deepening the concept of whole-course management of HCC, fully evaluating the general situation of patients, underlying liver disease, and biological characteristics of the tumor and based on which, formulating a reasonable and complete treatment regimen, dynamically evaluating the treatment response of patients, timely revising and constantly improving the treatment regimen, and carrying out multidisciplinary and individualized treatment can achieve a better survival outcome for HCC patients.

Suggested Reading

1. Finn RS, Qin S, Ikeda M, et al. Atezolizumab plus bevacizumab in unresectable hepatocellular carcinoma. N Engl J Med. 2020;382(20):1894–905.

2. Lovet JM, Ricci S, Mazzaferro V, et al. Sorafenib in advanced hepatocellular carcinoma. N Engl J Med. 2008;359:378–90.
3. Kudo M, Finn RS, Qin S, et al. Lenvatinib versus sorafenib in first line treatment of patients with unresectable hepatocellular carcinoma: a randomised phase 3 non-inferiority trial. Lancet. 2018;391(10126):1163–73.
4. Bruix J, Qin S, Merle P, et al. Regorafenib for patients with hepatocellular carcinoma who progressed on sorafenib treatment (RESORCE): a randomised, double-blind, placebocontrolled, phase 3 trial. Lancet. 2017;389:56–66.
5. Abou-Alfa GK, Meyer T, Cheng AL, et al. Cabozantinib in patients with advanced and progressing hepatocellular carcinoma. N Engl J Med. 2018;379:54–63.
6. Zhu AX, Kang YK, Yen CJ, et al. Ramucirumab after sorafenib in patients with advanced hepatocellular carcinoma and increased α-fetoprotein concentrations (REACH-2): a randomised, double-blind, placebo-controlled, phase 3 trial. Lancet Oncol. 2019;20:282–96.
7. Qin S, Li Q, Gu S, et al. Apatinib as second-line or later therapy in patients with advanced hepatocellular carcinoma (AHELP): a multicentre, double-blind, randomised, placebo-controlled, phase 3 trial. Lancet Gastroenterol Hepatol. 2021;6(7):559–68.
8. El-Khoueiry AB, Sangro B, Yau T, et al. Nivolumab in patients with advanced hepatocellular carcinoma (CheckMate 040): an open-label, non-comparative, phase 1/2 dose escalation and expansion trial. Lancet. 2017;389(10088):2492–502.
9. Finn RS, Ryoo BY, Merle P. Pembrolizumab as second-line therapy in patients with advanced hepatocellular carcinoma in keynote-240: a randomized, double-blind, phase III trial. J Clin Oncol. 2020;38(3):193–202.

Part VI

Radiation Therapy for Liver Cancer

Hepatocellular carcinoma (HCC) has become a serious life-threatening disease in China. For patients with unresectable HCC, the available treatments include Trans-arterial Chemo-Embolization (TACE), radiofrequency ablation (RFA), radiation therapy, systemic therapy, and so on. Radiation therapy is a local regional treatment using radiation to treat cancer, which is divided into external beam radiation therapy and internal radiation therapy. External beam radiation therapy uses a machine to generate radiation, which passes through the body surface and focuses on the tumor. Internal radiation therapy uses a radioisotope, which is implanted or enters into the tumor through the duct and generates particle rays to kill the tumor cells. External beam radiation therapy equipment includes a linear accelerator that produces high-energy X-ray, Gamma Knife, Cyberknife, tomotherapy (TOMO) system, proton and heavy ion accelerator, and so on. Internal radiation therapy includes iodine-131 particles and iodine-125 particles, isotope-labeled monoclonal antibodies, yttrium-90 glass microspheres, and so on. With the continuous progress of radiation therapy equipment, image-guided radiation therapy (IGRT) has been popularized, and the effect of radiation therapy for HCC has been greatly improved. It has become one of the important treatment choices for unresectable HCC.

21 Radiation Therapy for Liver Cancer

Xin Yin, Jing Sun, and Zhenggang Ren

Radiation therapy induces the death of tumor cells directly or indirectly through radiation. The radiation used for treatment includes photon and particle beams, which can destroy the double helix structure of tumor cell DNA, so that the cells cannot replicate and proliferate, thus achieving the therapeutic effects. Since the discovery of radiation 100 years ago, concretely, Roentgen reported the discovery of X-ray in 1895 and Marie Curie reported the discovery of radium in 1896, their biological effects were soon recognized and gradually applied to the treatment of some superficial tumors. The radiation therapy techniques for hepatocellular carcinoma have made great progress from initial whole liver radiation therapy and moving strip whole liver radiation therapy to three-dimensional conformal radiation therapy (3D-CRT) and intensity-modulated radiation therapy (IMRT), to current IGRT including stereotactic body radiation therapy (SBRT).

In 1956, Ariel reported the treatment of metastatic or primary liver cancer with a cobalt-60 machine. Due to the limitation of the irradiation technique, whole-liver radiation therapy was generally adopted at that time. However, the radiation dose for radical treatment of hepatocellular carcinoma should reach 60 Gy and above, which is the radiation dose for conventional fractionation, while the tolerance dose for whole liver irradiation is only 30 Gy. The normal liver is exposed to a large volume of radiation during the treatment, which not only fails to achieve the radical dose required to kill tumor cells but also easily causes radiation-induced liver injury. Therefore, radiation therapy for HCC was rarely applied.

In the early 1970s, radiation therapists began to treat HCC with the moving strip technique for whole liver irradiation. Moving strip irradiation controls the whole liver irradiation dose to a value for conventional fractionation equivalent to 30 Gy, which improves the tolerance of the liver to radiation therapy to some extent. Chinese Professor Erxin YU, et al. used moving strip radiation therapy combined with spleen-strengthening and Qi-regulating traditional Chinese medicine to treat HCC and retrospectively analyzed and reported 228 patients with HCC, showing 1-, 3-, and 5-year survival rates of 59%, 34%, and 25%. However, some scholars pointed out that the moving strip irradiation technique has serious defects in terms of radiobiology, whether in theory or practice. For example, both the tumor and normal liver tissue are irradiated due to poor selectivity; fractionated irradiation field on tumor tissue makes radiation dose distribution within the tumor uneven at the same time; radiation-induced damage in the tumor is also repaired as the normal liver tissue is repaired; the treatment

X. Yin · J. Sun · Z. Ren (✉)
ZhongShan Hospital Fudan University, Shanghai, China

X. Chen (ed.), *Diagnosis and Treatment of Liver Cancer in China*,
https://doi.org/10.1007/978-981-97-7969-7_21

cycle is long and the dose calculation is relatively complicated. Since the popularization of imaging techniques, the moving strip technique for whole liver irradiation has been gradually replaced by more advanced radiation therapy techniques such as 3D-CRT and IMRT.

Before the 1990s, radiation therapy for HCC showed poor efficacy and great damage to the liver due to the limitation of conventional two-dimensional radiation therapy techniques. As a result, most oncologists, including radiation therapists, have come to a pessimistic conclusion that radiation therapy is not suitable for HCC, and radiation therapy for HCC was only carried out in a few hospitals. After the mid-1990s, with the development and improvement of imaging techniques, the safety and efficacy of radiation therapy in patients with HCC have been greatly improved. For example, the application of 3D-CRT, IMRT, and IGRT has provided new opportunities for HCC treatment.

3D-CRT enables the reconstruction of three-dimensional structures by using computed tomography (CT) images. When co-planar or non-coplanar high-energy radiation beams are incident, the dose is adjusted according to the size and morphology of the tumor (by making a lead shielding or applying multi-leaf grating in the accelerator), so that the shape of the radiation field is the same as the geometric projection shape of the target volume in that direction. 3D-CRT has been popularized in most grass-roots radiation therapy units in China. Compared with two-dimensional radiation therapy, 3D-CRT can greatly reduce the radiation dose to normal tissues and increase the radiation dose to the tumor region, thus reducing the incidence of side effects and improving the efficacy of treatment.

IMRT, based on 3D-CRT, optimizes the weight of each beam in the radiation field so that the distribution of the high-dose region is consistent with the shape of the target volume in three dimensions, and the radiation dose distribution is reduced in normal tissues outside the target volume. Therefore, it can better protect the adjacent important tissues and organs and treat irregularly shaped tumors. IMRT has become the mainstream radiation therapy technique nowadays.

IGRT is developed based on IMRT with the addition of an image acquisition system to the radiation therapy equipment. Before each radiation treatment, the image of the patient's tumor layer is collected and compared with the image generated by the radiation treatment planning system. Only when the two images match accurately, radiation treatment will be applied, which greatly reduces the set-up error between treatments and further improves the precision of radiation therapy.

SBRT for HCC is an image-guided high-precision radiation therapy, with the characteristics of three-dimensionality, beam array focus, and fewer fractions. Compared with conventional radiation therapy techniques, SBRT has a higher single dose and fewer fractions, which can enable a higher bioequivalent dose to the tumor, and small field beam array focus can make the dose outside the target volume decrease rapidly, which can produce the effect of focal destruction to the tumor while minimizing the damage to normal tissues. SBRT has become the main development direction of radiation therapy for HCC due to shortened overall treatment time and increased patient compliance. In terms of clinical efficacy, SBRT is characterized by high local control rates for malignant tumors and relatively mild side effects. It has been reported that SBRT can be used as an alternative therapy for small HCC, as a bridging therapy before liver transplantation, or in combination with Trans-arterial Chemo-Embolization (TACE) for intrahepatic or extrahepatic lesions of some patients with unresectable HCC.

Suggested Reading

1. Ariel IM. The treatment of primary and metastatic cancer of the liver. Surgery. 1956;39(1):70–91.
2. Yu EX. A review of comprehensive radiation therapies for liver cancer. J Pract Oncol. 1997;12(2):57–8.
3. Li B, Yu J, Wang L, et al. Study of local three-dimensional conformal radiotherapy combined with transcatheter arterial chemoembolization for patients with stage III hepatocellular carcinoma. Am J Clin Oncol. 2003;26:e92.
4. Choi SH, Seong J. Strategic application of radiotherapy for hepatocellular carcinoma. Clin Mol Hepatol. 2018;24:114–34.

5. Sanuki N, Takeda A, Oku Y, et al. Stereotactic body radiotherapy for small hepatocellular carcinoma: a retrospective outcome analysis in 185 patients. Acta Oncol. 2014;53:399–404.
6. Li XL, Guo WX, Hong XD, et al. Efficacy of the treatment of transarterial chemoembolization combined with radiotherapy for hepatocellular carcinoma with portal vein tumor thrombus: a propensity score analysis. Hepatol Res. 2016;46:1088–98.
7. Moore A, Cohen-Naftaly M, Tobar A, et al. Stereotactic body radiation therapy(SBRT)for definitive treatment and as a bridge to liver transplantation in early stage inoperable hepatocellular carcinoma. Radiat Oncol. 2017;12:163.

22 Clinical Application of External Beam Radiation Therapy for Liver Cancer

Xin Yin, Jing Sun, and Zhenggang Ren

In recent years, with the progress of science and technology, radiation therapy techniques have also made rapid development and entered a new era of precise radiation therapy with precise positioning, precise planning, and precise implementation. Precise radiation therapy featured by IGRT significantly improves the efficacy of treating malignant tumors, greatly reduces the complications of normal tissues, prolongs the survival of patients with tumors, and improves the quality of survival.

Takahashi, a Japanese professor, first proposed the concept of conformal therapy in the 1960s. In the late 1990s, 3D-CRT was initially applied to patients with HCC and gradually became the mainstream technique of external beam radiation therapy for HCC. Professor Brahme, a Swedish radiation physicist, subsequently proposed the concept of intensity modulation. The IMRT equipment and technique enable relatively uniform doses at any point in the target volume by modulating the intensity of radiation in the target volume. However, due to the respiratory motion of the liver, there are still many uncertainties in the precision of intensity-modulated conformal radiation therapy for HCC, which needs to be combined with an image guidance technique and respiratory gating device to ensure the precision of treatment.

X. Yin · J. Sun · Z. Ren (✉)
ZhongShan Hospital Fudan University, Shanghai, China

SBRT for HCC uses special equipment and devices to focus many narrow radiation beams on the tumor target volume to deliver a relatively large dose of radiation, so that the tumor region can receive a sufficiently high treatment dose, resulting in local necrosis of the tumor with a significant increase in local control rate, and minimized damage to normal tissues, thus achieving the effect of radioactive ablation. To realize the SBRT technique, there must be guidance by four-dimensional imaging equipment and precise patient positioning fixation technique. Currently, many radiation therapy equipment including C-arm linear accelerators with image guidance, Cyberknife, and TOMO system can meet such requirements. SBRT is suitable for smaller lesions in the treatment of solid tumors and is currently used mainly for small HCC that are not suitable for surgical resection or ablation.

TOMO system enables high-precision radiation therapy for cancers through spiral CT scanning, image guidance function, and spiral irradiation. Precise tumor positioning and treatment are achieved by correcting the displacement of tumor target volume based on pre-treatment or on-treatment CT image data under real-time monitoring. Additionally, since the TOMO system itself is mounted on the spiral CT frame, the imaging source of CT image navigation is exactly the same as the 6 MV ray therapy source, and there is no deviation between the imaging isocenter and the therapy isocenter of the conventional accelerator.

X. Chen (ed.), *Diagnosis and Treatment of Liver Cancer in China*,
https://doi.org/10.1007/978-981-97-7969-7_22

Gamma Knife is also known as a gamma-ray stereotactic body therapy system. Gamma Knife enables precise SBRT for tumors by geometrically focusing high-dose gamma rays on tumor target volume to distribute high-dose radiation in the focal area and low-dose radiation in adjacent normal tissues, which can not only maximize the anti-tumor effect but also protect adjacent normal tissues, thus reducing the harm of radiation therapy and achieving the purpose of optimizing the short-term treatment effect. Gamma Knife was initially applied to treat single or multiple intracranial metastases (no more than 3) less than 3 cm in diameter. Due to the influence of respiratory motion of the liver and the lack of an image guidance system and respiratory tracking system in Gamma Knife, there is uncertainty during the whole course of radiation therapy for HCC. Nevertheless, there have been reports of the use of Gamma Knife to treat patients with unresectable small HCC or patients who refused to receive surgery. Zhixiong LONG et al. treated 20 cases of primary small HCC with body Gamma Knife, showing good efficacy with 1-, 3-, and 5-year survival rates of 95%, 68%, and 53%, respectively. Peng CAI et al. treated 52 cases of HCC patients with 60 lesions using Gamma Knife, showing an overall effective rate (PR + CR + SD) of 93.3%, a rate of decline in alpha-fetoprotein (AFP) of 82.7%, and a survival rate at 6 months or more of 90.4%, as well as significantly improved survival quality. However, current clinical studies are mostly limited to small sample, uncontrolled retrospective studies, which need to be confirmed by further prospective controlled studies.

There is a growing number of reports of image-guided SBRT for the treatment of small HCC. Recently, Kim et al. reviewed and compared multicenter studies on the treatment of HCC by SBRT and ablation, showing that SBRT had a better local tumor control rate than RFA, with a 3-year local recurrence rate of 21% and 28% ($P < 0.001$), respectively. A study on early-stage HCC (with diameter less than 3 cm and number of lesions less than 3) treated by a radiation therapy dose of 35–45 Gy/5–15 Fx showed a similar survival benefit with a 3-year overall survival rate of 70.4% for SBRT versus 69.1% for radiofrequency therapy. The 3-year local recurrence rates of tumors were 5.3% and 12.9%, respectively. Thus, SBRT was superior to radiofrequency therapy in local lesion control.

The application of proton and heavy ion in radiation therapy for HCC is still at an exploratory stage. The radiation of conventional radiation therapy comes from photon (e.g., high-energy X-ray and ^{60}Co ray), and the energy will be greatly attenuated before reaching the tumor target volume through human tissues, which not only affects the dose distribution in the tumor target volume but also causes relatively great radiation damage to surrounding tissues. In theory, little energy is released when proton and heavy ion radiation enter the human body, and when they reach the tumor target volume, all the energy should be released, forming a "Bragg peak," which enables the tumor target volume to receive a larger radiation dose, while the damage to surrounding tissues is rapidly reduced to a minimum. Heavy ion radiation therapy uses particle radiation (usually carbon ions) with higher energy than proton, which can effectively kill hypoxic or radiation therapy-resistant tumor cells, and has a killing effect on tumor cells in each phase of the cell cycle, and therefore has advantages over proton beam. Komatsu S et al. investigated the efficacy and safety in 343 patients with HCC treated with proton (242 patients) or heavy ion (101 patients). The results showed that patients treated with proton had a high local control rate of 90.8% and a 5-year survival rate of 38.2%, while patients treated with heavy ion had a local control rate of 93% and a 5-year survival rate of 36.3%, and there were no Grade 3 or 4 toxic effects or above.

Suggested Reading

1. Chino F, Stephens SJ, Choi S, et al. The role of external beam radiotherapy in the treatment of hepatocellular cancer. Cancer. 2018;124:3476–89.
2. Feng M, Suresh K, Schipper MJ, et al. Individualized adaptive stereotactic body radiotherapy for liver tumors in patients at high risk for liver damage. JAMA Oncol. 2018;4:40–7.

3. Li P, Xia T, Chang D. γ-Ray stereotactic body radiation therapy for patients with primary hepatic carcinoma of stage I/II. Int J Radiat Oncol Biol Phys. 2012;84:334–5.
4. Long ZX, Wang JG, Li WD, et al. A study on efficacy of body Gamma Knife in treating primary small hepatocellular carcinoma. Chin J Radiat Oncol. 2008;17(5):348–9.
5. Cai P, Sun JS, Yang SY. A study on short-term efficacy of whole-body Gamma Knife in 52 patients with primary liver cancer. Chin J Clin Oncol Rehab. 2002;9(5):97.
6. Zeng ZC, Seong J, Yoon SM, et al. Consensus on stereotactic body radiation therapy for small-sized hepatocellular carcinoma at the 7th Asia-Pacific primary liver cancer expert meeting. Liver Cancer. 2017;6:264–74.
7. Kim N, Cheng J, Jung I, et al. Stereotactic body radiation therapy vs. radiofrequency ablation in Asian patients with hepatocellular carcinoma. J Hepatol. 2020;73(1):121–9.
8. Hara K, Takeda A, Tsurugai Y, et al. Radiotherapy for hepatocellular carcinoma results in comparable survival to radiofrequency ablation: a propensity score analysis. Hepatology. 2019;69:2533–45.
9. Komatsu S, Fukumoto T, Demizu Y, et al. Clinical results and risk factors of proton and carbon ion therapy for hepatocellular carcinoma. Cancer. 2011;117:4890–904.

23 Clinical Application of External Beam Radiation Therapy in the Local Treatment of Liver Cancer

Xin Yin, Jing Sun, and Zhenggang Ren

In recent years, thanks to the development of radiation therapy techniques and the update of radiation therapy equipment, external beam radiation therapy has been applied in all stages of hepatocellular carcinoma (HCC). In 2009, external beam radiation therapy was recommended as one of the treatment options for HCC by the National Comprehensive Cancer Network (NCCN) Guidelines. The 2018 NCCN Guidelines clearly state that three-dimensional conformal radiation therapy, intensity-modulated radiation therapy, or stereotactic body radiation therapy (SBRT) are all applicable regardless of the location of the tumor. The 2019 NCCN Guidelines further recommend image-guided radiation therapy in the treatment of HCC. Chinese Society of Clinical Oncology Guidelines for the Diagnosis and Treatment of Primary Liver Cancer also recommend SBRT for the treatment of early-stage small HCC, and local radiation therapy combined with TACE for the treatment of intermediate stage HCC and extrahepatic metastases, according to different levels of evidence.

23.1 Consolidating the Treatment Effect of Interventional Therapy for Intrahepatic Tumor

Domestic retrospective data showed that the 2- and 3-year survival rates of TACE combined with external beam radiation therapy compared with TACE treatment alone were 42.3% and 26.5% and 24.0% and 11.1% ($P = 0.026$), respectively. A retrospective study in South Korea showed that the 2-year survival rates of TACE combined with external beam radiation therapy compared with TACE alone were 36.8% and 14.3% ($P = 0.001$), respectively. According to a meta-analysis study by Huo et al., interventional therapy combined with external beam radiation therapy compared with interventional therapy alone can significantly improve the overall survival (OS) of patients with intermediate or advanced stage HCC. However, the evidence obtained so far mainly comes from exploratory retrospective studies, which need to be further confirmed by prospective randomized controlled studies.

X. Yin · J. Sun · Z. Ren (✉)
ZhongShan Hospital Fudan University,
Shanghai, China

X. Chen (ed.), *Diagnosis and Treatment of Liver Cancer in China*,
https://doi.org/10.1007/978-981-97-7969-7_23

23.2 External Beam Radiation Therapy for HCC with Portal Vein/Inferior Vena Cava Tumor Thrombus

In a randomized controlled study conducted in South Korea, patients with tumor thrombus were randomly divided into the TACE+RT group and the sorafenib group. In the TACE+RT group, intrahepatic lesions were treated by TACE, while tumor thrombus and adjacent intrahepatic lesions (2 cm) were treated by radiation therapy at the dose of 45 Gy and 2.5–3 Gy/Fx. The results showed that the median OS (mOS) and median progression-free survival (mPFS) were significantly longer in the TACE+RT group than in the sorafenib group (mPFS: 30.0 weeks vs. 11.3 weeks, $P < 0.001$; mOS: 55.0 weeks vs. 43 weeks, $P = 0.04$). In a multicenter randomized controlled study by Shuqun CHENG and his team from Shanghai Eastern Hepatobiliary Surgical Hospital, patients with resectable HCC combined with portal vein tumor thrombus were randomly divided into two groups: preoperative neoadjuvant radiotherapy group (82 patients) and surgical resection-alone group (82 patients), with a preoperative radiotherapy dose of 18 Gy/6 Fx for tumor and portal vein tumor thrombus, and the surgery was performed about 4 weeks after radiation therapy. The results showed that the 1- and 2-year OS rates were significantly higher in the preoperative radiotherapy group (75.2%, 27.4%) than those in the surgical resection-alone group (43.1%, 9.4%).

23.3 Radiation Therapy for Early-Stage HCC

The treatment options for early-stage HCC mainly include surgery, liver transplantation, and radiofrequency ablation (RFA). When patients are not suitable for or refuse invasive surgery or RFA due to certain reasons, SBRT will be an alternative therapy. Recently, Kim et al. published a multicenter retrospective matching analysis method comparing the treatment effect of SBRT or RF for small HCC. The results showed that SBRT had a better local tumor control rate than RFA, with 3-year local recurrence rates of 21% and 28%, respectively. Researchers from the U.S. Mayo Clinic compared the efficacy of RFA and SBRT in non-surgical patients with TNM stage I or II HCC through propensity score matching analysis based on the National Cancer Database data. The results showed that the 5-year overall survival rates was 29.8% (95% confidence interval (CI): 24.5–35.3%) in the RFA group and 19.3% (95% CI: 13.5–25.9%, $P < 0.001$) in the SBRT group. A meta-analysis study by Lee et al. in South Korea compared the efficacy of RFA and SBRT for HCC, including a total of 11 studies and involving 2238 patients. The results showed that the SBRT group had a higher 2-year local tumor control rate (83.8%, 95% CI: 77.6–88.4%) than the RFA group (71.8%, 95% CI: 61.5–80.2%, $P = 0.024$). However, in terms of overall survival, patients in the RFA group had a better survival benefit, and the risk of death was 1.43 times higher in the SBRT group than in the RFA group (HR = 1.43, 95% CI: 1.05–1.95, $P = 0.023$). SBRT has shown a good local control rate and potential survival improvement in treating small HCC. However, most of the current studies have limited follow-up time and lack long-term survival data, and further prospective multicenter controlled studies are required to confirm the long-term efficacy.

23.4 External Beam Radiation Therapy as the Dominant Therapy for Extrahepatic Metastases

Extrahepatic metastases of HCC include metastases to lymph nodes, lung, bone, adrenal, and brain. In case of these conditions, comprehensive multidisciplinary treatment, including radiation therapy, is needed. A retrospective study conducted by Zhaochong ZENG et al. randomizedly allocated HCC patients with lymph node metastasis into two groups receiving external beam radiation therapy and not receiving external ream radiation therapy, showing a mOS of 9.4 months in the group receiving external beam radiation therapy and 3.3 months in the group not receiving radiation therapy. Both univariate and multivariate analyses showed significant survival differences ($P < 0.001$). Other studies have also shown that external beam radiation therapy is safe and effective for lymph node metastasis in HCC patients, which can achieve local control and symptom relief for metastatic tumors, thus obtaining survival benefits.

In conclusion, external beam radiation therapy for HCC plays an important role in the management of early, intermediate, and advanced HCC. For patients with small HCC not suitable for surgical resection or RFA, SBRT can be used as an alternative therapy. For patients with focal intrahepatic lesions, external beam radiation therapy can be supplementary to interventional therapy to improve the local control of intrahepatic tumors. Such combination therapies still warrant further exploration and research, especially for patients with portal vein tumor thrombus. For patients with advanced stage HCC with extrahepatic metastases (metastases to lymph nodes, bone, adrenal, lung, brain, etc.), external beam radiation therapy can effectively relieve symptoms or complications caused by local infiltration or compression of metastatic lesions and improve patients' survival quality. Although the evidence level for external beam radiation therapy in different stages of HCC is not very high so far, the potential survival benefits and improvement of quality of life for patients undergoing radiation therapy should be fully considered, and researchers should be encouraged to conduct high-level prospective clinical studies.

Suggested Reading

1. NCCN, National Comprehensive Cancer Network. NCCN clinical practice guidelines in oncology: hepatobiliary cancers (Version 4. 2018-October 22, 2018) [EB/OL]. https://www.nccn.org/.
2. Zeng ZC, Tang ZY, Fan J, et al. A comparison of chemoembolization combination with and without radiotherapy for unresectable hepatocellular carcinoma. Cancer J. 2004;10:307–16.
3. Shim SJ, Seong J, Han KH, et al. Local radiotherapy as a complement to incomplete transcatheter arterial chemoembolization in locally advanced hepatocellular carcinoma. Liver Int. 2005;25:1189–96.
4. Huo YR, Eslick GD. Transcatheter arterial chemoembolization plus radiotherapy compared with chemoembolization alone for hepatocellular carcinoma: a systematic review and meta-analysis. JAMA Oncol. 2015;1(6):756–65.
5. Yoon SM, Ryoo BY, Lee SJ, et al. Efficacy and safety of transarterial chemoembolization plus external beam radiotherapy vs sorafenib in hepatocellular carcinoma with macroscopic vascular invasion: a randomized clinical trial. JAMA Oncol. 2018;4:661–9.
6. Wei XB, Jiang YB, Zhang XP, et al. Neoadjuvant three-dimensional conformal radiotherapy for resectable hepatocellular carcinoma with portal vein tumor thrombus: a randomized, open-label, multicenter controlled study. J Clin Oncol. 2019;37:2141–51.
7. Kim N, Cheng J, Jung I, et al. Stereotactic body radiation therapy vs. radiofrequency ablation in Asian patients with hepatocellular carcinoma. J Hepatol. 2020;73(1):121–9.
8. Rajyagur U, Devalkumar J, Borger T, et al. Radiofrequency ablation versus stereotactic body radiotherapy for localized hepatocellular carcinoma in nonsurgically managed patients: analysis of the national cancer database. J Clin Oncol. 2018;36:600–8.
9. Lee J, Shin IS, Yoon WS, et al. Comparisons between radiofrequency ablation and stereotactic body radiotherapy for liver malignancies: meta-analyses and a systematic review. Radiother Oncol. 2020;145:63–70.
10. Zeng ZC, Tang ZY, Qin LX, et al. Consideration of the role of radiotherapy for lymph node metastases in patients with HCC-A retrospective analysis for prognostic factors from 125 patients. Int J Radiat Oncol Boil Phys. 2005;63:1067–76.
11. Kim K, Chie EK, Kim W, et al. Absence of symptom and intact liver function are positive prognosticators for patients undergoing radiotherapy for lymph node metastasis from hepatocellular carcinoma. Int J Radiat Oncol Biol Phys. 2010;78:729–34.
12. Yamashita H, Nakagawa K, Shiraishi K, et al. Radiotherapy for lymph node metastases in patients with hepatocellular carcinoma: retrospective study. J Gastroenterol Hepatol. 2007;22:523–7.
13. Zhou LY, Zeng ZC, Fan J, et al. Radiotherapy treatment of adrenal gland metastases from hepatocellular carcinoma: clinical features and prognostic factors. BMC Cancer. 2014;14:878.
14. He J, Zeng ZC, Tang ZY, et al. Clinical features and prognostic factors in patients with bone metastases from hepatocellular carcinoma receiving external-beam radiotherapy. Cancer. 2009;115:2710–20.
15. Jiang W, Zeng ZC, Zhang JY, et al. Palliative radiation therapy for pulmonary metastases from hepatocellular carcinoma. Clin Exp Metastasis. 2012;29:197–205.
16. Park Y, Kim KS, Kim K, et al. Nomogram prediction of survival in patients with brain metastases from hepatocellular carcinoma treated with whole-brain radiotherapy: a multicenter retrospective study. J Neuro-Oncol. 2015;125:377–83.

17. Radiation Oncology Branch of the Chinese Medical Association, Expert Committee on Liver Cancer and Digestive System of China Institute of Biomedical Engineering, Liver Cancer Research Group of Radiation Oncology Branch of China Research Hospital. Consensus on radiation therapy for primary liver cancer in 2016. Chin J Radiat Oncol. 2016;25(11):1150.

Internal Radiation Therapy for Liver Cancer

24

Xin Yin, Jing Sun, and Zhenggang Ren

Internal radiation therapy utilizes the natural body cavity or tissue space, or by means of intervention, to place the radioactive source in the body cavity gap adjacent to the tumor, or implant the radioactive source into the tumor site under image guidance so that the radiation can be concentrated in the tumor region. The internal radiation therapy implant can be permanent (radioactive particle implantation) and temporary (after-loading radiation therapy) according to the placement manner. Due to high targeting, the radiation intensity in the tumor region is much higher than that in normal tissues, thus achieving the purpose of effective killing of tumor cells.

For hepatocellular carcinoma (HCC), the current commonly used internal radiation is selective internal radiation therapy (SIRT), such as ^{90}Y microspheres, iodine-131-labeled monoclonal antibody, radioactive iodine-131-labeled iodized oil, iodine-125 particle implantation, and so on. Isotope-labeled lipiodol was first used in the treatment of HCC. Shimabukuro K first used iodine-131-labeled iodized oil in the treatment of HCC in 1984. The tumoraffin property of lipiodol allows iodine-131 to stay in the tumors for a long time, thus playing the dual role of local radiation therapy and blocking the blood supply of the tumors.

X. Yin · J. Sun · Z. Ren (✉)
ZhongShan Hospital Fudan University, Shanghai, China

Radioactive particle implantation brachytherapy is widely used in patients with HCC. It is characterized by the implantation of microradioactive source particles (iodine-131 particles) into the tumor tissue or into the lumen invaded by the tumor, such as in the portal vein with tumor thrombus, through an image-guided system. Low-dose persistent radiation is generated by radioactive particles for tumor treatment. Iodine-125 particle implantation therapy is mainly used for patients with intermediate or advanced stage HCC combined with portal vein tumor thrombus, usually combined with portal vein stent and Trans-arterial Chemo-Embolization (TACE). The radioactive particles are implanted directly into the portal vein lumen, which can significantly improve patient survival without increasing the side effects related to radiation therapy. However, there is no standardized consensus on the operation process and radiation dose, and there is also no commercialized radioactive particle stent and radiation treatment planning system, making it difficult to achieve absolute uniformity of radiation dose in the target volume. Moreover, there is a lack of high-level evidence to support its efficacy and strict normative guidance. Prospective studies evaluating the survival benefits of Iodine-125 particle implantation therapy are needed.

SIRT is a special technique of brachytherapy, in which radioactive microspheres are injected into the tumor site through the hepatic artery to

X. Chen (ed.), *Diagnosis and Treatment of Liver Cancer in China*,
https://doi.org/10.1007/978-981-97-7969-7_24

achieve selective internal radiation within the tumor. There are two different forms of the most commonly used radionuclide (yttrium-90), which are glass and resin microspheres. Yttrium-90 has a shorter half-life and emits β-rays, which is relatively safe and considered an ideal therapeutic radionuclide. Radionuclide-labeled microspheres are injected into the tumor through the hepatic artery, providing both an embolic effect and high-dose internal irradiation to the tumor while minimizing damage to adjacent normal tissue. A multicenter, open-label, randomized, controlled phase III trial (SARAH) conducted by Vilgrain V et al. in 25 centers in France explored the efficacy of SIRT versus sorafenib in the treatment of advanced HCC. The study enrolled 400 patients with Barcelona Clinic Liver Cancer classification, (BCLC) HCC. A total of 200 patients received radioembolization and 200 patients received sorafenib treatment. The median overall survival was 8 months in the SIRT group and 9.9 months in the sorafenib group, with no statistically significant difference. However, the study concluded that SIRT can significantly reduce the side effects of treatment, improve the quality of life of HCC patients, and thus benefit patients with intermediate or advanced stage HCC who cannot undergo surgical resection.

Recently, computed tomography-guided high-dose-rate brachytherapy (CT-HDRBT) based on an after-loading therapy technique has been applied for HCC in Western countries, with iridium-192 as the main radioactive source. The ESMO 2019 guidelines recommend that HDRBT can be used in patients with HCC who cannot undergo surgical resection, or replace TACE as a bridging therapy for liver transplantation. Some foreign studies have found that CT-HDRBT can achieve a better tumor response rate than conventional TACE. At present, since the clinical application and research of CT-HDRBT therapy are rarely carried out in China, there is still a lack of relevant clinical data on its efficacy and side effects.

The emergence of internal radiation therapy has become a new treatment option for HCC. With the development of clinical medicine, internal radiation therapy for HCC would gradually develop toward the precise localization of tumors. At present, the relevant technical specifications and guidelines for the clinical application of internal radiation therapy, especially for radioactive particle implantation, should be further improved. Prospective clinical studies should be conducted to explore the indication of radioactive microspheres versus conventional TACE, and how to select ideal candidates. It is believed that in the near future, internal radiation therapy for HCC will be further improved inefficacy and safety.

Suggested Reading

1. Kobayashi H, Nakajo M, Shimabukuro K, et al. Possibility of radiotherapy of hepatic cancer by transcatheter arterial embolization with radioactive lipiodol. Nippon Acta Radiol. 1984;44:96.
2. Sun H, Zhang M, Liu R, et al. Endovascular implantation of 125I seed combined with transcatheter arterial chemoembolization for unresectable hepatocellular carcinoma. Future Oncol. 2018;14:1165–76.
3. Zhang ZH, Zhang W, Gu JY, et al. Treatment of hepatocellular carcinoma with tumor thrombus with the use of iodine-125 seed strand implantation and transarterial chemoembolization: a propensity-score analysis. J Vasc Interv Radiol. 2018;29:1085–93.
4. Vilgrain V, Pereira H, Assenat E, et al. Efficacy and safety of selective internal radiotherapy with yttrium-90 resin microspheres compared with sorafenib in locally advanced and inoperable hepatocellular carcinoma (SARAH): an open-label randomised controlled phase 3 trial. Lancet Oncol. 2017;18:1624–36.
5. Vogel A, Cervantes A, Chau I, et al. Hepatocellular carcinoma: ESMO clinical practice guidelines for diagnosis, treatment and follow-up. Ann Oncol. 2019;30:871–3.
6. Denecke T, Stelter L, Schnapauff D, et al. CT-guided interstitial brachytherapy of hepatocellular carcinoma before liver transplantation: an equivalent alternative to transarterial chemoembolization? Eur Radiol. 2015;25:2608–16.

25 Application of Radiation Therapy in the Multimodality Treatment of Liver Cancer

Xin Yin, Jing Sun, and Zhenggang Ren

Hepatocellular carcinoma (HCC) is a systemic disease with high metastatic characteristics. Local treatment strategies such as surgery, interventional therapy, radiation therapy, as well as ablation therapy can achieve significant local response, but cannot prevent tumor recurrence and metastasis. Based on the new advances in molecular targeted therapy and immunotherapy in recent years, the treatment modality of HCC has changed significantly, and multimodality combination therapy has been widely used in the management of HCC. The *Guidelines for the Diagnosis and Treatment of Primary Liver Cancer* (2019 Edition) clearly states that attention should be paid to the comprehensive treatment of HCC, including combinations of local therapy with local therapy or local therapy with systemic therapy and other modalities to curb HCC progression and metastasis.

Trans-arterial Chemo-Embolization (TACE) is considered one of the major local treatments for patients with unresectable intermediate or advanced HCC. Given that HCC has a dual blood supply from the hepatic artery and portal vein, residual tumors can survive on blood supply from the portal vein after TACE treatment, resulting in poor tumor control. TACE combined with external beam radiation therapy can improve tumor control rate and prolong patient survival. A meta-analysis of TACE combined with radiation therapy versus TACE alone published in 2015 included 25 clinical studies (11 randomized controlled studies with small sample sizes and 14 non-randomized controlled studies), including 2577 HCC patients. The results showed that the proportion of patients achieving complete response or partial response was significantly higher in the radiation therapy plus TACE group than in the TACE-alone group ($P < 0.001$). The median survival of patients in the two groups was 22.7 and 13.5 months ($P < 0.001$), respectively. Subgroup analysis showed that the radiation therapy combined with TACE was significantly superior to TACE alone in 1-, 2-, and 3-year survival rates, regardless of the presence of portal vein tumor thrombus. However, the study proposed that radiation therapy combined with TACE not only improved patient survival but also increased the risk of gastrointestinal ulcers and risk of liver function damage. In a single-center randomized prospective clinical study by Yoon's team in South Korea, 90 patients with imaging-visible HCC with portal vein thrombus were enrolled, with 45 cases in each group. One group was given TACE combined with radiation therapy, and the other group was given sorafenib orally twice a day, 400 mg at each time. The median survival was 12.8 months in the TACE plus external beam radiation therapy group and 10.0 months in the

X. Yin · J. Sun · Z. Ren (✉)
ZhongShan Hospital Fudan University, Shanghai, China

X. Chen (ed.), *Diagnosis and Treatment of Liver Cancer in China*,
https://doi.org/10.1007/978-981-97-7969-7_25

sorafenib group, with a statistically significant difference ($P = 0.04$).

With regard to the study of radiation therapy combined with molecular targeted therapy, a European multicenter prospective clinical study (SORAMIC study) by Ricke J et al. explored the safety and efficacy of sequential therapy with sorafenib followed by Selective Internal Radiation Therapy (SIRT) virus sorafenib monotherapy for advanced stage HCC. With an 8.3-month follow-up, the preliminary findings revealed that the incidence of adverse drug events ≥3 in grade was similar between the combination therapy group and the monotherapy group. Patients were well tolerated sequential therapy of sorafenib followed by Selective Internal Radiation Therapy (SIRT), and the survival data are still being followed up. At the 2019 APPLE Annual Meeting, Chinese scholar Yongshun CHEN reported his clinical study: a total of 60 HCC patients with portal vein tumor thrombus were recruited in the study, and the preliminary results showed encouraging efficacy of apatinib combined with radiation therapy for advanced HCC, with an objective response rate (ORR) of 30.8% and a disease control rate of 90%.

In a study of external beam radiation therapy combined with chemotherapy for advanced HCC, Japanese scholar Kodama K retrospectively analyzed and compared the efficacy of hepatic arterial infusion chemotherapy combined with external beam radiation therapy versus sorafenib in the treatment of 108 HCC patients with Child-Pugh score ≤7 and main portal vein tumor thrombus. The results showed that 68 patients who received hepatic arterial infusion chemotherapy combined with radiation therapy had significantly longer overall survival (OS), progression-free survival (PFS), and post-progression survival (PPS) than patients in the sorafenib group (OS: 9.9 months vs. 5.3 months, $P = 0.002$; PFS: 3.9 months vs. 2.1 months, $P = 0.048$; PPS: 3.7 months vs. 1.9 months, $P = 0.02$). The study proposed that hepatic arterial infusion chemotherapy combined with local radiation therapy was superior to sorafenib monotherapy in patients with advanced HCC combined with main portal vein tumor thrombus and compensated liver function.

Studies have indicated that when local tumor lesions are treated with external beam radiation therapy, distant untreated metastatic tumors might also shrink, which is known as the "abscopal effect." According to the available data, the abscopal effect caused by local radiation therapy occurs only in a few HCC patients. Theoretically, tumor antigen release induced by radiation therapy can help trigger the activation of the immune-killing effect, and combination therapy with Programmed death-1 (PD-1) antibodies will have a synergistic effect to improve tumor control. A phase I prospective clinical trial including a total of 79 patients with metastatic solid tumors demonstrated the efficacy and safety of Stereotactic Body Radiotherapy (SBRT) combined with (PD-1) antibodies in metastatic solid tumors. The metastatic lesions were treated with stereotactic body radiation, followed by (PD-1) antibody (pembrolizumab monotherapy) within 7 days after radiation therapy. Among the 68 patients who underwent follow-up imaging, the ORR was 13.2%, PFS was 3.1 months (95% confidence interval (CI): 2.9–3.4 months) and OS was 9.6 months (95% CI: 6.5 months to not achieved). So far, the clinical study on radiation therapy combined with immunotherapy for HCC is still at the initial stage. The first domestic "clinical study on carbon ion radiation therapy combined with anti-PD-1 antibody (SHR-1210) for metastatic hepatocellular carcinoma" and the clinical study on "sintilimab combined with radiation therapy for advanced hepatocellular carcinoma with main portal vein tumor thrombus" are currently recruiting subjects. More studies on radiation therapy combined with immunotherapy are expected to obtain encouraging results in the future.

With the continuous development of radiation therapy technology, radiation treatment modalities are becoming diversified, and radiation therapy technology is becoming more precise. Radiation therapy is more and more widely used in early, intermediate, and advanced HCC. This clinical applied technology will be more perfect, and the indications will be more standardized.

Particularly, radiation therapy is expected to play a more important role in the comprehensive treatment of HCC with the promotion and application of stereotactic body radiation therapy. In addition to the improvement and refinement of radiation therapy technology, more carefully designed prospective studies on indications of its application are required to obtain high-level evidence support. Since HCC is a systemic disease, the combination of radiation therapy with systemic therapy (chemotherapy, molecular targeted therapy, or immunotherapy) will be the development trend of HCC treatment in the future. In the process of combination therapy, the dose, fraction method, and combination method of radiation therapy should be explored in multiple prospective clinical trials to achieve the optimal efficacy of combination therapy.

Suggested Reading

1. Huo YR, Eslick GD. Transcatheter arterial chemoembolization plus radiotherapy compared with chemoembolization alone for hepatocellular carcinoma: a systematic review and meta-analysis. JAMA Oncol. 2015;1:756–65.
2. Yoon SM, Ryoo BY, Lee SJ, et al. Efficacy and safety of transarterial chemoembolization plus external beam radiotherapy vs sorafenib in hepatocellular carcinoma with macroscopic vascular invasion. JAMA Oncol. 2018;4(5):4661–9.
3. Ricke J, Bulla K, Kolligs F, et al. Safety and toxicity of radioembolization plus sorafenib in advanced hepatocellular carcinoma: analysis of the European multicentre trial SORAMIC. Liver Int. 2015;35:620–6.
4. Kodama K, Kawaoka T, Aikata H, et al. Comparison of outcome of hepatic arterial infusion chemotherapy combined with radiotherapy and sorafenib for advanced hepatocellular carcinoma patients with major portal vein tumor thrombosis. Oncology. 2018;94:215–22.
5. Lumniczky K, Sáfrány G. The impact of radiation therapy on the antitumor immunity: local effects and systemic consequences. Cancer Lett. 2015;356:114–25.
6. Dovedi SJ, Adlard AL, Lipowska-Bhalla G, et al. Acquired resistance to fractionated radiotherapy can be overcome by concurrent PD-L1 blockade. Cancer Res. 2014;74:5458–68.
7. Luke JJ, Lemons JM, Karrison TG, et al. Safety and clinical activity of pembrolizumab and multisite stereotactic body radiotherapy in patients with advanced solid tumors. J Clin Oncol. 2018;36:1611–8.

Part VII

Multimodality Treatment for Liver Cancer

26 Development and Changes in the Guidelines for Diagnosis and Treatment of Primary Liver Cancer (From 2011 Edition to 2017 Edition)

Lin Chen

26.1 Background

In the past half-century, there has been great advancement in the surgical treatment of primary hepatocellular carcinoma (HCC). Liver surgery techniques have evolved remarkably, enabling the resection of tumors in previously inaccessible regions. Huge HCC and those located in critical areas (close to the first, second, and third porta hepatis or inferior vena cava) can all be safely resected. Liver transplantation has demonstrated favorable outcomes for HCC patients meeting the Milan or University of California, San Francisco (UCSF) criteria. Beyond surgery, emerging local therapies—including transarterial chemoembolization Trans-Arterial Chemo-Embolization (TACE), ablation techniques (radiofrequency, microwave, cryotherapy, and ethanol injection), stereotactic body radiation therapy, and internal radiotherapy—have been integrated into clinical practice. Upon entering the twenty-first century, there has been a breakthrough in the systemic treatment of HCC as tyrosine kinase inhibitors (TKIs) led to positive outcomes in unresectable patients with advanced HCC. Furthermore, immune checkpoint inhibitors represented by anti-programmed death-1 (PD-1) antibody combined with TKI have also demonstrated promising efficacy in the treatment of advanced HCC. While expanding therapeutic options offer hope, optimizing treatment selection to maximize patient benefit remains a clinical priority.

L. Chen (✉)
Tongji Hospital Affiliated to Tongji Medical College, Huazhong University of Science & Technology, Wuhan, China

26.2 Selection of Surgical Treatments for HCC: The First Guideline for the Diagnosis and Treatment of HCC in China

In 1999, the German Society of Digestive and Metabolic Diseases published the world's first first HCC treatment guidelines. Subsequent guidelines emerged from France, the UK, South Korea, and others (Table 26.1). As surgical treatment was the primary treatment regimen during this time, diagnosis and treatment guidelines were also mainly developed by surgeons. The development of consensus on the diagnosis and treatment of HCC started early in China. In 2000, the Sixth Chinese National Conference of Liver Surgery, led by Professor Chen Xiaoping, drafted the "Selection of Surgical Treatments for Primary Liver Cancer," which was then adopted by the Section of Hepatic Surgery, Branch of Surgery, Chinese Medical Association in October 2000, and published in several authoritative Chinese journals in 2001 (Table 26.1). Since a breakthrough had not been made in the system-

X. Chen (ed.), *Diagnosis and Treatment of Liver Cancer in China*,
https://doi.org/10.1007/978-981-97-7969-7_26

Table 26.1 Summary of guidelines for the diagnosis and treatment of HCC in various countries

Guidelines	Country	Time	Institution
Guidelines of the German Society of Digestive and Metabolic Diseases for diagnosis and therapy of HCC	Germany	1999	German Society of Digestive and Metabolic Diseases
Selection of surgical treatments for primary liver cancer	China	2001	Liver Surgery Study Group, Branch of Surgery, Chinese Medical Association
HCC	France	2001	French National Federation of Cancer
Guidelines for the diagnosis and treatment of HCC in adults	United Kingdom	2003	British Society of Gastroenterology
BASL guidelines for the surveillance, diagnosis, and treatment of HCC	Belgium	2004	BASL HCC working group and BASL steering committee
Practice guidelines for diagnosis and treatment of HCC	South Korea	2004	KoreanPrimary Liver Cancer Study Group and National Cancer Center
Management of HCC	United States	2005	Practice Guidelines Committee, American Association for the Study of Liver Diseases
Clinical practice guidelines for HCC: The first evidence-based guidelines from Japan	Japan	2006	The Japanese Ministry of Health, Labour and Welfare

atic treatment of *primary liver cancer* at that time, this guideline systematically discussed the indications for surgery, ablation, TACE, and radiotherapy in the treatment of *primary liver cancer*. In 2004, the Section of Hepatic Surgery revised the guideline for the first time according to the latest advances in *primary liver cancer* treatment. The revisions mainly included (1) a change of the evaluation criteria for liver function to the globally accepted modified Child-Pugh scoring system; (2) an expansion of the indications for radical resection of *primary liver cancer*, which includes radical resection of a single tumor, irrespective of its size, as long as there is the sufficient residual liver volume (except for tumors in segments 4, 5, and 8 in the central region of the liver), and radical resection of caudate lobe tumors; and (3) addition of surgical indications for liver transplantation in *primary liver cancer*.

In 2008, the Section of Hepatic Surgery revised the guideline for the second time. The revisions mainly included (1) substitution of "*primary liver cancer*" with the internationally used term HCC; (2) standardization of HCC classification by maximum diameter, including micro-liver cancer (≤2.0 cm), small HCC (>2.0 cm, ≤5.0 cm), large HCC (>5.0 cm, ≤10 cm), and huge HCC (>10 cm); (3) proposition of the criteria for radical resection of HCC; (4) proposition of the treatment rules for recurrent HCC; (5) proposition of indications for the resection of unresectable HCC after downstaging; and (6) addition of surgical indications for laparoscopic hepatectomy. As factors such as tumor size, quantity, and liver function status need to be considered when selecting the treatment for HCC, the "FlowChart for the Diagnosis and Treatment of Hepatocellular Carcinoma" was developed by Professor Chen Xiaoping in order to facilitate understanding and wide application. This flow chart has been discussed and revised by all members of the Section of Hepatic Surgery, Branch of Surgery, Chinese Medical Association as well as other renowned liver surgeons in China and can be used as a reference for clinicians in the diagnosis and treatment of HCC. Compared with foreign guidelines for the treatment of HCC, the greatest advantage of the three versions of the "Selection of Surgical Treatments for HCC" (2001, 2004, and 2008 editions) is that it recapitulates the actual conditions in China: China has the highest number of HCC patients and nearly 80% of them have a history of HBV infection. Most patients have cirrhosis and portal hypertension, and they are often in the middle and late stages when HCC is diagnosed, accompanied by portal vein tumor thrombus or bile duct tumor thrombus. Due to the lack of experience in the surgical treatment of these patients and the view that they have surgical contraindications, non-surgical treatments are generally recommended abroad. If such foreign practices were adopted in China, many of these patients would lose the opportunity for surgery. "Selection of Surgical Treatments for HCC" provides a detailed discussion of the treatments for middle- to late-stage HCC, HCC with cirrhosis, and HCC with portal hypertension based on the extensive experience of Chinese scholars in the surgical treatment of HCC and serves as a reference for the treatment of HCC in China. This manuscript fills the gap in this field and has been widely acclaimed.

26.3 Guidelines for the Diagnosis and Treatment of HCC: Comprehensive Guideline for the Diagnosis and Treatment of HCC

In 2008, sorafenib, a TKI, was approved as the first-line treatment for unresectable HCC. It is the world's first first-line targeted therapy for HCC and has paved the way for systemic treatment of HCC. In addition to surgical resection, the advancement in intervention, ablation, radiotherapy, chemotherapy, and other new techniques has not only provided additional treatment options but also facilitated the comprehensive treatment of HCC through multidisciplinary cooperation. The development of imaging, laboratory testing, and pathology provided more choices for the screening and early diagnosis of HCC. However, a surgical treatment guideline is obviously far from enough. In order to improve HCC diagnosis and treatment in China, a scientific and authoritative comprehensive evidence-based guideline must be developed to standardize the whole process of HCC screening, diagnosis, staging, and treatment. In 2011, the Ministry of Health of the People's Republic of China issued the Guidelines for the Diagnosis and Treatment of HCC (2011 Edition) (hereinafter referred to as the "2011 Edition Guideline"), the first comprehensive guideline for diagnosis and treatment of HCC in China. The 2011 Edition Guideline, which was developed using evidence-based medicine, provides a systematic description of the diagnostic process, staging, grading, liver function assessment, and treatment strategies for HCC. This Guideline consist of nine sections: (1) Overview; (2) Diagnostic Techniques and Applications, which mainly discusses the monitoring and screening of high-risk population, clinical manifestations of HCC, auxiliary examinations, selection of imaging methods, diagnostic process, differential diagnosis, and pathological classification; (3) Classification and Staging of HCC: Pathological Classification of Liver Tumors (WHO 2005), which focuses on commonly used HCC staging methods in the world (TNM and BCLC staging) and methods of liver reserve function evaluation; (4) Surgical Treatments, which mainly summarizes the indications and contraindications for hepatectomy and liver transplantation and highlights the "Selection of Surgical Treatments for HCC"; (5) Local Treatments, which includes the indications, contraindications, and general technical requirements for ablation and TACE and focuses on the selection of local ablation therapy and surgery for tumors ≤ 5 cm; (6) Radiotherapy, which includes the indications and technical requirements for radiotherapy as well as common postoperative complications and treatments; (7) Systemic Treatments, which mainly introduces the application and contraindications for the TKI sorafenib and systemic chemotherapy (arsenic trioxide and FOLFOX regimen) in advanced HCC according to the latest research; (8) Suggestions for Multidisciplinary Treatment of HCC, which emphasizes on multidisciplinary standardized comprehensive treatment due to the particularity of HCC (most common in chronic liver disease or liver cirrhosis) and advocates personalized treatment for different patients and same patient in different stages; and (9) Follow-Up, which discusses follow-up periods and specifics. The 2011 Edition Guideline retained the contents on surgery, liver transplantation, local ablation, and TACE in the "Selection of Surgical Treatments for HCC" and added the screening and diagnosis, staging, radiotherapy, and molecular targeted and systemic chemotherapy for HCC. This Guideline advocates the development of personalized systematic treatment through multidisciplinary cooperation based on the patients' actual conditions and emphasizes the monitoring and screening of high-risk populations.

The "Guidelines for the Diagnosis and Treatment of HCC" (2017 Edition) (hereinafter referred to as the "2017 Edition Guideline") was issued in 2017. By following the principles of "combining detail and principle, making use of advanced foreign practices, emphasizing on Chinese characteristics, and highlighting key points," this edition was updated with the latest evidence-based medical research, namely, the application of associating liver partition and portal vein ligation for staged hepatectomy (ALPPS), and results of the EACH study of oxaliplatin-containing FOLFOX regimen in the treatment of advanced HCC and other publications. The 2017 Edition Guideline is an advanced version of the 2011 Edition Guideline and better reflects the clinical practice in China.

Main updates in the 2017 Edition Guideline include:

1. **Epidemiology**
   (a) 2011 Edition Guideline: HCC accounts for over 90% of HCCs;
   (b) 2017 Edition Guideline: HCC accounts for 85–90% of HCCs.
2. **Diagnostic techniques and applications**
   (a) Added "CT-based three-dimensional liver volume and tumor volume measurement."
   (b) Emphasized that magnetic resonance imaging (MRI) combined with hepatocyte-specific contrast medium can improve the detection rate of HCC ≤1.0 cm in diameter and the accuracy of HCC diagnosis and differential diagnosis.
   (c) 2011 Edition Guideline: The sensitivity and specificity of PET/CT in the clinical diagnosis of HCC need to be further improved, and this technique is not recommended as a routine examination method for HCC diagnosis.

   The 2017 Edition Guideline deleted the negative opinion on PET/CT and provided detailed descriptions and substantiating evidence on its important role in the diagnosis and treatment of HCC.
   (d) Liver biopsy: It was clearly stated that "patients with space-occupying lesions with typical imaging features of HCC who meet the clinical diagnostic criteria for HCC usually do not require liver biopsy for the purpose of diagnosis."
   (e) Defined pathological diagnosis specifications, including specimen processing, specimen sampling ("seven-point" baseline sampling method), pathological examination, and pathology report (emphasis on the grading of microvascular invasion to assess the risk of HCC recurrence and to serve as an important reference for the selection of treatment regimens).
3. **Staging: Proposed criteria for HCC staging reflecting national conditions and clinical practice in China as well as treatment strategies according to tumor stage (see Figs. 4.1–4.3).**
4. **Treatments**
   (a) Surgery
   - The 2017 Edition Guideline deleted the concept of palliative resection and defined the basic principles of hepatectomy: (a) Complete tumor resection without residual tumor at the resection margin and (b) Safety: Preservation of sufficient liver tissue for postoperative liver function compensation to reduce surgical mortality and surgical complications.
   - More accurate description of indications: Stages IA, IB, IIA, and IIB patients with adequate liver functional reserve; some stage IIIA and IIIB patients.
   - Refined preoperative evaluation criteria of liver functional reserve: Child-Pugh A, ICG retention rate at 15 minutes (ICG15) <20–30% and residual liver accounting for over 40% of the standard liver volume (patients with cirrhosis) or over 30% (patients

without cirrhosis) as the prerequisites for surgical resection.

- Expanded the indications for laparoscopic surgery: Added the following in addition to lesions located in Couinaud 2, 3, 5, and 6 segments: (a) The size of the lesion does not affect the dissection of the first and second hila (generally not more than 10 cm); and (b) Doctors with extensive experience may consider laparoscopic hemihepatectomy, trilobal resection, and Couinaud 1-, 7-, and 8-segment hepatectomy.
- Defined radical resection criteria: Intraoperative judgment criteria: (a) Absence of macroscopic tumor thrombus in the hepatic vein, portal vein, bile duct, and inferior vena cava; (b) Absence of adjacent organ invasion and hilar lymph nodes or distant metastasis; and (c) Liver resection margin >1 cm from the tumor boundary (if the resection margin is <1 cm, there should be no residual tumor cells in the histological examination of the resected liver section, namely, a negative resection margin).

  Postoperative judgment criteria: (a) Absence of tumor lesion confirmed by ultrasound, computed tomography (CT), or MRI (at least two imaging techniques) 2 months after operation; and (b) if alpha-fetoprotein (AFP) is elevated before operation, AFP quantitative determination is required 2 months after operation, and AFP level should be within the normal range (very few patients require more than 2 months for AFP to decrease to normal).
- Improved the resectability of HCC: Added the application of preoperative TACE, portal vein embolization or portal vein ligation, and ALPPS.
- Emphasized the prevention and treatment of postoperative metastasis and recurrence: Postoperative prophylactic TACE, and postoperative transportal chemotherapy combined with TACE and interferon in patients with portal vein tumor thrombus.

(b) Liver transplantation: Clearly recommended the use of UCSF criteria for liver transplant indications, emphasized the prevention of recurrence after liver transplantation, recommended reduced dosage of calcineurin inhibitors in the early stage after transplantation, and advised immunosuppressive regimen using mTOR inhibitors.

(c) Local ablation: Compared with the 2011 Edition Guideline, the 2017 Edition Guideline continued to emphasize surgical resection as the first choice for HCC and ablation combined with other therapies is encouraged for patients with unresectable HCC.

(d) Interventional therapy
  - Added renal dysfunction as a criterion in the contraindications for interventional therapy, that is, TACE is not recommended for patients with creatinine >2 mg/dL or creatinine clearance <30 mL/min.
  - Highlighted local therapy and combination of local therapy and systemic therapy: (a) TACE combined with ablation (radiofrequency ablation and microwave ablation); (b) TACE combined with radiotherapy as the primary treatment following interventional therapy for main portal vein tumor thrombus, venous tumor thrombus, and localized large HCC; (c) TACE combined with two-step hepatectomy: Liver resection is recommended when large or massive HCC shrinks after TACE therapy; and (d) TACE combined with systemic therapy, including combination with molecular targeted drug (i.e., arsenic trioxide), targeted radioimmunotherapy, and gene therapy.

(e) Immunotherapy: Added "Immune checkpoint inhibitors" (i.e., CTLA-4 inhibitor and PD-1/PD-L1 inhibitor), tumor vaccines (i.e., dendritic cell vaccines), cellular immunotherapy (cytokine-induced killer cells, i.e., CIK), and other immunotherapies in addition to immunomodulators.

(f) Radiotherapy: The 2017 Edition Guideline affirmed the efficacy of radiotherapy by stating that radiotherapy can shrink or downstage the tumor and provide the chance of surgical resection in some stage IIIA and IIIB patients with portal vein/inferior vena cava tumor thrombus or extrahepatic metastasis.

(g) Symptomatic and supportive treatment: (a) Added details on symptomatic and supportive treatment: "Moderate rehabilitation exercise can enhance the immunity. Symptomatic and supportive treatment should be strengthened, including active analgesia, correction of anemia, correction of hypoalbuminemia, and enhanced nutritional support in patients with advanced HCC, blood glucose control in diabetes patients, as well as treatment of accompanying symptoms such as ascites, jaundice, hepatic encephalopathy, and gastrointestinal hemorrhage." (b) Added the need to care for the psychological status of patients and their families: "Positive measures should be taken to change the negative mentality of advanced HCC patients and their families, and palliative care should be provided to reduce their depression and anxiety and to feel safe and comfortable."

There has been significant progress in the clinical treatment and basic research of HCC in recent years, including an increased number of new treatment regimens, closer cooperation between disciplines, and further standardization in the application of various treatments. However, how to develop the best personalized treatment regimen based on the specific conditions of the patients still requires more clinical experience in addition to the new guidelines. Exchanges among treatment centers and various disciplines need to be strengthened, more multicenter randomized controlled clinical and basic research should be carried out, and existing HCC diagnosis and treatment standards need to be further improved in order to jointly improve the level of diagnosis and treatment of HCC in China.

Suggested Reading

1. Caselmann WH, Blum HE, Fleig WE, et al. Guidelines of the German Society of Digestive and Metabolic Diseases for diagnosis and therapy of hepatocellular carcinoma. German Society of Digestive and Metabolic Diseases. Z Gastroenterol. 1999;37(5):353–65.
2. Giovannini M, Elias D, Monges G, et al. French National Federation of Cancer (FNCLCC). Hepatocellular carcinoma. Br J Cancer. 2001;84(Suppl 2):74–7.
3. Ryder SD, British Society of Gastroenterology. Guidelines for the diagnosis and treatment of hepatocellular carcinoma (HCC) in adults. Gut. 2003;52(Suppl 3):1–8.
4. Van Vlierberghe H, Borbath I, Delwaide J, et al. BASL guidelines for the surveillance, diagnosis and treatment of hepatocellular carcinoma. Acta Gastroenterol Belg. 2004;67(1):14–25.
5. Park JW, Korean HCC Study Group and National Cancer Center. Practice guideline for diagnosis and treatment of hepatocellular carcinoma. Korean J Hepatol. 2004;10(2):88–98.
6. Bruix J, Sherman M, Practice Guidelines Committee. Management of hepatocellular carcinoma. Hepatology. 2005;42(5):1208–36.
7. Makuuchi M, Kokudo N. Clinical practice guidelines for hepatocellular carcinoma: the first evidence based guidelines from Japan. World J Gastroenterol. 2006;12(5):828–9.
8. Liver Surgery Study Group, Branch of Surgery, Chinese Medical Association. Selection of surgical treatments for HCC. Chin J Surg. 2001;39(10):762–3.
9. Liver Surgery Study Group, Branch of Surgery, Chinese Medical Association. Selection of surgical treatments for HCC. Chin J Hepatol. 2001;9(3):134–6.
10. Liver Surgery Study Group, Branch of Surgery, Chinese Medical Association. Selection of surgical treatments for HCC. Chin J Oncol. 2001;23(2):172–4.
11. Liver Surgery Study Group, Branch of Surgery, Chinese Medical Association. Selection of surgical treatments for HCC (first revision in 2004). Chin J Gen Surg. 2005;20(4):262–4.
12. Liver Surgery Study Group, Branch of Surgery, Chinese Medical Association. Selection of surgical treatments for hepatocellular carcinoma (revised in 2008, 3rd edition). Chin J Surg. 2009;47(3):222–4.
13. Liver Surgery Study Group, Branch of Surgery, Chinese Medical Association. Selection of surgical

treatments for hepatocellular carcinoma (revised). Chin J Surg. 2012;50(6):505–6.
14. Ministry of Health of the People's Republic of China. Guidelines for the diagnosis and treatment of HCC (2011 edition). J Clin Oncol. 2011;16(10):929–46.
15. Bureau of Medical Administration, Health and Family Planning Commission of the People's Republic of China. Guidelines for the diagnosis and treatment of HCC (2017 edition). Chin J Gastrointest Surg. 2017;16(7):635–47.

27 Molecular Mechanisms and Multimodality Treatments for Liver Cancer Recurrence and Metastasis

Zeyang Ding and Bixiang Zhang

Currently, surgical resection is the predominant treatment of liver cancer, especially in those with early stage. However, recurrence and metastasis after surgery are the primary issues that affect the prognosis of liver cancer. Therefore, studies exploring the molecular mechanism of liver cancer recurrence and metastasis provide a theoretical basis for the development of new targeted therapy drugs for liver cancer, promote advancement in the treatment measures and treatment concept of the disease, and improve the efficacy of multimodality treatment for liver cancer.

The dissemination of cancer cells from the primary tumor to distant organs and tissues is a continuous process of invasion and metastasis. This process generally includes the following six main steps: (1) Shedding: Cancer cells detach from the main tumor and invade the surrounding extracellular matrix (ECM) and stromal tissue; (2) Intravasation: Cancer cells invade and enter the vasculature such as blood vessels, lymphatic vessels, and bile duct; (3) Shuttling: Cancer cells are shuttled and transported through the vasculature, which has been further corroborated by the recently discovered cancer self-seeding theory; (4) Implantation: Cancer cells reach distant tissues or target organs and adapt to new environments; (5) Colonize: Cancer cells form metastatic clones and micro-metastases and can remain in dormancy for months or even years; and (6) cancer cells proliferation and form macro-metastases at the sites of metastasis. Hepatocellular carcinoma (HCC) metastasis can be either distant metastasis or intrahepatic recurrence (i.e., intrahepatic metastasis). Liver cancer cells can metastasize to other parts of the liver through the portal vein, then to distant sites through the hepatic vein, or to adjacent tissues and organs through the lymphatics or direct invasion. In recent years, there has been great progress in the precise mechanism of liver cancer recurrence and metastasis.

27.1 Genomic Alterations: Drivers of HCC Recurrence and Metastasis

Numerous multi-omics studies of HCC and corresponding functional analyses showed that the development, recurrence, and metastasis of HCC are accompanied by abnormal genomic changes that affect the biological behaviors associated with HCC recurrence and metastasis, such as abnormal amplification of chromosomes 6p21 (VEGFA), 11q13 (FGF19/CCND1), 1q21 (CHD1L/ALC1), and 1q24 (MAEL), as well as homozygous deletion of chromosome 9, which is associated with HCC metastasis. In addition, mutations in the coding region of genes are also common in HCC. For

Z. Ding · B. Zhang (✉)
Tongji Hospital Affiliated to Tongji Medical College, Huazhong University of Science & Technology, Wuhan, China

X. Chen (ed.), *Diagnosis and Treatment of Liver Cancer in China*,
https://doi.org/10.1007/978-981-97-7969-7_27

example, mutations in the TP53 gene, TERT gene, and CTNNB1 gene are common in HCC and they affect the biological behaviors of HCC such as invasion and metastasis. Low-frequency (<10%) mutations in the coding regions of some genes (e.g., AXIN1, ARID1A, TSC1/TSC2, KEAP1, JAK1, and WNK2) are also closely related to HCC invasion and metastasis. Furthermore, epigenetic changes including abnormal DNA methylation and hydroxymethylation levels, abnormal histone acetylation levels, functional changes in chromatin remodeling complexes, and abnormal expression changes in non-coding RNAs, can also be seen in HCC and are closely associated with HCC invasion and metastasis. In China, hepatitis B virus (HBV) infection is the predominant pathogenic factor in the development of HCC. Excessive activation of proto-oncogenes caused by the integration of HBV DNA into the host hepatocyte genome is the primary pathogenesis of HCC and plays an important role in HCC invasion and metastasis. These changes in turn induce corresponding changes in the activity of signaling pathways closely related to HCC recurrence and metastasis, such as the MAPK pathway, β-catenin pathway, TGF-β pathway, Hippo pathway, Notch pathway, JAK-Stat pathway, Hedgehog pathway, and PI3K-AKT pathway, which ultimately lead to a series of biological behavioral changes related to HCC recurrence and metastasis, such as epithelial–mesenchymal transition, adhesion changes, vascular invasion, enhanced proliferative capacity, increased tumor angiogenesis, anoikis evasion, and immune escape.

27.2 Spatial and Temporal Heterogeneity of HCC: Key Factors in HCC Recurrence and Metastasis

HCC recurrence and metastasis are multistep complex processes involving multiple regulatory factors. Among them, spatial and temporal heterogeneity of HCC plays a critical role in HCC recurrence and metastasis. HCC heterogeneity is caused by the generation of progeny with different phenotypes and biological behaviors due to the unstable genome of HCC or by multicentric HCC. As a result, it is difficult for targeted therapeutic drugs to thoroughly kill heterogeneous HCC and leads to drug resistance to HCC. In addition, HCC cells of different phenotypes and functions can work together to help HCC adapt to environmental changes during metastasis and ultimately create favorable conditions for successful colonization. The existence of spatial and temporal heterogeneity of HCC has been confirmed by several studies, including intratumoral heterogeneity of HCC, heterogeneity between primary tumor and recurrent foci, heterogeneity between circulating tumor cells and primary tumor, heterogeneity of microenvironment, and metabolic reprogramming in HCC progression. Moreover, the same molecule may play a different role at different stages of HCC progression due to temporal heterogeneity. For example, TIF1γ, an inhibitory molecule in the TGF-β pathway, inhibits the proliferation-inhibiting effect of the TGF-β pathway in early HCC and facilitates the invasion and metastasis effects of the TGF-β pathway in advanced HCC due to the loss of the proliferation-inhibiting effect of the TGF-β pathway and further downregulation of TIF1γ expression as a result of hypermethylation of its promoter. Another example is that the ARID1A gene can induce the generation of reactive oxygen species (ROS) and promote the development of HCC in the early stage of HCC progression. However, ARID1A can also inhibit invasion and metastasis by enhancing the accessibility of chromatin through chromatin remodeling and inducing the expression of corresponding proteins. Hence, ARID1A may lose its property of inhibiting metastasis in advanced HCC due to mutation or deletion. In summary, spatial and temporal heterogeneity of HCC is a critical factor in HCC invasion and metastasis and poses a great challenge for the treatment of HCC.

27.3 HCC Microenvironment: The "Soil" for Recurrence and Metastasis

In 1889, Paget first proposed the seed and soil hypothesis of tumor metastasis by arguing that tumor metastasis is the result of the interaction and mutual adaptation of specific tumor cells (seeds) with their surrounding microenvironment (soil). This hypothesis has been continuously verified and proven in recent decades. For HCC, the microenvironment (niche) is a complex system and structure composed of various inflammatory mediators, cytokines, neovascularization, ROS, fibrous stroma, inflammatory immune cells, and tumor-associated fibroblasts. Chronic inflammation of the liver, cirrhosis, and HCC cells all play an important role in the final formation of the HCC microenvironment. There is mounting evidence showing that during the metastasis and recurrence of HCC, HCC cells continue to adapt to and modify the microenvironment, and the HCC microenvironment in turn supports HCC cells throughout their metastasis. Specifically, HCC can act on stellate cells and cancer-associated fibroblasts (CAFs), tumor-associated macrophages (TAMs), tumor-associated neutrophils, regulatory T cells (Treg cells), myeloid-derived suppressor cells, and other mesenchymal and immune cells in the microenvironment through various secreted proteins and chemokines or exosomes to activate stellate cells or fibroblasts and induce TAM polarization. These activated cells in turn secrete various molecules to promote the proliferation, invasion, metastasis, and stem cell characteristics of HCC cells and induce immunosuppression. In addition, HCC can promote neovascularization by secreting several molecules such as VEGF, PDGF, TGF-β1, angiopoietin-1, and angiopoietin-2 and can even metastasize directly by vascular mimicry or formation of vessels encapsulating tumor clusters. Other components in the microenvironment such as CAFs and TAMs also play an important supporting role in these metastasis processes and modes. In addition, the fibrous stroma and ECM have also been reported to promote HCC invasion and metastasis. Increased interstitial stiffness due to cirrhosis leads to enhanced mechanical signals, which can directly enhance the invasiveness of HCC. HCC can in turn secrete various molecules to increase interstitial stiffness. Furthermore, ECM can directly activate FAK and AKT through the integrin family molecules on the surface of HCC to promote HCC invasion and metastasis. Recent studies have explored the effect of the intestinal microbiota on HCC recurrence and metastasis and showed that the microbiota can alter bile acid metabolism and bile components, induce the secretion of inflammatory mediators, and promote the invasion and metastasis of HCC and intrahepatic cholangiocarcinoma. In summary, interactions among multiple components in the HCC microenvironment and HCC cells and the formation of feedback loops supporting the invasion and metastasis of HCC are important targets for the research and development of anti-metastatic drugs.

27.4 HCC Stem Cells: "Seeds" and Executors of Recurrence and Metastasis

The cancer stem cell (CSC) theory postulates that CSCs act as initiating cells or "seed" cells during the development, recurrence, and metastasis of tumors. CSCs are a small population of cells with self-renewing capacity and unlimited proliferative potentials. These cells maintain the growth of tumors and have self-renewal potential. Insensitivity to chemotherapeutic drugs is also one of the characteristics of CSCs. Early studies of HCC have identified various cell subpopulations with specific markers (e.g., CD133, CD90, CD24, CD44s, CD13, EpCAM, OV-6, Nanog, and other positive liver cancer cell populations) that have the biological characteristics of liver CSCs, such as strong self-renewal capability, non-anchor growth, single cell tumorigenicity, resistance to chemotherapeutic drugs, and induction of tumor angiogenesis. In addition, there is also heterogeneity in HCC stem cells involving multiple HCC stem cell populations with different markers that are heterogeneous in phenotype, function, and expression profile. For example, $EpCAM^+$ $CD133^+$ HCC stem cells have epithelial cell phenotype and strong self-renewal capability and tumorigenicity, but weak migration and metastasis. $CD44^+$ HCC stem cells are phenotypically reminiscent of mesenchymal cells, whereas $CD90^+$ HCC stem cells are phenotypically reminiscent of endothelial cells. These two groups of cells are less proliferative and have weaker self-renewal capacity and tumorigenicity but stronger metastasis capability than $EpCAM^+$ HCC stem cells. $CD24^+$ HCC stem cells have strong self-renewal and tumorigenic abilities but weak in vitro proliferation. $CD13^+$ HCC stem cells have weak proliferation and self-renewal capacity but are resistant to chemotherapeutic drugs and are considered to be a type of dormant HCC stem cell. Moreover, when $CD90^+$ cells are co-cultured with $EpCAM^+$ cells, $CD90^+$ cells can significantly enhance the migration and metastasis of $EpCAM^+$ cells to the lungs. This indicates that HCC stem cell populations with different phenotypes often coexist, have complementary advantages, and together play important roles in the progression, recurrence, and metastasis of liver cancer. Numerous proteins and non-coding RNAs can regulate HCC recurrence and metastasis by regulating the stem cell characteristics of HCC cells including their self-renewal, resistance to chemotherapeutic drugs, dormancy, and activation. Further in-depth study of the role and regulatory mechanism of HCC stem cells in HCC evolution is of great significance for the development of therapeutic agents that target HCC stem cell populations.

27.5 Multimodality Treatments for Liver Cancer Recurrence and Metastasis

Traditional treatments for HCC recurrence and metastasis include transarterial chemoembolism (TACE), ablation therapy, radiotherapy, intraperitoneal hyperthermic chemoperfusion, and re-resection. In-depth studies on the mechanisms of liver cancer recurrence and metastasis and the development of new cancer drugs have shown that anti-angiogenic therapy predominated by tyrosine kinase inhibitors (TKIs) and immunotherapy based on immune checkpoint inhibitors (ICIs) have promising clinical application prospects in advanced liver cancer. The combination of these treatments is also a major direction of clinical application.

Repeated liver resection of recurrent lesions is an option for recurrent HCC. However, timing for the repeated resection after the first resection is important, for that it is associated with the prognosis of recurrent HCC. A previous study from the Hepatic Surgery Center of Wuhan Tongji Hospital reported that both the short interval between repeated resection and the first operation (less than 18 months), or recurrent HCC with microvascular invasion are independent risk factors for the overall survival of patients.

TACE has always been the treatment of choice for unresectable HCC patients with acceptable liver function. A randomized controlled clinical trial showed that in locally advanced HCC patients when compared with systemic therapy of sorafenib, TACE improved the progression-free survival (PFS), but not overall survival (OS). Another small-cohort phase II clinical trial of HCC patients with vascular invasion showed that external beam radiotherapy combined with TACE could improve the PFS and OS of patients. Other studies have also shown that preoperative neoadjuvant radiotherapy can improve the postoperative OS of patients with HCC and branch portal vein tumor thrombus.

Sorafenib is the first multi-target (VEGFR1–3, B-Raf, and PDGFRα) oral TKI approved as the first-line oral targeted therapy for advanced HCC. A phase III clinical trial of sorafenib showed that patients in the sorafenib arm had significantly longer survival than those in the placebo arm (mOS 10.7 months vs. 7.9 months, risk ratio 0.69, 95% confidence interval (CI): 0.55–0.87, $P < 0.001$). Lenvatinib, a multi-target oral TKI targeting VEGFR1–3, FGFR1–4, RET, KIT, and PDGFRα, was demonstrated to be non-inferior to sorafenib in a multicenter, randomized, open-label, non-inferiority head-to-head phase III clinical trial (REFLECT study) with OS as the primary endpoint. Based on the results of this study, lenvatinib was approved as a first-line treatment for advanced liver cancer in 2018.

Second-line targeted therapies for advanced HCC include regorafenib (VEGFR, TIE2, angiopoietin-1 receptor, KIT, and RET kinase inhibitors), cabozantinib (VEGFR2, Met, and Axl kinase inhibitors), and ramucirumab (VEGF2R monoclonal antibody). Compared with placebo, both regorafenib (RESORCE study) and cabozantinib (CELESTIAL study) have been shown to improve the OS of advanced HCC patients who progressed after first-line sorafenib treatment. In addition, ramucirumab improved the OS of HCC patients who progressed after sorafenib treatment and had alpha-fetoprotein ≥400 ng/mL (REACH-2 study).

ICIs including inhibitors of programmed cell death protein 1 (PD-1) and ligand 1 (PD-L1) have been widely used in the treatment of various advanced malignancies. Based on the results of the CheckMate-040 and Keynote-224 trials, both PD-1 inhibitors nivolumab and pembrolizumab have been approved as the second-line treatments for HCC patients with progressive disease after sorafenib treatment, respectively. However, in the CheckMate-459 and Keynote-240 trials of nivolumab and pembrolizumab as first-line treatments, both PD-1 inhibitors failed to achieve the primary endpoint of improving OS in advanced HCC patients compared with sorafenib, but both showed OS benefits in the patients. The combination of ICIs with TKIs and chemotherapy is also a promising regimen for clinical application. The phase III clinical study IMbrave150 showed that atezolizumab (anti-PD-L1 monoclonal antibody) combined with bevacizumab (anti-VEGF monoclonal antibody) achieved the co-primary endpoints of providing statistically significant and clinically significant improvements in both the OS and PFS of advanced HCC patients compared with sorafenib. In addition, there are several other ongoing clinical trials of combination regimens for advanced HCC, including nivolumab combined with sorafenib (NCT02576509), PD-1/PD-L1 monoclonal antibodies (tislelizumab, camrelizumab, spartalizumab, durvalumab, avelumab, or tremelimumab) combined with TKIs (regorafenib, apatinib, cabozantinib, or sorafenib), PD-1 monoclonal antibody combined with FOLFOX4 chemotherapy, and PD-1 monoclonal antibody combined with CTLA-4 monoclonal antibody (ipilimumab). In HCC, PD-1 monoclonal antibody combined with VEGFR-2 blocker not only promotes normalization of tumor angiogenesis but also enhances tumor antigen exposure and tumor immune responses. In summary, despite the great progress in multimodality treatment and the therapeutic potential of combination therapies in HCC, there are still many shortcomings in multimodality treatment that need to be addressed. For example, molecular markers of effective or ineffective treatment response will need to be identified to help with the development of more precise personalized treatments. In addition, whether there are new and more effective treatment regimens will need to be further investigated.

HCC recurrence and metastasis are multi-step cascades involving many factors. Mutation, amplification, and rearrangement of the genome or insertion of viral genes may lead to dysregulation of pathways related to recurrence and metastasis and hence provide the molecular basis for cancer recurrence and metastasis. Spatial and temporal heterogeneity of tumor cells constitute the biological characteristics of HCC invasion and metastasis, and the tumor microenvironment provides a hotbed for HCC recurrence and metastasis. Further study of the molecular mechanisms of HCC recurrence and metastasis can provide a theoretical basis and new insights into effective clinical treatments for HCC. We believe that HCC can be ultimately cured by a better understanding of the molecular mechanisms of HCC recurrence and metastasis, further improvement of recurrence prediction models, continuous discovery of new anti-cancer targets, advancement of multimodality treatments, and development of tumor vaccines that induce active immunity.

Suggested Reading

1. Siegel RL, Miller KD, Jemal A. Cancer statistics, 2019. CA Cancer J Clin. 2019;69(1):7–34.
2. Villanueva A. Hepatocellular carcinoma. N Engl J Med. 2019;380(15):1450–62.
3. Gupta GP, Massague J. Cancer metastasis: building a framework. Cell. 2006;127(4):679–95.
4. Kim MY, Oskarsson T, Acharyya S, et al. Tumor self-seeding by circulating cancer cells. Cell. 2009;139(7):1315–26.
5. Schulze K, Imbeaud S, Letouze E, et al. Exome sequencing of hepatocellular carcinomas identifies new mutational signatures and potential therapeutic targets. Nat Genet. 2015;47(5):505–11.

6. Zhou SL, Zhou ZJ, Hu ZQ, et al. Genomic sequencing identifies WNK2 as a driver in hepatocellular carcinoma and a risk factor for early recurrence. J Hepatol. 2019;71(6):1152–63.
7. Kan Z, Zheng H, Liu X, et al. Whole-genome sequencing identifies recurrent mutations in hepatocellular carcinoma. Genome Res. 2013;23(9):1422–33.
8. Qiu Z, Li H, Zhang Z, et al. A pharmacogenomic landscape in human liver cancers. Cancer Cell. 2019;36(2):179–93.e111.
9. Chen L, Chan TH, Yuan YF, et al. CHD1L promotes hepatocellular carcinoma progression and metastasis in mice and is associated with these processes in human patients. J Clin Invest. 2010;120(4):1178–91.
10. Liu L, Dai Y, Chen J, et al. Maelstrom promotes hepatocellular carcinoma metastasis by inducing epithelial-mesenchymal transition by way of Akt/GSK-3beta/Snail signaling. Hepatology. 2014;59(2):531–43.
11. Zucman-Rossi J, Villanueva A, Nault JC, et al. Genetic landscape and biomarkers of hepatocellular carcinoma. Gastroenterology. 2015;149(5):1226–39.e1224.
12. Qiao Y, Wang J, Karagoz E, et al. Axis inhibition protein 1 (Axin1) deletion-induced hepatocarcinogenesis requires intact beta-catenin but not Notch cascade in mice. Hepatology. 2019;71(6):1152–63.
13. Sun X, Wang SC, Wei Y, et al. Arid1a has context-dependent oncogenic and tumor suppressor functions in liver cancer. Cancer Cell. 2018;33(1):151–2.
14. Ho DWH, Chan LK, Chiu YT, et al. TSC1/2 mutations define a molecular subset of HCC with aggressive behaviour and treatment implication. Gut. 2017;66(8):1496–506.
15. Shen J, Chen M, Lee D, et al. Histone chaperone FACT complex mediates oxidative stress response to promote liver cancer progression. Gut. 2019;69(2):329–42.
16. Li GX, Ding ZY, Wang YW, et al. Integrative analysis of DNA methylation and gene expression identify a six epigenetic driver signature for predicting prognosis in hepatocellular carcinoma. J Cell Physiol. 2019;234(7):11942–50.
17. Li G, Xu W, Zhang L, et al. Development and validation of a CIMP-associated prognostic model for hepatocellular carcinoma. EBioMedicine. 2019;47:128–41.
18. Lu M, Zhu W, Wang X, et al. ACOT12-dependent alteration of acetyl-CoA drives hepatocellular carcinoma metastasis by epigenetic induction of epithelial-mesenchymal transition. Cell Metab. 2019;29(4):886–900.e885.
19. Chen WX, Zhang ZG, Ding ZY, et al. MicroRNA-630 suppresses tumor metastasis through the TGF-beta-miR-630-Slug signaling pathway and correlates inversely with poor prognosis in hepatocellular carcinoma. Oncotarget. 2016;7(16):22674–86.
20. Zhou SJ, Deng YL, Liang HF, et al. Hepatitis B virus X protein promotes CREB-mediated activation of miR-3188 and Notch signaling in hepatocellular carcinoma. Cell Death Differ. 2017;24(9):1577–87.
21. Leng C, Zhang ZG, Chen WX, et al. An integrin beta4-EGFR unit promotes hepatocellular carcinoma lung metastases by enhancing anchorage independence through activation of FAK-AKT pathway. Cancer Lett. 2016;376(1):188–96.
22. Longerich T, Endris V, Neumann O, et al. RSPO2 gene rearrangement: a powerful driver of beta-catenin activation in liver tumours. Gut. 2019;68(7):1287–96.
23. Chen J, Zhu H, Liu Q, et al. DEPTOR induces a partial epithelial-to-mesenchymal transition and metastasis via autocrine TGFbeta1 signaling and is associated with poor prognosis in hepatocellular carcinoma. J Exp Clin Cancer Res. 2019;38(1):273.
24. Chang L, Azzolin L, di Biagio D, et al. The SWI/SNF complex is a mechanoregulated inhibitor of YAP and TAZ. Nature. 2018;563(7730):265–9.
25. Song J, Zhang X, Liao Z, et al. 14-3-3zeta inhibits heme oxygenase-1 (HO-1) degradation and promotes hepatocellular carcinoma proliferation: involvement of STAT3 signaling. J Exp Clin Cancer Res. 2019;38(1):3.
26. Zhang ZQ, Chen J, Huang WQ, et al. FAM134B induces tumorigenesis and epithelial-to-mesenchymal transition via Akt signaling in hepatocellular carcinoma. Mol Oncol. 2019;13(4):792–810.
27. Huang A, Zhao X, Yang XR, et al. Circumventing intratumoral heterogeneity to identify potential therapeutic targets in hepatocellular carcinoma. J Hepatol. 2017;67(2):293–301.
28. Duan M, Hao J, Cui S, et al. Diverse modes of clonal evolution in HBV-related hepatocellular carcinoma revealed by single-cell genome sequencing. Cell Res. 2018;28(3):359–73.
29. Zhang Q, Lou Y, Yang J, et al. Integrated multiomic analysis reveals comprehensive tumour heterogeneity and novel immunophenotypic classification in hepatocellular carcinomas. Gut. 2019;68(11):2019–31.
30. Ding ZY, Jin GN, Wang W, et al. Reduced expression of transcriptional intermediary factor 1 gamma promotes metastasis and indicates poor prognosis of hepatocellular carcinoma. Hepatology. 2014;60(5):1620–36.
31. Liu Q, Zhang H, Jiang X, et al. Factors involved in cancer metastasis: a better understanding to "seed and soil" hypothesis. Mol Cancer. 2017;16(1):176.
32. Liu C, Liu L, Chen X, et al. LSD1 stimulates cancer-associated fibroblasts to drive Notch3-dependent self-renewal of liver cancer stem-like cells. Cancer Res. 2018;78(4):938–49.
33. Zhu Y, Yang J, Xu D, et al. Disruption of tumour-associated macrophage trafficking by the osteopontin-induced colony-stimulating factor-1 signalling sensitises hepatocellular carcinoma to anti-PD-L1 blockade. Gut. 2019;68(9):1653–66.
34. Li YW, Qiu SJ, Fan J, et al. Intratumoral neutrophils: a poor prognostic factor for hepatocellular carcinoma following resection. J Hepatol. 2011;54(3):497–505.
35. Zhou SL, Dai Z, Zhou ZJ, et al. Overexpression of CXCL5 mediates neutrophil infiltration and indicates poor prognosis for hepatocellular carcinoma. Hepatology. 2012;56(6):2242–54.

36. Gao Q, Zhao YJ, Wang XY, et al. CXCR6 upregulation contributes to a proinflammatory tumor microenvironment that drives metastasis and poor patient outcomes in hepatocellular carcinoma. Cancer Res. 2012;72(14):3546–56.
37. Chiu DK, Tse AP, Xu IM, et al. Hypoxia inducible factor HIF-1 promotes myeloid-derived suppressor cells accumulation through ENTPD2/CD39L1 in hepatocellular carcinoma. Nat Commun. 2017;8(1):517.
38. Zhou SL, Zhou ZJ, Hu ZQ, et al. Tumor-associated neutrophils recruit macrophages and t-regulatory cells to promote progression of hepatocellular carcinoma and resistance to sorafenib. Gastroenterology. 2016;150(7):1646–58.e1617.
39. Zhou SL, Yin D, Hu ZQ, et al. A positive feedback loop between cancer stem-like cells and tumor-associated neutrophils controls hepatocellular carcinoma progression. Hepatology. 2019;70(4):1214–30.
40. Sun T, Sun BC, Zhao XL, et al. Promotion of tumor cell metastasis and vasculogenic mimicry by way of transcription coactivation by Bcl-2 and Twist1: a study of hepatocellular carcinoma. Hepatology. 2011;54(5):1690–706.
41. Renne SL, Woo HY, Allegra S, et al. Vessels encapsulating tumor clusters (VETC) is a powerful predictor of aggressive hepatocellular carcinoma. Hepatology. 2019;71(1):183–95.
42. Dou C, Liu Z, Tu K, et al. P300 acetyltransferase mediates stiffness-induced activation of hepatic stellate cells into tumor-promoting myofibroblasts. Gastroenterology. 2018;154(8):2209–21.e2214.
43. Wong C, Tse AP, Huang YP, et al. Lysyl oxidase-like 2 is critical to tumor microenvironment and metastatic niche formation in hepatocellular carcinoma. Hepatology. 2014;60(5):1645–58.
44. Dapito DH, Mencin A, Gwak GY, et al. Promotion of hepatocellular carcinoma by the intestinal microbiota and TLR4. Cancer Cell. 2012;21(4):504–16.
45. Jia X, Lu S, Zeng Z, et al. Characterization of gut microbiota, bile acid metabolism, and cytokines in intrahepatic cholangiocarcinoma. Hepatology. 2019;71(3):893–906.
46. Hanahan D, Weinberg RA. Hallmarks of cancer: the next generation. Cell. 2011;144(5):646–74.
47. Hainaut P, Plymoth A. Targeting the hallmarks of cancer: towards a rational approach to next-generation cancer therapy. Curr Opin Oncol. 2013;25(1):50–1.
48. Adorno-Cruz V, Kibria G, Liu X, et al. Cancer stem cells: targeting the roots of cancer, seeds of metastasis, and sources of therapy resistance. Cancer Res. 2015;75(6):924–9.
49. Yamashita T, Wang XW. Cancer stem cells in the development of liver cancer. J Clin Invest. 2013;123(5):1911–8.
50. Shan J, Shen J, Liu L, et al. Nanog regulates self-renewal of cancer stem cells through the insulin-like growth factor pathway in human hepatocellular carcinoma. Hepatology. 2012;56(3):1004–14.
51. Yamashita T, Ji J, Budhu A, et al. EpCAM-positive hepatocellular carcinoma cells are tumor-initiating cells with stem/progenitor cell features. Gastroenterology. 2009;136(3):1012–24.
52. Liu S, Li N, Yu X, et al. Expression of intercellular adhesion molecule 1 by hepatocellular carcinoma stem cells and circulating tumor cells. Gastroenterology. 2013;144(5):1031–41.e1010.
53. Zheng H, Pomyen Y, Hernandez MO, et al. Single cell analysis reveals cancer stem cell heterogeneity in hepatocellular carcinoma. Hepatology. 2018;68(1):127–40.
54. Yamashita T, Honda M, Nakamoto Y, et al. Discrete nature of EpCAM+ and CD90+ cancer stem cells in human hepatocellular carcinoma. Hepatology. 2013;57(4):1484–97.
55. Mima K, Okabe H, Ishimoto T, et al. CD44s regulates the TGF-beta-mediated mesenchymal phenotype and is associated with poor prognosis in patients with hepatocellular carcinoma. Cancer Res. 2012;72(13):3414–23.
56. Malfettone A, Soukupova J, Bertran E, et al. Transforming growth factor-beta-induced plasticity causes a migratory stemness phenotype in hepatocellular carcinoma. Cancer Lett. 2017;392:39–50.
57. Lee TK, Castilho A, Cheung VC, et al. CD24(+) liver tumor-initiating cells drive self-renewal and tumor initiation through STAT3-mediated NANOG regulation. Cell Stem Cell. 2011;9(1):50–63.
58. Haraguchi N, Ishii H, Mimori K, et al. CD13 is a therapeutic target in human liver cancer stem cells. J Clin Invest. 2010;120(9):3326–39.
59. Wang Y, He L, Du Y, et al. The long noncoding RNA lncTCF7 promotes self-renewal of human liver cancer stem cells through activation of Wnt signaling. Cell Stem Cell. 2015;16(4):413–25.
60. Yarchoan M, Agarwal P, Villanueva A, et al. Recent developments and therapeutic strategies against hepatocellular carcinoma. Cancer Res. 2019;79(17):4326–30.
61. Huang ZY, Liang BY, Xiong M, et al. Long-term outcomes of repeat hepatic resection in patients with recurrent hepatocellular carcinoma and analysis of recurrent types and their prognosis: a single-center experience in China. Ann Surg Oncol. 2012;19(8):2515–25.
62. Mazzaferro V, Sposito C, Bhoori S, et al. Yttrium-90 radioembolization for intermediate-advanced hepatocellular carcinoma: a phase 2 study. Hepatology. 2013;57(5):1826–37.
63. Yoon SM, Ryoo BY, Lee SJ, et al. Efficacy and safety of transarterial chemoembolization plus external beam radiotherapy vs sorafenib in hepatocellular carcinoma with macroscopic vascular invasion: a randomized clinical trial. JAMA Oncol. 2018;4(5):661–9.
64. Wei X, Jiang Y, Zhang X, et al. Neoadjuvant three-dimensional conformal radiotherapy for resectable hepatocellular carcinoma with portal vein tumor thrombus: a randomized, open-label, multicenter controlled study. J Clin Oncol. 2019;37(24):2141–51.

65. Llovet JM, Ricci S, Mazzaferro V, et al. Sorafenib in advanced hepatocellular carcinoma. N Engl J Med. 2008;359(4):378–90.
66. Kudo M, Finn RS, Qin S, et al. Lenvatinib versus sorafenib in first-line treatment of patients with unresectable hepatocellular carcinoma: a randomised phase 3 non-inferiority trial. Lancet. 2018;391(10126):1163–73.
67. Abou-Alfa GK, Meyer T, Cheng AL, et al. Cabozantinib in patients with advanced and progressing hepatocellular carcinoma. N Engl J Med. 2018;379(1):54–63.
68. El-Khoueiry AB, Sangro B, Yau T, et al. Nivolumab in patients with advanced hepatocellular carcinoma (CheckMate 040): an open-label, non-comparative, phase 1/2 dose escalation and expansion trial. Lancet. 2017;389(10088):2492–502.
69. Shigeta K, Datta M, Hato T, et al. Dual programmed death receptor-1 and vascular endothelial growth factor receptor-2 blockade promotes vascular normalization and enhances antitumor immune responses in hepatocellular carcinoma. Hepatology. 2019;71(4):1247–61.

28 Molecular Targeted Therapy-Based Multimodality Treatments for Liver Cancer

Shuai Xiang

28.1 Background

The success of the Sorafenib Hepatocellular Carcinoma Assessment Randomized Protocol (SHARP) and Asia-Pacific studies marked a new era of molecular targeted therapy for hepatocellular carcinoma (HCC). Since the approval of sorafenib as a first-line treatment for advanced liver cancer by the Food and Drug Administration (FDA) in 2008, more and more advanced liver cancer patients have benefited from sorafenib treatment. In the following decade, a large number of clinical trials had been conducted to explore more effective drugs and treatments. However, none of these trials were able to find a more effective drug than sorafenib. Regorafenib, cabozantinib, ramucirumab, and sunitinib can be used as second-line treatments when sorafenib is intolerable or when the disease progresses after sorafenib treatment. Lenvatinib was shown to be non-inferior to sorafenib in the 2018 Study Assessing the Efficacy and Safety of Lenvatinib in Subjects With Unresectable Hepatocellular Carcinoma (REFLECT) study and was hence approved by the FDA as a first-line treatment for HCC.

According to statistics, less than 20% of HCC patients are suitable for radical surgery at the time of diagnosis, and the 5-year liver cancer recurrence rate after radical resection is up to 60–80%. Therefore, HCC treatment must be a multimodality treatment predominated by surgery. Multimodality treatment is defined as the combination of two or more treatment modalities. There are several treatments for liver cancer, including local therapy and systemic chemotherapy such as surgery, ablation, local radiotherapy, regional chemotherapy, and arterial embolization, as well as systemic therapies such as molecular targeted therapy, immunotherapy, and traditional Chinese medicine treatment. The most common mode of HCC metastasis is transportal dissemination, followed by lung metastasis and bone metastasis. Liver cancer should be considered a systemic disease once it metastasizes, and systemic therapy should play an important role at this stage. The approval of HCC as an indication for sorafenib marks the arrival of a brand new era, and molecular targeted therapy has been actively promoting the development of multimodality treatment for HCC in the past decade.

S. Xiang (✉)
Tongji Hospital Affiliated to Tongji Medical College, Huazhong University of Science & Technology, Wuhan, China

X. Chen (ed.), *Diagnosis and Treatment of Liver Cancer in China*,
https://doi.org/10.1007/978-981-97-7969-7_28

28.2 Exploration of Molecular Targeted Therapy Combined with Interventional Therapy for Liver Cancer

Given the high risk of postoperative recurrence, it is particularly important to seek postoperative adjuvant therapy to reduce the risk of recurrence and improve survival. Sorafenib can be used as a postoperative adjuvant therapy for patients with a high risk of recurrence to inhibit tumor cell proliferation and angiogenesis. Transarterial Chemoembolization (TACE) is an important local treatment for unresectable liver cancer. This procedure blocks the blood supply of a tumor, resulting in tumor ischemic necrosis, and chemotherapeutic drugs are then directly administered to kill the tumor. TACE can prolong the survival of patients despite the difficulty in eradicating the tumor after multiple TACE treatments.

Embolization leads to hypoxia and induces the release of factors related to tumor formation, angiogenesis, and fibrosis. There is evidence indicating that the serum concentrations of major proangiogenic factors such as vascular endothelial growth factor (VEGF) and fibroblast growth factor (FGF) are increased after TACE treatment. Since tumors can still progress and metastasize after TACE and the survival rate of patients is not high, these phenomena may be related to the upregulation of these factors. Given that molecular targeted therapy can improve the overall survival (OS) of advanced liver cancer patients by targeting signal transduction, whether the combination of TACE and anti-angiogenic drugs can improve treatment efficacy has become an important topic of research. However, all clinical trials trying to find the best combination regimen have so far failed.

Orantinib is an oral multikinase inhibitor that targets VEGFR-2 and Platelet-Derived Growth Factor Receptor-β (PDGFR-β). A phase II clinical study showed that orantinib combined with a single TACE may prolong progression-free survival (PFS) despite that the observation was not statistically significant and the OS rate was not improved. A phase III clinical study by Kudo et al. A randomized, double-blind, placebo-controlled phase III clinical study of orantinib combined with TACE in the treatment of unresectable HCC (ORIENTAL) in Japan evaluated the efficacy of orantinib combined with TACE in the treatment of unresectable HCC. This randomized, double-blind, placebo-controlled phase III clinical study was performed across 75 sites in Japan, South Korea, and Taiwan. The interim analysis showed that the combination therapy did not achieve the intended purpose, and the study was considered ineffective and was prematurely terminated. The results indicated that there was no significant difference in OS between the orantinib arm and the placebo arm.

Brivanib, an oral selective dual inhibitor of VEGF and FGF, showed anti-proliferative and anti-angiogenic activities and preliminary efficacy in a phase II clinical trial of advanced liver cancer patients. Another phase III clinical trial by Kudo et al. evaluated whether brivanib combined with TACE can improve the OS rate of HCC patients. This was a multicenter, randomized, double-blinded, placebo-controlled, prospective study of 870 patients with inoperable HCC across 83 medical centers in 12 countries. Since both BRISK-FL and BRISK-PS, phase III clinical trials evaluating brivanib as a first-line and second-line treatment for HCC, respectively, failed to achieve their primary endpoint (i.e., benefiting patients in OS), Kudo et al. terminated the trials 2 years early. By the time of termination, the study had screened 734 patients and randomized 502 patients. The trial results showed that brivanib combined with TACE did not improve the OS of patients compared with TACE alone.

Failure of the phase III clinical study of brivanib monotherapy in HCC seemed to serve as an explanation for the failure of brivanib and TACE combination therapy. The ORIENTAL study of orantinib combined with TACE was also terminated prematurely due to inefficacy. This then raises the question of whether sorafenib, the first-line treatment for advanced liver cancer, can achieve better efficacy in combination with TAC. Researchers have performed extensive research on this topic and conducted numerous large-scale clinical studies in the past decade. Although the conclusions are inconsistent, TACE combined with molecular targeted drugs nevertheless plays an important role in the multimodality treatment of HCC.

The Sorafenib or Placebo Plus Transarterial Chemoembolization With Doxorubicin-Eluting Beads for Intermediate Stage Hepatocellular Carcinoma (SPACE) trial is the first global multicenter, prospective, randomized-controlled, double-blinded phase II clinical study. A total of 307 patients with intermediate-stage HCC were enrolled and randomized into the Drug-Eluting Bead-TACE Plus Sorafenib Versus TACE Alone for the Treatment of Hepatocellular Carcinoma (DEB-TACE) plus sorafenib arm and placebo arm. TACE treatment was given at weeks 1, 9, 25, and 49 and then every 24 weeks thereafter. The primary endpoint of this trial was time to progression (TTP), and the secondary endpoints were OS, time to microvascular invasion or extrahepatic spread, and time to untreatable progression (TTUP) with TACE. The trial failed to achieve the expected TTP and OS, and this failure was thought to be attributed to inappropriate treatment caused by regular TACE, which in turn affected the patient's liver function, and caused the patients to miss the best time for treatment. However, subgroup analysis showed that the Asian population was more likely to benefit from the combination therapy than the non-Asian population, possibly due to the longer duration of medication in the Asian population.

TACTICS, a randomized, open-label, multicenter phase II clinical study led by Japanese investigators, evaluated the efficacy and safety of TACE combined with sorafenib versus TACE alone in the treatment of HCC. In this study, patients with unresectable early-stage and intermediate-stage HCC were enrolled and randomized 1:1 into the TACE arm and TACE plus sorafenib arm. In the combination therapy arm, patients were first given 400 mg/day sorafenib for 2–3 weeks before the first TACE to block angiogenesis-related pathways, and the dose of sorafenib was then increased to 800 mg/day during TACE treatment until TTUP. The primary endpoints of the study were PFS and OS. PFS events were defined as death or time to TTUP. TTUP was defined as the time from the start of oral sorafenib until evidence rendering TACE impossible (untreatable tumor progression, worsening of liver function to Child Pugh C, or vascular invasion/extrahepatic metastasis). The TACTICS study produced encouraging results as PFS was significantly prolonged to 25.2 months in the TACE plus sorafenib arm compared with 13.5 months in the TACE arm (hazard ratio (HR) = 0.59, 95% confidence interval (CI): 0.41–0.87, $P = 0.006$). However, OS benefit was not observed. The study also showed that the combination therapy significantly improved the time to vascular invasion and extrahepatic metastasis. The combination therapy prolonged the time to vascular invasion from 4.0 to 31.3 months (HR = 0.26, 95% CI: 0.09–0.75, $P = 0.008$) and to extrahepatic metastasis from 6.9 to 15.7 months (HR = 0.21, 95% CI: 0.06–0.70, $P = 0.006$). In addition, TACE combined with sorafenib significantly prolonged the TACE treatment interval (21.1 weeks vs. 16.9 weeks, $P = 0.018$). These findings seem to indicate that oral administration of targeted drugs before the start of TACE to maximize exposure to the molecular targeted drugs is the key to patient benefits.

Researchers in China have also dedicated tremendous efforts to exploring effective multimodality regimens for HCC. A multicenter phase III clinical trial led by Professor Shi Ming was conducted at the Sun Yat-sen University Cancer Center. A total of 818 inoperable HCC patients with portal vein invasion were screened and randomized 1:1 into the Folinic Acid, Fluorouracil, and Oxaliplatin (FOLFOX) hepatic arterial infusion chemotherapy plus sorafenib arm and sorafenib monotherapy arm. The results of the study showed that the combination therapy arm had significantly longer mOS (13.37 months vs. 7.13 months, HR = 0.35, $P < 0.001$) and mPFS (7.03 months vs. 2.6 months, $P < 0.001$) compared with the monotherapy arm. The incidence of treatment-related adverse events was overall similar between the two arms.

28.3 Exploration of Molecular Targeted Therapy Combined with Immune Checkpoint Inhibitors in the Treatment of Liver Cancer

A decade after the first clinical application of molecular targeted drugs, increasing attention has been placed on the immune checkpoint inhibitors (ICIs) programmed cell death-ligand 1 (PD-L1)/programmed cell death protein 1 (PD-1) antibodies. Tumor cells can evade immune surveillance by expressing PD-L1 that binds to PD-1 on T cells and inhibiting the transcription of genes and cytokines required for T cell activation and thereby continue to proliferate. As an ICI, PD-1 antibody can block the binding of PD-L1 on tumor cells to PD-1 on T cells, allowing T cells to restore their tumor-killing ability and restart the immune system. Since 2017, nivolumab and pembrolizumab have been successively approved by the FDA as second-line treatments for advanced liver cancer.

Since molecular targeted drugs can inhibit certain signaling pathways and create an immunosuppressive microenvironment, a combination of ICIs and molecular targeted agents can modulate the tumor microenvironment and thereby promote the infiltration of cytotoxic T cells into the tumor tissue. Lenvatinib has demonstrated potent antitumor activity in animals as it can reduce tumor-associated macrophages, increase the percentage of activated $CD8^+$ T cells, and promote the secretion of IFN-γ and granzyme B. Lenvatinib combined with pembrolizumab can further increase the proportion of T cells, especially $CD8^+$ T cells, among CD45+ cells and the frequency of IFN-γ^+ granzyme B^+ $CD8^+$ T cells. The combination therapy arm showed a more robust antitumor activity than the monotherapy arm.

In April 2019, the American Association for Cancer Research published the results of KEYNOTE-524, a phase Ib trial of lenvatinib combined with pembrolizumab in the treatment of advanced liver cancer. Six patients without other appropriate treatment regimens were first enrolled to evaluate dose-limiting toxicity after treatment cycle 1. After establishing the tolerability of lenvatinib combined with pembrolizumab, the second part of the study was performed in 24 systemic therapy-naive patients with unresectable HCC. The patients were treated with lenvatinib (12 mg for ≥60 kg and 8 mg for <60 kg) once daily plus 200 mg/3 weeks of pembrolizumab. Radiographic assessment by an independent third party showed that the overall objective response rate (ORR) was 60.0%, disease control rate was 93.3%, mPFS was 9.7 months, and mOS was 14.6 months. In comparison, the ORR of lenvatinib in the REFLECT study was 24.1%, and the response rate appeared to be significantly improved by lenvatinib and pembrolizumab combination therapy.

On July 23, 2019, the FDA approved lenvatinib plus pembrolizumab with a breakthrough therapy designation (BTD) as a first-line treatment for patients with advanced liver cancer who are not suitable for loco-regional therapy or surgical resection. Although this approval is an affirmation of the efficacy and safety of lenvatinib + K drug (pembrolizumab), it should be noted that this combination therapy has not received the final approval of the FDA. In May 2020, the American Society of Clinical Oncology released updated data showing a 46% ORR and 88% DCR in 100 patients, indicating good treatment efficacy. The value and safety of this combination therapy will need to be further assessed using a larger sample size and a longer follow-up period. The phase III LEAP-002 trial is currently ongoing, and the results are eagerly awaited.

On May 14, 2020, the complete data of the IMbrave150 study were officially published in the New England Journal of Medicine. In the IMbrave150 study, atezolizumab (a PD-L1 inhibitor) combined with bevacizumab (anti-angiogenic targeted drug), namely, the "T+A" regimen, was used as the treatment for advanced liver cancer. The data showed that this regimen significantly prolonged patient OS and PFS, with a 12-month survival rate of 67.2%. This is the first new therapy confirmed by phase III clinical trial to be superior to the existing first-line drug sorafenib in the past decade. Chinese researchers have also made great contributions to this study.

Of the 501 systemic therapy-naive patients with unresectable HCC, 194 were from China. Data from the Chinese subgroup also suggested that the "T+A" regimen may be more suitable for Chinese patients. Chinese patients as a whole have several poor prognostic factors including a high incidence of hepatitis B virus infection, macrovascular invasion/extrahepatic metastasis, and an alpha-fetoprotein ≥400 ng/mL. The study data showed that the HR of OS of Chinese patients was 0.44, and the 6-month survival rate of patients was up to 86.6%, demonstrating that the efficacy of the combination therapy was better in Chinese patients than in the overall study population. The "T+A" regimen is now recommended by many global guidelines as one of the first-line treatment regimens for advanced liver cancer.

A prefix for drug numbers developed by Jiangsu Hengrui Medicine Co., Ltd. (SHR-1210: carrelizumab) SHR-1210 (carrelizumab) is a humanized IgG4 monoclonal antibody drug that acts as a multi-target ICI that targets PD-1 and PD-L1/PD-L2. Basic research showed that SHR-1210 can simultaneously block PD-1 and VEGF receptor 2 in vivo and exhibit synergistic antitumor effects when used in combination with apatinib. In 2018, the results of NCT02942329 led by Chinese researchers were presented for the first time at the annual meeting of the American Society of Clinical Oncology. The phase I clinical trial explored the combined use of SHR-1210 and apatinib in advanced liver cancer, gastric cancer, and esophagogastric junction cancer and achieved encouraging results.

The NCT02942329 study was divided into two phases (Ia and Ib), and the study population was patients with advanced liver cancer who failed sorafenib treatment, as well as patients with gastric cancer and gastroesophageal junction cancer. The purpose of the phase Ia study was to explore the maximum tolerated dose of the combination therapy and provide a basis for the dosage in the phase II trial. The ascending doses of apatinib were set at 125, 250, and 500 mg/day. SHR-1210 was administered at a fixed dose of 200 mg once every 2 weeks. A total of 15 patients were enrolled in the phase Ia study, with 5 patients in each dose arm. Due to the observation of three cases of dose-limiting toxicity in the 500 mg/day dose arm, all of which being grade 3 pneumonia, the subsequent recommended dosages were changed to 250 mg/day of apatinib and 200 mg of SHR-1210 once every 2 weeks. The phase Ib study was aimed to explore the efficacy and safety of the drugs and the results were encouraging. All 18 HCC patients were infected with HBV, including 17 patients in Barcelona Clinic Liver Cancer staging system (BCLC) stage C and 1 in stage B. The 16 HCC patients with evaluable response had 50% ORR, 93.8% disease control rate, 3.4 months of mean wait time for response, and 5.8 months of mPFS. The response rate of liver cancer patients was not more than 10% to apatanib and about 10% to PD-1 antibody. However, the ORR of apatinib and PD-1 combination therapy was 50% in advanced liver cancer, indicating that the combination therapy has a two-way synergistic effect. This efficacy was comparable to that in the KEYNOTE-524 study. It is worth noting that Barcelona Clinic Liver Cancer staging system (BCLC) stage C patients accounted for up to 94.4% in this study but only 70% in KEYNOTE-524. In addition, the incidence of serious adverse events was lower in this study than in KEYNOTE-524, and no treatment-related deaths were observed. The global multicenter phase III study (NCT03764293) of SHR-1210 combined with apatinib as the first-line treatment for advanced liver cancer has now been approved, and further confirmation of the efficacy and safety of this combination therapy is highly anticipated.

It is expected that the combination of ICI and molecular targeted agents will play an important role in the multimodality treatment of advanced liver cancer. However, how to identify biomarkers that predict the efficacy of molecular targeted drugs combined with immunotherapy remains unresolved in HCC immunotherapy, and further studies are warranted.

28.4 Summary

Molecular targeted therapy has brought increasing hope to advanced liver cancer patients since its development over the past decade. However, the efficacy of molecular targeted therapy is still limited and far from meeting the needs of patients. Multimodality treatment combining molecular targeted therapy has improved this situation. After extensive exploration, the TACTICS study finally established the efficacy of TACE combined with sorafenib in the treatment of liver cancer. The efficacy of ICIs in the treatment of liver cancer has gained increasing attention in recent years. There is growing evidence suggesting that the combination of ICIs and molecular targeted agents will play an important role in the multimodality treatment of advanced liver cancer.

Suggested Reading

1. Lee JH, Lee JH, Lim YS, et al. Sustained efficacy of adjuvant immunotherapy with cytokine-induced killer cells for hepatocellular carcinoma: an extended 5-year follow-up. Cancer Immunol Immunother. 2019;68:23–32.
2. Takayama T, Sekine T, Makuuchi M, et al. Adoptive immunotherapy to lower postsurgical recurrence rates of hepatocellular carcinoma: a randomised trial. Lancet. 2000;356:802–7.
3. Lee JH, Lee JH, Lim YS, et al. Adjuvant immunotherapy with autologous cytokine-induced killer cells for hepatocellular carcinoma. Gastroenterology. 2015;148:1383–91.
4. Park JW, Finn RS, Kim JS, et al. Phase II, open-label study of brivanib as first-line therapy in patients with advanced hepatocellular carcinoma. Clin Cancer Res. 2011;17:1973–83.
5. Finn RS, Kang YK, Mulcahy M, et al. Phase II, open-label study of brivanib as second-line therapy in patients with advanced hepatocellular carcinoma. Clin Cancer Res. 2012;18:2090–8.
6. Kudo M, Han G, Finn RS, et al. Brivanib as adjuvant therapy to transarterial chemoembolization in patients with hepatocellular carcinoma: a randomized phase III trial. Hepatology. 2014;60:1697–707.
7. Lencioni R, Llovet JM, Han G, et al. Sorafenib or placebo plus TACE with doxorubicin-eluting beads for intermediate stage HCC: the SPACE trial. J Hepatol. 2016;64:1090–8.
8. He M, Li Q, Zou R, et al. Sorafenib plus hepatic arterial infusion of oxaliplatin, fluorouracil, and leucovorin vs sorafenib alone for hepatocellular carcinoma with portal vein invasion: a randomized clinical trial. JAMA Oncol. 2019;5:953–60.
9. Kato Y, Tabata K, Kimura T, et al. Lenvatinib plus anti-PD-1 antibody combination treatment activates CD8+ T cells through reduction of tumor-associated macrophage and activation of the interferon pathway. PLoS One. 2019;14:e0212513.
10. Finn RS, Qin S, Ikeda M, et al. Atezolizumab plus bevacizumab in unresectable hepatocellular carcinoma. N Engl J Med. 2020;382:1894–905.
11. Xu J, Zhang Y, Jia R, et al. Anti-PD-1 antibody SHR-1210 combined with apatinib for advanced hepatocellular carcinoma, gastric, or esophagogastric junction cancer: an open-label, dose escalation and expansion study. Clin Cancer Res. 2019;25:515–23.

29 Active Roles of Underlying Liver Disease Management, Liver Function Protection, and Traditional Chinese Medicine Treatment in the Multimodality Treatment of Liver Cancer

Binhao Zhang

Surgical resection is still the treatment of choice for liver cancer patients. In fact, surgical resection and liver transplantation are currently the only curative options for liver cancer. However, not all patients are suitable for surgical treatment since liver cancer generally develops from cirrhosis, and patients with severe cirrhosis are prone to liver failure after surgical resection. Furthermore, underlying liver disease in some patients is far more life-threatening than liver cancer itself. Therefore, in addition to invasive treatments such as surgery, transcatheter arterial chemoembolization (TACE), ablation, targeted therapy, and immunotherapy, underlying liver disease management, liver function protection, and traditional Chinese medicine (TCM) treatment are also important for patients with liver cancer. These treatments can improve the general conditions of patients and provide them with more opportunities for liver cancer treatments. Perioperative treatment of surgical patients, multimodality treatment of non-surgical patients, and palliative treatment of end-stage patients are all significant effective means.

B. Zhang (✉)
Tongji Hospital Affiliated to Tongji Medical College, Huazhong University of Science & Technology, Wuhan, China

29.1 Management of Underlying Liver Diseases

Chronic liver diseases such as hepatitis B virus (HBV) and hepatitis C virus (HCV) infections as well as cirrhosis are the main risk factors for the development of liver cancer (Table 29.1). These underlying liver diseases have a significant impact on the development, progression, and prognosis of liver cancer. Aside from liver cancer treatments, treatments for underlying liver diseases are important in reducing the development of liver cancer and controlling postoperative recurrence. The top priority for the treatment of underlying liver disease is to control the cause, such as providing antiviral therapy for viral infections. Long-term treatments to control of inflammation and fibrosis are also required.

Antiviral therapies such as nucleos(t)ide analogs are important for patients with HBV infection and active viral replication. The use of potent drugs with a low risk of resistance, such as entecavir, tenofovir disoproxil, or telbivudine, is recommended. For HCV-related liver cancer, pegylated interferon-α combined with ribavirin or antiviral therapy is recommended. Administration of antiviral drugs before the start of surgery or TACE is recommended as these therapies may cause active HBV replication. Since antiviral therapy can reduce the postopera-

X. Chen (ed.), *Diagnosis and Treatment of Liver Cancer in China*,
https://doi.org/10.1007/978-981-97-7969-7_29

Table 29.1 Epidemiological data of hepatectomy for liver cancer across 112 sites in China

	Value (n = 18,275)
Age (years)	51.7 ± 11.94
Sex (male), no. (%)	15,351 (84)
HBsAg positive, no. (%)	12,838 (80.50)
HCV, no. (%)	503 (3.84)
Liver cirrhosis, no. (%)	
Without	2756 (19.88)
Slight	23 (42.95)
Moderate	35 (28.33)
Severe	29 (8.85)
Portal hypertension, no. (%)	1203 (8.00)
Number of tumors, no. (%)	
0	10 (0.10)
1	11,238 (80.73)
2	1956 (14.05)
≥3	716 (5.14)
AFP, no. (%)	
<20	5217 (38.11)
20–400	4756 (34.74)
≥400	3718 (27.16)
Modified Child-Pugh stage, no. (%)	
A	14,165 (88.59)
B	1750 (10.94)
C	75 (0.47)

Source: Zhang B, Zhang Z, Huang Z, et al. 42573 cases of hepatectomy in China: a multicenter retrospective investigation. Sci China Life Sci, 2018, 61:660–670

tive recurrence rate, it is recommended throughout the course of liver cancer treatment.

29.2 Antiviral Therapy for HBV Infection

HBV infection is the main cause of liver cancer in China and is prevalent in over 80% of liver cancer patients (Table 29.1). In China, there are about 300,000 new HBV-related liver cancer patients each year. Approximately 60% of liver cancer cases in the world are caused by HBV infection.

The progression of chronic hepatitis B depends on the host and viral conditions, and hepatitis B patients are at risk of developing cirrhosis and liver cancer. Liver fibrosis, liver cirrhosis, and portal hypertension caused by hepatitis B are important factors that must be considered in the treatment of liver cancer. Many clinical studies have been conducted in recent years to investigate the timing and duration of antiviral therapy and the role of perioperative antiviral therapy in liver cancer patients with HBV infection. Control of HBV infection helps control the development and progression of liver cancer. For patients undergoing surgical resection, control of hepatitis B is also helpful in reducing postoperative recurrence and improving prognosis. Lifelong antiviral therapy is currently recommended for liver cancer patients with HBV infection. For perioperative management of liver cancer patients, HBV needs to be controlled within a safe range. Surgical treatment should be performed with caution in patients with a high viral load as HBV outbreak may lead to liver failure.

High HBV viral load and liver inflammation are closely associated with post-hepatectomy liver failure. Hepatectomy may activate HBV replication in patients with HBV infection, especially in those who have not received antiviral therapy. Postoperative HBV outbreak may lead to irreversible liver failure even in those with good preoperative liver function.

Alanine aminotransferase generally increases quickly after hepatectomy and then gradually decreases to the preoperative level. An acute outbreak of chronic HBV may occur if alanine aminotransferase continues to rise after surgery and HBV DNA load is >10^4 copies/mL for more than 2 weeks. These in turn may lead to liver failure, hepatic encephalopathy, hepatorenal syndrome, hepatopulmonary syndrome, or death-causing co-infections. Clinical studies have shown that active hepatitis, preoperative HBV load >10^4 copies/mL, and no preoperative antiviral therapy are independent risk factors for post-hepatectomy complications in liver cancer (Tables 29.2 and 29.3). For liver cancer patients with HBV infection, postoperative liver function recovery is significantly worse in those who did not receive perioperative antiviral therapy than in those who did. Postoperative viral DNA load may significantly increase in patients without preoperative

Table 29.2 Relationship between anti-HBV therapy and incidence of post-hepatectomy complication in liver cancer

Variable	Antiviral group (n = 72)	Control group (n = 40)	P value
Type of hepatectomy, n (%)			0.535
Left lateral hepatectomy	15 (20.8)	7 (17.5)	
Left hepatectomy	12 (16.7)	6 (15.0)	
Right hepatectomy	26 (36.1)	14 (35.0)	
Bi/Trisegmentectomy	19 (26.4)	13 (32.5)	
Surgery duration (min)	216 ± 57	226 ± 54	0.445
Intraoperative blood loss (mL)	389 ± 214	374 ± 182	0.719
Blood transfusion, n (%)	7 (9.7)	3 (7.5)	0.961
Packets red cell (mL)	642 ± 269	1000 ± 529	0.258
Postoperative complications, n (%)	25 (34.7)	30 (75.0)	<0.01
Exacerbation of chronic hepatitis B	0 (0)	6 (15.0)	<0.01
Hepatic insufficiency	1 (1.4)	5 (12.5)	<0.05
Hepatic encephalopathy	1 (1.4)	4 (10.0)	<0.05
Hepatorenal syndrome	0 (0)	3 (7.5)	<0.05
Ascites	17 (23.6)	24 (60.0)	<0.01
Bile leakage	4 (5.6)	2 (5.0)	0.913
Hemorrhage/reoperation	0 (0)	0 (0)	
Other complications/case	2 (2.8)	3 (7.5)	0.246
Classification of surgical complication			<0.05
Grade I	19	9	
Grade II	5	14	
Grade III	1	7	
Hospital stay (days)	16 ± 3	24 ± 8	<0.05

Source: Zhang B, Xu D, Wang R, et al. Perioperative antiviral therapy improves safety in patients with hepatitis B related HCC following hepatectomy. Int J Surg, 2015, 15:1–5

Table 29.3 Multivariate analysis of factors associated with complications

	Odds ratio (95% CI)	P value
$G_{3–4}S_{1–4}$ staging	10.89 (3.74–31.71)	<0.01
Preoperative HBV DNA >10^4 copies/mL	1.68 (0.34–8.27)	0.521
No antiviral therapy	5.25 (1.33–20.72)	<0.05

Source: Zhang B, Xu D, Wang R, et al. Perioperative antiviral therapy improves safety in patients with hepatitis B related HCC following hepatectomy. Int J Surg, 2015, 15:1–5

antiviral therapy, suggesting HBV activation or even an outbreak. These phenomena may be attributed to the inhibitory effect of major surgery on the immune functions of patients, which in turn may lead to HBV activation.

Hepatitis B treatment is aimed to prolong survival and improve quality of life by controlling HBV titer and preventing HBV-induced liver cancer. In addition, the treatment also prevents mother-to-child transmission, HBV activation, and extrahepatic symptoms. The selection of treatment regimens depends on various factors such as the natural course of viral infection, stage of disease development, and age of the patient. Treatments for HBV-related liver cancer are described below.

For HBV-related liver cancer, the purpose of antiviral therapy with nucleotide analogs is to first stabilize HBV-induced liver fibrosis and prevent its progression by inhibiting viral replication, and second to reduce the risk of recurrence after liver cancer treatment. It is worth noting that stabilizing HBV-induced liver fibrosis and preventing its progression are prerequisites for the safety and efficacy of liver cancer treatment. For patients with acute or subacute hepatitis B, the primary objective is to prevent and treat liver failure. The European Association for the Study of the Liver (EASL) and the American Association for the Study of Liver Diseases (AASLD) have established specific requirements for HBV antiviral therapy in terms of viral DNA load, transaminase level, degree of liver fibrosis, HBV surface antigen expression, extrahepatic symptoms, and medical history. However, treatments for HBV-related liver cancer have the following characteristics: (1) Most patients have varying degrees of liver cirrhosis; (2) treatment of liver cancer requires treatment of underlying liver diseases to provide assurance in safety and efficacy, and hepatitis B treatment is not only an etiological treatment but also a prerequisite for liver cancer treatment; (3) the systemic and immune effects liver cancer treatments have may potentially activate HBV or even cause hepatitis outbreak, leading to liver failure and treatment failure; (4) liver cancer patients often have a history of standard or non-standard antiviral therapy at the time of diagnosis, but for hepatitis B patients with a low viral DNA load, antiviral therapy can still reduce the recurrence of liver cancer; and (5) surgical resection is the most important and effective treatment for liver cancer, and the importance of perioperative antiviral therapy is gradually being recognized. In summary, lifelong antiviral therapy is recommended for liver cancer patients with HBV infection.

Treatments for hepatitis B patients mainly include oral nucleos(t)ide analogs and interferon for injection. Nucleos(t)ide analogs mainly include lamivudine, adefovir dipivoxil, entecavir, telbivudine, tenofovir disoproxil fumarate, and tenofovir alafenamide fumarate. Entecavir, tenofovir disoproxil fumarate and tenofovir alafenamide fumarate have a strong barrier, while lamivudine, adefovir dipivoxil, and telbivudine have a weak barrier to HBV drug resistance. For liver cancer patients with HBV infection, oral nucleos(t)ide analogs are recommended as antiviral therapy in the "Guidelines for the Diagnosis and Treatment of Primary Liver Cancer (2019 Edition)" of China. Use of potent drugs with a low risk of resistance such as entecavir, tenofovir disoproxil, or telbivudine, is recommended. Entecavir and tenofovir disoproxil are the recommended first-line anti-hepatitis B drugs due to their low drug resistance and high potency in viral control. Due to their potent antiviral effects, these two drugs can effectively improve liver function and reduce or delay the development of HBV-related liver diseases.

It is important to monitor disease progression and perform drug resistance testing during the course of antiviral therapy. HBV drug resistance is closely related to the high baseline level of HBV DNA, a slow decline in DNA load, and previous use of low-grade nucleoside analogs. Appropriate adjustments to the regimen should be made based on the results of HBV DNA detection and drug-resistant mutation.

29.3 Treatment of HCV Infection

Hepatitis C is one of the leading causes of chronic liver disease in the world. There are currently over 71 million chronic hepatitis C cases worldwide, and many of these cases are not aware that they are HCV carriers. As liver damage caused by chronic hepatitis C can develop into cirrhosis or even liver cancer, hepatitis C treatment is important in the treatment of underlying diseases of liver cancer. HCV has a higher chronicity rate than HBV. Hepatitis C may cause extrahepatic damage in addition to liver damage, including insulin resistance and diabetes. In addition, there may still be extrahepatic clinical manifestations after HCV clearance. Since alcohol consumption may accelerate the progression of cirrhosis, ethanol intake should be limited in hepatitis C patients. All patients suspected of HCV infection should be tested for serum anti-HCV antibodies and further tested for HCV RNA. The degree of liver fibrosis should be assessed in hepatitis C patients, including liver biopsy, measurement of fibrosis parameters, ultrasound, and liver elasticity measurement.

The primary treatment for HCV infection is antiviral therapy as hepatitis C is nowadays a curable disease. The World Health Organization expects to eliminate hepatitis C worldwide by 2030, but current hepatitis C treatments are still faced with the problems of high cost and drug resistance. The primary goal of hepatitis C treatment is to control viral infection and achieve sustained virological response (SVR), which is the absence of HCV RNA at 12 weeks (SVR12) and 24 weeks (SVR24) after treatment. A further goal of treatment is to prevent the development of liver injury, liver fibrosis, and liver cancer. Antiviral therapy is required for patients who are positive for the quantitative HCV test (HCV RNA quantification). Interferon combined with ribavirin is the typical treatment for hepatitis C. Interferons, including general interferon and long-acting interferon, can effectively cure hepatitis C, but the disease may recur in some patients after interferon treatment. In addition, interferons have greater side effects in some special patients, which affects the wide application of this regimen.

New drugs approved for marketing in Europe and the United States in recent years include protease inhibitors, such as boceprevir, telaprevir, and simeprevir, and NS5B nucleotide polymerase inhibitors, such as sofosbuvir. The use of new oral anti-HCV drugs has increased SVR from 40% to 70%. Early viral clearance helps shorten the treatment course and improve the response rate of patients who previously failed interferon plus ribavirin combination therapy. These direct-acting antivirals have improved the SVR to genotype 1 to over 90%. Continuous HCV clearance also indicates that hepatitis C is cured etiologically. Sofosbuvir requires only 12 weeks of treatment to achieve viral clearance and is equally effective against genotypes 1, 2, 3, and 4.

However, since these new drugs have not yet been marketed in China, the main treatment for hepatitis C is still the typical interferon plus ribavirin combination regimen. Attention should be paid to drug resistance and side effects during HCV treatment. Follow-up of liver diseases and detection of liver fibrosis should be performed. Patients should undergo regular ultrasound and computed tomography examination to facilitate early detection of cirrhosis and liver cancer.

29.4 Treatment of Cirrhosis

The natural course of cirrhosis is characterized by a transition from the compensated stage to a decompensated stage, and the disease is typically manifested as ascites, gastrointestinal bleeding, jaundice, and hepatic encephalopathy. Approximately 5–7% of cirrhosis patients progress from the compensated stage to the decompensated stage every year, resulting in dysfunction of multiple organs or systems. Treatment in the decompensated stage is aimed to control cirrhosis progression rather than to merely control corresponding complications. The ultimate goal of treatment is to protect the intactness of the liver structure by controlling the etiology, reducing inflammation, stopping liver fibrosis, and restoring cell function and number. However, there is currently no treatment regimen that can achieve these objectives. A few anti-inflammatory and anti-fibrotic drugs have demonstrated some efficacy in animals, but there is still no effective drug for clinical application. Therefore, cirrhosis treatments mainly include treatments for the cause of the disease and treatments for factors related to the progression of cirrhosis.

Effective control of etiology may improve the outcome of compensated cirrhosis and prevent the occurrence of decompensated cirrhosis. For hepatitis B-related cirrhosis, effective antiviral therapy can improve the prognosis of some cirrhosis patients, but it is not effective for all patients. Similarly, while antiviral therapy can improve liver function, mitigate portal hypertension, and improve the outcome of hepatitis C-related cirrhosis, it is only effective in some patients. For alcoholic cirrhosis, the cause of the disease needs to be eliminated by quitting in order to mitigate cirrhosis progression. Whether other etiological treatments can improve cirrhosis progression is unknown, but treatment of autoimmune liver disease may be helpful.

Treatments for factors related to cirrhosis progression mainly include: (1) Antibiotics for intestinal and hepatic circulation disorders (e.g., rifaximin); rifaximin has been reported in some retrospective studies and case reports to improve other complications of cirrhosis except hepatic encephalopathy; (2) long-term albumin infusion to improve circulatory and renal functions; (3) use of statins to reduce the inflammatory response and decrease portal venous pressure in order to improve the survival of patients with advanced liver cirrhosis; and (4) use of β-blockers to potentially benefit patients with decompensated cirrhosis by reducing portal venous pressure. Theoretically, anticoagulation therapy can reduce the risk of portal vein thrombosis and reduce portal venous pressure. However, due to the particularity of the risk of gastrointestinal bleeding in patients with cirrhosis, this treatment is still controversial.

Other treatments for cirrhosis are mainly aimed at the treatment of complications of cirrhosis, including control of ascites, management of gastrointestinal bleeding, treatment of jaundice, and mitigation of hepatic encephalopathy. These symptomatic treatments do not have a substantial effect on the process of cirrhosis but are mainly aimed to improve the quality of life of patients and provide an opportunity for treatment. For liver cancer patients with cirrhosis, treatment of decompensated cirrhosis is often more difficult than treatment of tumors.

29.5 Protection of Liver Function

Focus should be placed on the protection of live function in liver cancer patients as they may have abnormal liver function during the natural course of the disease or during treatment. A good lifestyle is also important in addition to the use of liver-protecting drugs. Liver cancer patients should avoid heavy physical labor, especially those with superficial liver tumors due to the risk of tumor rupture and bleeding after heavy physical work. These patients can engage in lighter activities. Patients should get enough rest after hepatectomy, maintain good sleep quality, and avoid excessive physical exertion. Patients should consume a bland diet with low sugar, high vitamins, and the appropriate amount of high-quality protein, avoid foods that are irritating, hard, and rough, and refrain from using liver-damaging drugs.

As invasive treatment for liver cancer is based on sufficient liver function reserve, liver function protection is an important basis for liver cancer treatment. Liver function protection is also critical in reducing the incidence of perioperative complications and mortality in hepatectomy. For surgical treatments of liver cancer, including surgical resection, ablation, and TACE, strict preoperative evaluation, precise intraoperative procedures, and active treatment of postoperative complications are the safety guarantees for surgical treatments. Liver function protection should be implemented through the perioperative period.

There are a wide variety of hepatoprotective drugs, including: (1) anti-inflammatory hepatoprotective drugs, such as glycyrrhizic acid preparations; (2) phospholipid drugs, such as polyene phosphatidylcholine; (3) detoxification drugs, such as glutathione and glucuronic acid; (4) cholagogues, such as ademetionine and ursodeoxycholic acid; (5) drugs that improve liver energy metabolism, such as vitamins and coenzymes; (6) aminotransferase-lowering drugs, such as bifendate and bicyclol; and (7) biological agents, such as hepatocyte growth factors. These drugs can protect liver function, increase treatment safety, reduce complications, and improve quality of life.

29.6 Traditional Chinese Medicine

TCM treatment can improve symptoms, increase the body's immunity, reduce the side effects of chemotherapy or radiation therapy, and improve the quality of life. In addition to the use of traditional syndrome differentiation and treatment as well as decoctions, China has approved a number of modern TCM preparations for the treatment of liver cancer, all of which have shown good efficacy, patient adherence, safety, and tolerability. TCM treatments have gained increasing attention in recent years, and there are clinical reports with high levels of evidence worldwide. Many studies have confirmed that TCM has its unique advantages in liver protection and fibrosis prevention and can play an effective role in the treatment of primary liver cancer-related underlying liver diseases. There are also several reports on the role and biological mechanism of TCM-based anti-tumor therapy, including the regulation of signaling pathways, tumor angiogenesis, cell cycle regulation, invasion and migration, tumor immune regulation, and cancer stem cells.

TCM has a long history of being used as an anti-tumor treatment, and the guidelines for TCM diagnosis and treatment of tumors have been developed using international standards and applied to modern clinical treatment. Recurrence and metastasis of liver cancer are the main causes of death after invasive treatments, especially surgical treatments. Even for early liver cancer, the 5-year recurrence rate is as high as 70%. TCM plays an important role in the multimodality treatment of liver cancer due to its advantages in systemic conditioning, low toxicity, liver protection, and fibrosis prevention.

Liver cancer is a malignant disease characterized by a deficiency of qi and blood in the viscera as the root cause, and mutual interactions among phlegm, heat, blood stasis, and toxicity as the syndrome, along with tangible nodules in the liver that lead to liver dysfunction manifested as swelling and pain in the right flank, weight loss, loss of appetite, fatigue, and even jaundice, coma, and mass in the right flank.

Similar records about liver cancer can be found as early as in "The Yellow Emperor's Inner Canon" and the disease was described as a lump in the left hypochondrium, jaundice, pneumatosis, abdominal mass, and tympanites in ancient China. The symptoms described are similar to those of liver cancer, and there were meticulous observations on the difficulty in early diagnosis of liver cancer, rapid clinical progression, cachexia in the advanced stage, and poor prognosis. For treatment, emphasis was laid not only on the principle of medication based on syndrome differentiation but also on disease differentiation and flexibility.

29.6.1 Syndrome Differentiation and Treatment

1. Key points of syndrome differentiation
   (a) Differentiation of deficiency and excess: Deficiency in origin and excess in superficiality are extremely obvious in the patient. Deficiency in origin is manifested as fatigue and lassitude, gradual weight loss, sallow complexion, shortness of breath, and laziness to speak. Excess in superficiality is manifested as hard masses in the right flank and even jaundice, and abdominal distension.
   (b) Differentiation of critical syndrome: Coma, hematemesis, hematochezia, hydrothorax, and ascites can be observed in the advanced stage.
2. Principle of treatment: Given the root cause of deficiency of qi and blood in viscera and symptoms of mutual interactions among phlegm, heat, blood stasis, and toxicity, treatment should strengthen the body's immunity, eliminate pathogenic factors, and target both symptoms and root causes to restore liver function, ensure smooth qi and blood circulation, and discharge dampness-heat and stasis in order to improve and alleviate the condition. Treatments for symptoms are aimed to soothe the liver and regulate qi, promote blood circulation and remove blood stasis, clear away heat and dampness, purge fire and detoxify, and eliminate accumulation and dissipate mass. The rational combination of liver soothing and qi-regulating treatments should be considered. On the contrary, treatments for root causes are aimed to invigorate the spleen and supplement qi, nourish blood, soothe the liver, and supplement yin fluid. The relations between "vital qi" and "evil qi" and between "attack" and "supplement" should be properly balanced based on the course of disease and the general conditions of the patient. What also needs to be noted is that attacking medicines such as toxic products from insects should not be used too much. Otherwise, although it may be quick to relieve the disease, it may deplete vital qi and aggravate the condition. The use of Chinese herbal medicines with anti-liver cancer effect is preferred on top of syndrome differentiation and treatment in order to strengthen the specificity of treatments.

29.6.2 Differentiation of Syndromes

29.6.2.1 Stagnation of Liver Qi

Symptoms: Distending pain and mass in the right flank, chest tightness, deep sighing, poor appetite, occasional diarrhea, irregular menstruation, thin greasy tongue coating, and taut pulse.

Treatment: Sooth liver, invigorate spleen, promote blood circulation, and remove blood stasis.

Prescription: Chaihu Shugan powder.

In the prescription, radix bupleuri, fructus aurantii, rhizoma cyperi, and pericarpium citri reticulatae are for soothing the liver and rectifying qi; Rhizoma chuanxiong is for promoting blood circulation and removing blood stasis; and radix paeoniae alba and radix glycyrrhizae are for calming the liver and relieving tension. Radix curcumae and corydalis tuber may be added to promote blood circulation and relieve pain if the latter is obvious. If there are masses in the right blank, curcuma zedoary, peach kernel, pinellia, and *Fritillaria thunbergii* may be added to remove blood stasis and resolve hard lumps. For those with a poor appetite, codonopsis pilosula, atractylodes macrocephala, semen coicis, and shenqu may be added to promote appetite and invigorate the spleen.

29.6.2.2 Qi Stagnation and Blood Stasis

Symptoms: Tremendous right flank pain (dull and stabbing pain) especially at night that can extend to the shoulders and back; large and hard lumps in the right flank or even in the left flank; and sallow complexion, fatigue, abdominal distension, yellow skin, exposed veins, loss of appetite, loose stool, irregular menstruation, dark purple tongue with petechiae, and taut and sluggish pulse.

Treatment: Promote qi, activate blood circulation, and disperse blood stasis.

Prescription: Fuyuan Huoxue Decoction.

Peach kernel, safflower, and rhubarb for promoting blood circulation and dispersing blood stasis; Radices trichosanthis for "eliminating blood stasis"; Angelica for invigorating and nourishing blood; Radix bupleuri for promoting qi and soothing the liver; Pangolin for clearing the liver veins; and licorice for relieving pain. *Rhizoma sparganii*, curcuma zedoary, corydalis tuber, radix curcumae, hirudo, and Chinese Polyphaga may be added to enhance blood circulation, relieve pain, and disperse blood stasis. Biejiajian Pills or Dahuang Zhechong Pills may be added to remove qi stagnation.

For patients with bulging abdominal distension, sallow complexion, and exposed veins, euphorbia kansui, euphorbia pekinensis, and lilac daphne flower bud may be added to create a purging drink or a nutrient-regulating drink can be used to promote blood circulation, remove blood stasis, activate qi and excrete water.

29.6.2.3 Damp Heat and Toxins

Symptoms: Right flank pain that extends to the shoulders and back, right flank lumps, yellow eyes, dry mouth and bitter taste, upset and irritable, poor appetite, abdominal fullness and distention, dry and hard stool, scanty dark urine, red tongue, yellow greasy tongue coating, taut, and slippery pulse.

Treatment: Clear heat, promote bile flow, purge fire, and remove toxin.

Prescription: Yinchenhao Decoction.

Capillary artemisia, *Gardenia jasminoides*, and *Rheum officinale* can clear away heat and dampness, promote bile flow, and reduce jaundice. *Hedyotis diffusa*, *Scutellaria baicalensis*, and dandelion are often added to clear heat, purge fire, and detoxify. For patients with obvious pain, radix bupleuri, rhizoma cyperi, and rhizoma corydalis can be added to soothe the liver, regulate qi, promote blood circulation, and relieve pain.

29.6.2.4 Deficiency of Liver Yin

Symptoms: Hypochondriac pain, hard flank lumps, upset, tidal fever and night sweating, dizziness, loss of appetite, abdominal distension, and even hematemesis, hematochezia, subcutaneous bleeding, red tongue with little coating, and thin and weak pulse.

Treatment: Nourish blood, soothe liver, and remove pathogenic heat from the blood and toxins from the body.

Prescription: Yiguan Decoction.

Rhizome of rehmannia, angelica sinensis, and matrimony vine are for nourishing the yin and blood in the liver and kidney; *Adenophora stricta* and *Ophiopogon japonicus* are for nourishing the yin of the lung and stomach; and szechwan Chinaberry fruit is for dispersing stagnated liver qi and relieve depression. In the case of bleeding, *Agrimonia pilosa*, *Rhizoma imperatae*, and cortex moutan may be added to cool blood and stop bleeding. For patients with jaundice, Yinchenhao decoction may be used in conjunction to promote bile flow and reduce jaundice.

For those with long-term liver yin deficiency affecting kidney yin, turtle shell, tortoise plastron, glossy privet fruit, and *Eclipta alba* may be added to nourish kidney yin and clear asthenic fever. For those with long-term kidney yin deficiency resulting in yin-yang deficiency, which is manifested as intolerance to cold, abdominal distension, edema, backache, and knee weakness, Jinkui Shenqi Pills may be used to nourish kidney yang.

Chinese herbal medicines with anti-liver cancer effect should be used on top of syndrome differentiation and treatment, including *Hedyotis diffusa*, *Scutellaria barbata*, Chinese lobelia, *Polygonum bistorta*, Indian strawberry, verbena, phoenix-tail fern, lithospermum, radix *Sophorae flavescentis*, dandelion, Paris polyphylla, wild chrysanthemum flower, herba sarcandrae, selfheal, and so on to clear away heat and toxic materials; setose thistle, china root greenbrier, euonymus alatus, Chinese Polyphaga, *Polygonum cuspidatum*, *Salvia miltiorrhiza*, *Rhizoma sparganii*, fructus polygoni orientalis, and leech to promote blood circulation and remove blood stasis. Seaweed, selfheal, and oyster and be used to resolve hard lumps.

For patients who are complicated with blood syndrome, jaundice, coma, or abdominal distension, syndrome differentiation and treatment can be performed by referring to the relevant chapters. Patients who are critically ill must be treated through the integration of TCM and Western medicine.

Suggested Reading

1. Ercolani G, Grazi GL, Ravaioli M, et al. Liver resection for hepatocellular carcinoma on cirrhosis: univariate and multivariate analysis of risk factors for intrahepatic recurrence. Ann Surg. 2003;237:536–43.
2. Dusheiko G. Candidates for therapy: HBV. J Hepatol. 2006;44:S84–9.
3. Chen CJ, Yang HI, Su J, et al. Risk of hepatocellular carcinoma across a biological gradient of serum hepatitis B virus DNA level. JAMA. 2006;295:65–73.
4. Zhang B, Zhang Z, Huang Z, et al. 42573 cases of hepatectomy in China: a multicenter retrospective investigation. Sci China Life Sci. 2018;61:660–70.
5. Lai CL, Ratziu V, Yuen MF, et al. Viral hepatitis B. Lancet. 2003;362:2089–94.
6. European Association for the Study of the Liver. EASL 2017 clinical practice guidelines on the management of hepatitis B virus infection. J Hepatol. 2017;67:370–98.
7. Grazi GL, Cescon M, Ravaioli M, et al. Liver resection for hepatocellular carcinoma in cirrhotics and noncirrhotics. Evaluation of clinicopathologic features and comparison of risk factors for long-term survival and tumour recurrence in a single centre. Aliment Pharmacol Ther. 2003;17(Suppl 2):119–29.
8. Fuster J, Garcia-Valdecasas JC, Grande L, et al. Hepatocellular carcinoma and cirrhosis. Results of surgical treatment in a European series. Ann Surg. 1996;223:297–302.
9. Zhang B, Xu D, Wang R, et al. Perioperative antiviral therapy improves safety in patients with hepatitis B related HCC following hepatectomy. Int J Surg. 2015;15:1–5.
10. Huang G, Lau WY, Wang ZG, et al. Antiviral therapy improves postoperative survival in patients with hepatocellular carcinoma: a randomized controlled trial. Ann Surg. 2015;261:56–66.
11. Huang G, Li P, Lau WY, et al. Antiviral therapy reduces hepatocellular carcinoma recurrence in patients with low HBV-DNA levels: a randomized controlled trial. Ann Surg. 2018;268:943–54.
12. Yin J, Li N, Han Y, et al. Effect of antiviral treatment with nucleotide/nucleoside analogs on postoperative prognosis of hepatitis B virus-related hepatocellular carcinoma: a two-stage longitudinal clinical study. J Clin Oncol. 2013;31:3647–55.
13. Kubota KM, Kusaka K, Kobayashi T, et al. Measurement of liver volume and hepatic functional reserve as a guide to decision-making in resectional surgery for hepatic tumors. Hepatology. 1997;26:1176–81.
14. Shimada MT, Akazawa K, Kamakura T, et al. Estimation of risk of major complications after hepatic resection. Am J Surg. 1994;167:399–403.

15. Yamanaka NOE, Kuwata K, Tanaka N. A multiple regression equation for prediction of posthepatectomy liver failure. Ann Surg. 1984;200:658–63.
16. Hung IF, Poon RT, Lai CL, et al. Recurrence of hepatitis B-related hepatocellular carcinoma is associated with high viral load at the time of resection. Am J Gastroenterol. 2008;103:1663–73.
17. Huang L, Li J, Lau WY, et al. Perioperative reactivation of hepatitis B virus replication in patients undergoing partial hepatectomy for hepatocellular carcinoma. J Gastroenterol Hepatol. 2012;27:158–64.
18. Thia TJ, Ooi L, Chung YF, et al. A study into the risk of exacerbation of chronic hepatitis B after liver resection for hepatocellular carcinoma. J Gastrointest Surg. 2007;11:612–8.
19. Terrault NA, Bzowej NH, Chang KM, et al. AASLD guidelines for treatment of chronic hepatitis B. Hepatology. 2016;63:261–83.
20. Feng ZQ, Wu LC, Shen MH, et al. Clinical observation on Babaodan combined with interventional therapy for primary liver cancer with heat toxin and blood stasis. Chin J Trad Chin Med. 2007;25(11):2404–7.
21. European Association for the Study of the Liner. EASL clinical practice guidelines: management of chronic hepatitis B virus infection. J Hepatol. 2012;57:167–85.
22. Lok AS, Brown RS Jr, Wong JB, et al. Antiviral therapy for chronic hepatitis B viral infection in adults: a systematic review and meta-analysis. Hepatology. 2016;63:284–306.
23. Health and Family Planning Commission of the People's Republic of China. Guidelines for the diagnosis and treatment of primary liver cancer (2017 edition). J Clin Hepatob Dis. 2017;33(8):1419–31.
24. Lok AS. Chronic hepatitis B: update 2009. Hepatology. 2009;50:661–2.
25. Chang T, Kew YS, Lee S, et al. Entecavir treatment for up to 5 years in patients with hepatitis B e antigen-positive chronic hepatitis B. Hepatology. 2010;51:422–30.
26. Schiff E, Lee WM, Chao YC, et al. Efficacy and safety of entecavir in patients with chronic hepatitis B and advanced hepatic fibrosis or cirrhosis. Am J Gastroenterol. 2008;103:2776–83.
27. Shim JH, Kim KM, Lim YS, et al. Efficacy of entecavir in treatment-naïve patients with hepatitis B virus-related decompensated cirrhosis. J Hepatol. 2010;52:176–82.
28. Tenney DJ, Baldick CJ, Pokornowski KA, et al. Long-term monitoring shows hepatitis B virus resistance to entecavir in nucleoside-naive patientsis rare through 5 years of therapy. Hepatology. 2009;49:1503–14.
29. LimYS, YooBC, ByunKS, et al. Tenofovirmonotherapy versus tenofovir and entecavir combination therapy in adefovir-resistant chronic hepatitis B patients with multiple drug failure: results of a randomised trial. Gut. 2016;65:1042–51.
30. Zoulim F, Locarnini S. Management of treatment failure in chronic hepatitis B. J Hepatol. 2012;56(Suppl 1):112–22.
31. Petersen J, Buti M, Janssen HL, et al. Entecavir plus tenofovir combination as rescue therapy in pre-treated chronic hepatitis B patients: an international multicenter cohort study. J Hepatol. 2012;56:520–6.
32. Polaris Observatory HCV Collaborators. Global prevalence and genotype distribution of hepatitis C virus infection in 2015: a modelling study. Lancet Gastroenterol Hepatol. 2017;2(3):161–76.
33. European Association for the Study of the Liver. EASL recommendations on treatment of hepatitis C 2018. J Hepatol. 2018;69:461–511.
34. European Association for the Study of the Liver. EASL clinical practice guidelines: management of hepatitis C virus infection. J Hepatol. 2011;55:245–64.
35. van der Meer AJ, Bereiguer M. Reversion of disease manifestations after HCV eradication. J Hepatol. 2016;65:S95–S108.
36. Mahale P, Li R, Torres HA, et al. The effect of sustained virological response on the risk of extrahepatic manifestations of hepatitis C virus infection. Gut. 2018;67:553–61.
37. Negro F, Crax A, Sulkowski MS, et al. Extrahepatic morbidity and mortality of chronic hepatitis C. Gastroenterology. 2015;149:1345–60.
38. European Union HCV Collaborators. Hepatitis C virus prevalence and level of intervention required to achieve the WHO targets for elimination in the European Union by 2030: a modelling study. Lancet Gastroenterol Hepatol. 2017;2(5):325–36.
39. Martinot-Peignoux MSC, Maylin S, Ripault MP, et al. Twelve weeks posttreatment follow-up is as relevant as 24 weeks to determine the sustained virologic response in patients with hepatitis C virus receiving pegylated interferon and ribavirin. Hepatology. 2010;51:1122–6.
40. D'Amico G, Pagliaro L. Natural history and prognostic indicators of survival in cirrhosis: a systematic review of 118 studies. J Hepatol. 2006;44:217–31.
41. Bernardi M, Angeli P, Schnabl B. Mechanisms of decompensation and organ failure in cirrhosis: from peripheral arterial vasodilation to systemic inflammation hypothesis. J Hepatol. 2015;63:1272–84.
42. European Association for the Study of the Liver. EASL clinical practice guidelines for the management of patients with decompensated cirrhosis. J Hepatol. 2018;69:406–60.
43. Cheung MCM, Walker AJ, Hudson BE, et al. Outcomes after successful direct-acting antiviral therapy for patients with chronic hepatitis C and decompensated cirrhosis. J Hepatol. 2016;65:741–7.
44. Lens SA, Mari OZ, Londo OMC, et al. Effects of all-oral anti-viral therapy on hvpg and systemic hemodynamics in patients with hepatitis C virus-associated cirrhosis. Gastroenterology. 2017;153:1273–83.

45. Kang SH, Lee JH, Nam JY, et al. Rifaximin treatment is associated with reduced risk of cirrhotic complications and prolonged overall survival in patients experiencing hepatic encephalopathy. Aliment Pharmacol Ther. 2017;46:845–55.
46. Caraceni P, Riggio O, Angeli P, et al. Long-term albumin administration in decompensated cirrhosis (ANSWER): an open-label randomised trial. Lancet. 2018;391:2417–29.
47. Sola E, Sole C, Simon-Talero M, et al. Midodrine and albumin for prevention of complications in patients with cirrhosis awaiting liver transplantation. A randomized placebo-controlled trial. J Hepatol. 2018;69:1250–9.
48. Abraldes JG, Albillos A, Bañares R, et al. Simvastatin lowers portal pressure in patients with cirrhosis and portal hypertension: a randomized controlled trial. Gastroenterology. 2009;136:1651–8.
49. Abraldes JG, Aracil C, Turnes J, et al. Addition of simvastatin to standard therapy for the prevention of variceal rebleeding does not reduce rebleeding but increases survival in patients with cirrhosis. Gastroenterology. 2016;150:1160–70.
50. Abraldes JG, Turnes J, Garcia-Pagan JC, et al. Hemodynamic response to pharmacological treatment of portal hyper-tension and long-term prognosis of cirrhosis. Hepatology. 2003;37:902–8.
51. Huang X, Tang J, Cai H, et al. Anti-inflammatory effects of monoammonium glycyrrhizinate on lipopolysaccharide-induced acute lung injury in mice through regulating nuclear factor-kappa b signaling pathway. Evid Based Complement Alternat Med. 2015;2015:272474.
52. Garg M, Singhal T, Sharma H. Cardioprotective effect of ammonium glycyrrhizinate against doxorubicin-induced cardiomyopathy in experimental animals. Indian J Pharmacol. 2014;46:527–30.
53. Shi JR, Mao LG, Jiang RA, et al. Monoammonium glycyrrhizinate inhibited the inflammation of LPS-induced acute lung injury in mice. Int Immunopharmacol. 2010;10:1235–41.
54. Yan T, Bi XY, Fang Y, et al. Effect of Huaier granule on postoperative long-term survival of patients with primary liver cancer. Chin J Hepatobiliary Surg. 2012;18(2):99–102.
55. Gao JL. Prospective, randomize-controlled clinical study of ganfule prescription in the treatment of advanced primary liver cancer. Chin J Tradit Chin Med. 2014;39(2):236–9.
56. Chen Q, Laurence AD, Chen Y, et al. Effect of Huaier granule on recurrence after curative resection of HCC: a multicentre, randomised clinical trial. Gut. 2018;67:2006–16.
57. Sun N, Sun FX, Li XL, et al. Significance of treatment of underlying liver disease in the treatment of primary liver cancer. Chin J Hepatol (Electronic Version). 2018;10(1):11–4.
58. Zou Y, Xiong H, Xiong H, et al. A polysaccharide from mushroom Huaier retards human hepatocellular carcinoma growth, angiogenesis, and metastasis in nude mice. Tumour Biol. 2015;36:2929–36.
59. Liu J, Wang S, Zhang Y, et al. Traditional Chinese medicine and cancer: history, present situation, and development. Thorac Cancer. 2015;6:561–9.
60. Wasser SP. Medicinal mushrooms as a source of antitumor and immunomodulating polysaccharides. Appl Microbiol Biotechnol. 2002;60:258–74.
61. Schepetkin IA. Botanical polysaccharides: macrophage immunomodulation and therapeutic potential. Int Immunopharmacol. 2006;6:317–33.
62. Bao H, Liu P, Jiang K, et al. Huaier polysaccharide induces apoptosis in hepatocellular carcinoma cells through p38 MAPK. Oncol Lett. 2016;12:1058–66.
63. Hu Z, Yang A, Su G, et al. Huaier restrains proliferative and invasive potential of human hepatoma SKHEP-1 cells partially through decreased Lamin B1 and elevated NOV. Sci Rep. 2016;6:31298.
64. Yan L, Liu X, Yin A, et al. Huaier aqueous extract inhibits cervical cancer cell proliferation via JNK/p38 pathway. Int J Oncol. 2015;47:1054–60.
65. Wang Y, Hu Y. Optimization of polysaccharides extraction from Trametes robiniophila and its antioxidant activities. Carbohydr Polym. 2014;111:324–32.
66. Lei JY, Yan LN, Zhu JQ, et al. Hepatocellular carcinoma patients may benefit from postoperative huaier aqueous extract after liver transplantation. Transplant Proc. 2015;47:2920–4.
67. Forner A, Llovet JM, Bruix J. Hepatocellular carcinoma. Lancet. 2012;379:1245–55.
68. Lu LC, Cheng AL, Poon RT. Recent advances in the prevention of hepatocellular carcinoma recurrence. Semin Liver Dis. 2014;34:427–34.
69. Wang BH, Zhao B, Yan L, et al. Discussion on the treatment of cancer pain from the heart, liver and spleen theory of Huangdi Neijing. Chin J Tradit Chin Med Inform. 2013;10(10):88–90.
70. Sun D, Ye LH. Professor Zhou Zhongying's clinical experience in treating liver cancer. J Zhejiang Chin Med Univ. 2017;41(11):860–2.
71. Cao W, Huo JG, Fang J, et al. Zhou Min's experience in the diagnosis and treatment of liver cancer. Jiangsu J Tradit Chin Med. 2019;51(7):18–21.
72. Li DQ, Sun L, Lin JH. Effect of local topical application of Wuwei Shuangbai powder on pain relief in primary liver cancer and its effect on hemorheological parameters. J Guangzhou Univ Tradit Chin Med. 2017;34(2):177–80.
73. Xie JR, Liang GY, Li M, et al. Study on the effect of Yiqi Huoxue Huayu law on caspase 3 and tissues of rats with liver cancer. Inform Tradit Chin Meds. 2009;26(1):68–9.

Part VIII

Prospects on Multimodality Treatment for Liver Cancer

30 Innovations and Progress in Surgical Treatments for Liver Cancer

Jiahong Dong and Sheng Ye

Since the beginning of the 21st century, the dissemination and integration of modern technology into traditional surgical practice has profoundly changed the surgical landscape, as well as surgical concepts and paradigms. In the past, traditional surgery was full of uncertainty, which was mainly based on the surgeons experiences, knowledge and intuition. Nowadays, modern science and technology has enabled greater practical certainty in surgical management across multiple dimensions and entire processes. Collectively, these advances ensure that empirical surgery shifted towards precision surgery, based on deterministic practice, with the aim of significantly improving patient outcomes. During the process of optimizing our surgical practice for complex hepatobiliary diseases in the past 20 years, we have found that current technology has empowered modern surgery with brand new concepts. Consequently, we believe that it is necessary to redefine 21st century surgery with the distinct characteristics of this modern era.

J. Dong (✉) · S. Ye
Beijing Tsinghua Changgung Hospital,
Beijing, China
e-mail: dongjiahong@mail.tsinghua.edu.cn

30.1 The Concept of "Precision Liver Surgery" Has Been Widely Recognized by International Peers

"Precision liver surgery" is the practical embodiment of the concept of precision surgery in hepatobiliary surgery. This novel surgical concept has been widely recognized and promptly adopted in the field of hepatobiliary surgery worldwide. At the same time, many scholars of other medical fields have also found that this concept has significant application value and development potential when adapted to their respective specialties. We were invited to write a review in 2013 entitled "Precision Liver Surgery" for the Liver Surgery volume of the internationally renowned journal *Seminars in Liver Disease*, which was listed as the leading article. This was the first time that the concept, strategy, and technical characteristics of "Precision Liver Surgery" were comprehensively discussed in an international setting. The main characteristics of precision liver surgery are certainty, predictability, controllability, integration, standardization, and individualization. Jean C. Emond, the executive editor of the journal and a professor at Columbia University, gave high appraisal in the introduction of the concept of precision liver surgery and the level of liver surgery in China.

X. Chen (ed.), *Diagnosis and Treatment of Liver Cancer in China*,
https://doi.org/10.1007/978-981-97-7969-7_30

The hepatic artery, hepatic vein, portal vein, and bile duct are four interwoven vascular systems that constitute the complex anatomical structure of the liver. Various functions of the liver, including metabolite synthesis, detoxification, coagulation, immunity, and digestion contribute to the complexity and diversity of liver diseases. Precision liver surgery is an anatomic surgery that relies on a precise and accurate understanding of the surgical anatomy of the liver. The goal of this technique is to completely remove the target lesion while ensuring the integrity of the remaining liver vasculature. The compensatory and regenerative potential of the liver are the physiological basis for precision liver surgery. Before liver resection, the safe resection volume of liver parenchyma should be accurately controlled based on the precise assessment of hepatic functional reserve and liver regeneration capacity in order to avoid postoperative liver insufficiency or even liver failure. In addition, the nature, lesion characteristics, and pathological features of different liver diseases are the basis for the selection of appropriate surgical methods, extent of reasonable resection, and adjunctive therapy. As an example, hepatocellular carcinoma often spreads in the tumor-bearing liver segment along the portal vein branch, while hepatolithiasis is characterized by a segmental distribution in the liver along the biliary tree. This helps determine that the anatomic resection of the liver segment is an ideal surgical treatment for the above lesions.

The continuous development of modern imaging technology, establishment of a digital surgical platform, and improvement of hepatic functional reserve monitoring and surgical techniques have laid a solid technical foundation for the realization of precision liver surgery. This combination of medical imaging and computer technology gave rise to modern digital surgery, shifting medical imaging to image fusion and 3D visualization. The establishment of a digital surgical platform enables the true evolution of preoperative evaluation and surgical planning from the previous experience-based practice to precise and objective decision-making. Clinical application of the indocyanine green (ICG) test and galactosyl human serum albumin (GSA) technique in combination with a dynamic single-Photon emission computed tomography (SPECT) scan provides a reliable basis for the accurate determination of the patient's pre-surgical hepatic functional reserve and tolerable hepatectomy volume. In addition, intraoperative ultrasound, hepatic vascular inflow occlusion, living donor liver transplantation, precise hepatic vascular reconstruction, and robot-assisted laparoscopy have greatly guided the movement of liver surgery toward precision surgery.

At present, more and more surgeons realize that precision liver surgery can reduce postoperative complications and improve patient prognosis, optimize surgical safety, treatment efficacy and minimally invasive intervention, and provide optimal liver surgery practice and maximum patient recovery based on evidence-based surgical decision-making and precise and controllable technology.

30.2 Digitalization of Surgical Treatments for Liver Cancer

In traditional surgery, surgeons perform surgical mental simulations prior to surgery and then operate based on their preconceived three-dimensional visualizations. The quality of such surgical methods often depends on the individual surgeon's clinical experience and operating skills. However, it is often difficult for members of the same surgical team to share the same conception of the entire procedure formed in the mind of any given surgeon.

Through the continued development of science and technology, computer graphics, and data visualization technology, these improved computer image processing and analysis methods have helped surgeons to construct 3D visualization models from 2D imaging data. This clearly displays the complex course, distribution, and spatial relationship of the vascular system in models, allows quantitative analysis of the image data, and provides additional information such as the diameter and length of the blood vessels as well as regions of organ parenchyma.

A virtual reality-based surgery, virtual surgery (VS), was further developed based on the use of 3D visualization technology and is a new interdisciplinary research field that integrates medicine, biomechanics, mechanics, materials science, computer graphics, computer vision, mathematical analysis, and robotics. Its purpose is to use preexisting human investigative skills to navigate and manipulate objects in the virtual world, thus providing intuitive and natural real-time perception of sight, sound, and touch through various sensing devices. VS gives participants an immersive feeling of interactive simulation to simulate various processes and timeframes (preoperative, intraoperative, and postoperative) involved in the surgical procedure. Other purposes of VS include surgical plan design, surgical rehearsals, surgical teaching, surgical skills training, intraoperative guidance, and postoperative rehabilitation.

In recent years, a variety of virtual surgical simulators have been developed to enable trainers to be in a 3D virtual surgical environment generated by a computer and to practice surgical operations with virtual surgical instruments. This technology not only provides the trainer with 3D visualization but also simulates force and tactile feedback so that the trainer can learn and improve surgical skills in a virtual reality environment.

3D visualization model construction and VS are tools for precise preoperative evaluation and planning. In real surgery, computer-assisted surgery (CAS), an intraoperative navigation technology, is required to combine preoperative evaluation and planning with the actual operation. The basic principle of CAS is to use an external tracking device to measure the position of the surgical instrument relative to the operating object in real time and then display the position on the medical image so that the surgeon can see the current position of the surgical instrument in real-time and make judgment and decision on the surgical procedures. Surgical navigation is very similar to global positioning system (GPS). At present, CT/magnetic resonance imaging (MRI) navigation has been widely used in clinical practice. However, with the increasingly high demand for surgical quality in modern surgery, the registration error between the preoperative image and the surgical object inherent in this navigation method has become a problem that cannot be ignored. Therefore, some scholars began to study the introduction of CT or MRI equipment into the operating room and the use of intraoperative real-time tomography images for surgical navigation.

The use of surgical robots emerged in the late 1980s. In 1997, the US company Intuitive Surgical introduced the Da Vinci system, which was approved for use by the U.S. Food and Drug Administration in 2000. This system adopts a master/slave operation mode to improve the man–machine interaction interface, which is more in line with the operational habits of surgeons. It provides the surgeon with a true, precise, magnified, and high-definition surgical field of vision through a high-resolution 3D image processing system. The surgical actions of the surgeon are then precisely translated from the console into the robotic arms, which function like the surgeon's extended hands and wrists. Consequently, the movements of the surgeon's hands are transformed into more precise movements of the robotic arms, resulting in greater precision, stability, and flexibility in surgical operations. Robotic surgery has been widely used in cardiothoracic surgery and general surgery, which on the whole has greatly promoted the development of digital medical instruments.

The combination of surgical robot use with that of virtual technology, broadband network, and high-speed communication transmission technology can also allow remote surgical treatment. The direct driving force behind the emergence of telesurgery systems comes from the surgical treatment of emergency casualties on the front lines of the battlefield (where experienced surgeons are often scarce), as well as the treatment of space astronauts and workers in nuclear radiation environments. However, the development of telesurgery is currently facing many problems. First, any network-related time delay must be reduced to below what can be effectively sensed by humans in order to develop a sense of presence in an operation. Second, network security must be improved so that network communication in order for optimal and efficient surgical data transmission and network transmission.

Problems such as data loss, virus, and data variation must be overcome to improve surgical safety.

At present, digital surgical technology is developing rapidly in various surgical fields such as orthopedics and neurosurgery, and many projects have already entered the stage of clinical application. Due to the complex anatomical structure of the liver and the lack of bony landmarks, the construction of digital surgical platforms has been especially difficult in the field of hepatobiliary surgery and is thus widely considered to be a frontier topic in international research. Since 2000, we have pioneered the exploration of 3D reconstruction and the VS of the liver, gallbladder, and pancreas. The teams of Academician Dong Jiahong and Academician You Zheng from Tsinghua University have led the development of a precise hepatobiliary surgical planning system. This system can rapidly perform high – precision intelligent 3D reconstruction of the liver, biliary tract, and blood vessels. It also features adaptive Couinaud iiver segment segmentation, volume calculation, and subspecialty surgical planning functions. At present, 3D visualizationmodels of the liver and biliary system have beenestablished, and the virtual hepatectomy of a liver model has been discussed. An internationalresearch initiative between Japan and Germany developed computer-aided liver resection planning systems, which have already entered clinical practice. Our clinical studies indicate that the digital surgical planning system helps to improve the precision and safety of hepatectomy.

While Yttrium-90 (Y-90) radioembolization has been a clinically established therapeutic intervention for liver cancer treatment, modern advanced Y-90 radioembolization requires precise preoperative treatment planning, accurate intraoperative navigation, and postoperative efficacy evaluation.

Through an intelligent qualitative and quantitative analysis (IQQA) digital surgery platform, multi-modality imaging data, such as CT, MRI, PET/SPECT, DSA/CBCT, and Ultrasound, can be fully quantified and fused to facilitate precision treatment planning, intraoperative guidance for optimizing therapeutic delivery, as well as postprocedural evaluation.

During the preprocedural planning phase, by generating an IQQA 3D electronic organ map (eOrganM), the platform enables precise volumetric quantification of hepatic parenchyma, tumor lesions, vessels, functional vascular supply territories, and other vital anatomies.

Further, the platform provides quantitative dynamic arterial perfusion evaluation to simulate Y-90 treatment mapping and help identify optimal Y-90 microsphere injection sites to maximize tumor-targeted radiation dosimetry while preserving functional hepatic parenchyma.

Based on the current development of digital surgical technologies such as virtual reality, image navigation, and robotic surgery, the construction of a digital surgical platform in the field of hepatobiliary surgery is not only completely feasible and in line with the development of modern surgery but also has broad application prospects.

30.3 Preoperative Digital Platform in Precision Surgery for Liver Cancer

30.3.1 Construction of a Digital Liver

The liver is a parenchymal organ comprised of complex anatomical structures, physiological functions, and pathological changes, which to date are still poorly understood. Constructing a digital liver for hepatobiliary surgery is a new approach to comprehensively and systematically understanding the liver in the twenty-first century. Digital techniques such as multimedia and virtual reality are used to demonstrate the anatomical morphology, tissue architecture, physiological function, and pathological features of the liver in a multi-dimensional manner, so as to construct a digital liver with spatial, digital, networked, intelligent, and visual characteristics.

30.3.2 Quantifiable Liver Function Assessment Techniques

Regional stereoscopic quantitative assessment of liver function: Segmental quantitative evaluation of liver functional volume is performed by multimodal 3D reconstruction image fusion using

^{99m}Tc-GSA SPECT-CT and enhanced CT images. Based on the precise preoperative quantitative evaluation method for whole liver functional reserve and segmental liver reserve, the individualized evaluation and decision system and clinical technical standards for safe liver resection are established for different patients according to the liver volume essential for maintaining liver function and the safe limits of hepatectomy.

30.3.3 Digital Precise Intelligent Surgical Planning System for Hepatobiliary Surgery

Using pre-existing 3D visualization and virtual reality technology, the system transforms 2D image data of individual cases into 3D digital views of the liver to allow real-time virtual cutting and geometric quantitative analysis of surgical information such as liver anatomical structure, dominant regions of the vasculature, boundary of the liver segment, and distribution of lesions and the deformation and displacement they cause in adjacent vasculature, thereby serving as a highly precise and efficient auxiliary tool for surgical planning and optimization. The system applies 3D reconstruction and 3D printing technology to precisely analyze the stereoconformation and anatomical classification of the four groups of liver vasculature, which serves as the basis for designing the path, procedure, and injury control methods for hepatobiliary and pancreatic surgery.

30.3.4 Research and Development of Virtual Hepatobiliary Surgery System

We are developing a virtual hepatobiliary surgery system using real-time 3D graphics generation, virtual reality, multi-sensor interaction, and high-resolution display technologies. This system allows us to study the digital 3D view of the hepatobiliary system of individual patients. The system simulates surgery in a virtual computer-generated surgical environment that demonstrates the surgical process and predicts potentially complex and dangerous situations that may occur during the surgery, thus helping to meet the goal of improving the success rates of complex hepatobiliary surgery.

30.4 Intraoperative Digital Technology for Precision Surgery in Liver Cancer

30.4.1 Digital Image Navigation and Information Navigation Surgical System

By using digital medical imaging technology, the system fuses intraoperative ultrasound images of individual patients with their preoperative CT/MRI images and 3D liver images to precisely identify the spatial localization of the lesions and adjacent anatomical structures during the surgery and precisely guide the operation in real time. On the basis of anatomical image-guided surgery, the system further integrates liver function considerations and pathological factors into the development of an information-guided surgery approach, providing more comprehensive and precise information guidance for preoperative evaluation and intraoperative operation.

30.4.2 Visual Liver Surgery Technology

The technique uses ICG near-infrared fluorescence imaging to visualize the liver segment. ICG is injected into the portal vein branch of the target liver segment to reveal the 3D anatomical boundary of the liver segment, thus guiding precise anatomical resection of the liver segment. In addition, visual tracer-based optical fluorescence quantitative technology can also be developed using specific antibodies to hepatobiliary tumors to clearly display the pathological boundary of tumors and improve the precision radical resection rate of hepatobiliary tumors.

30.4.3 Robotic Remote Surgical System

The further development of various human–machine interface technologies for data and information exchange among surgeons, robots, and patients can allow reasonable, precise, and efficient communication of visual, tactile, and sound information between the planning end and the operation end, thereby facilitating the construction of a robotic remote surgical system. The surgeon can maneuver the handle according to real-time image feedback from the video sensor and precisely control the movement of all instruments at the robot operation terminal.

30.5 Perioperative Digital Management of Precision Surgery for Liver Cancer

Enhanced Recovery After Surgery (ERAS) is a patient-centered care pathway aimed to maximize the benefit of the patients during hospitalization. Any measures that are beneficial to the patient's postoperative recovery can be applied and continuously optimized. The clinical application of ERAS is a systematic process, including preoperative preparation, intraoperative and postoperative fluid management, selection of anesthesia methods, and intraoperative bleeding and temperature control, each of which seeks to maximize the benefit of the patient. ERAS requires active cooperation from physicians and nurses, adequate perioperative management, and individualized treatment regimens to achieve rapid recovery. The ERAS concept is safe and effective for the perioperative management of hepatectomy patients. It can alleviate surgical stress and promote early recovery of patients, providing a high clinical application value.

Precise preoperative quantitative metabolic assessment can provide reliable support for the risk, safety, and survival of patients undergoing surgery. Some studies have confirmed that preoperative branched-chain amino acid/tyrosine ratio <5 and anaerobic threshold in cardiopulmonary exercise testing (CPET) <11.5 mL/(min·kg) are independent prognostic factors for hepatectomy in patients with chronic liver injury. Body mass index (BMI) and waist circumference are also independent prognostic factors for long-term survival after hepatectomy for liver cancer, and waist circumference is more accurate than BMI in predicting postoperative disease-free survival. Preoperative CPET also plays a role in surgical risk assessment, collaborative surgical decision-making, individualized monitoring, and monitoring interventions and guides patients' postoperative recovery from multiple perspectives, all of which are important in ERAS.

Therefore, it is through the guidance of the theory of precision hepatobiliary surgery that the integration, innovation, and optimization of traditional hepatobiliary surgery technology and modern technologies such as digital medical imaging, computer image recognition and processing, virtual reality, information navigation, and robotics can be achieved with the help of the digital platform. This will greatly promote the improvement of technical precision and effectiveness of hepatobiliary surgery and unify treatment efficacy, surgical safety, and minimally invasive intervention in the treatment of hepatobiliary surgery.

Suggested Reading

1. Yoshida M, Beppu T, Shiraishi S, et al. ^{99m}Tc-GSA SPECT/CT fused images for assessment of hepatic function and hepatectomy planning. Ann Transl Med. 2015;3(2):17.
2. Taniguchi M, Okizaki A, Watanabe K, et al. Hepatic clearance measured with ^{99m}Tc-GSA single-photon emission computed tomography to estimate liver fibrosis. World J Gastroenterol. 2014;20(44):16714–20.
3. Zein NN, Hanounehi A, Bishop PD, et al. Three-dimensional print of a liver for preoperative planning in living donor liver transplantation. Liver Transpl. 2013;19:1304–10.
4. Oshiro Y, Yano H, Mitani J, et al. Novel 3-dimensional virtual hepatectomy simulation combined with real-time deformation. World J Gastroenterol. 2015;21(34):9982–92.

5. Miyata A, Ishizawa T, Kamiya M, et al. Photoacoustic tomography of human hepatic malignancies using intraoperative indocyaninegreen fluorescence imaging. PLoS One. 2014;9(11):e112667.
6. Chi C, Du Y, Ye J, et al. Intraoperative imaging-guided cancer surgery: from current fluorescence molecular imaging methods to future multi-modality imaging technology. Theranostics. 2014;4(11):1072–84.
7. Hughes MJ, McNally S, Wigmore SJ, et al. Enhanced recovery following liver surgery: a systematic review and meta-analysis. HPB (Oxford). 2014;16:699–706.
8. Hall TC, Dennison AR, Bilku DK, et al. Enhanced recovery programmes in hepatobiliary and pancreatic surgery: a systematic review. Ann R Coll Surg Engl. 2012;94:318–26.
9. Kaibori M, Ishizaki M, Matsui K, et al. Assessment of preoperative exercise capacity in hepatocellular carcinoma patients with chronic liver injury undergoing hepatectomy. BMC Gastroenterol. 2013;13:119–22.
10. Liu X, Xu J. Body mass index and waistline are predictors of survial for hepatocellular carcinoma after hepatectomy. Med Sci Monit. 2015;21:2203–9.
11. Levett DZ, Grocott MP. Cardiopulmonary exercise testing, prehabilitation, and Enhanced Recovery After Surgery(ERAS). Can J Anesth. 2015;62:131–42.

31 Prospects on Molecular Targeted Therapy and Immunotherapy for Liver Cancer

Jiahong Dong and Lin Zhang

The uses of molecular targeted therapy and immunotherapy are without a doubt the hottest topics of therapeutic research for the treatment of hepatocellular carcinoma (HCC) in recent years and are expected to continue in the near future. In 2007, sorafenib became the first-line therapy for progressive HCC, while, after nearly a decade of extensive exploration in 2018, lenvatinib became the second approved first-line treatment for progressive HCC in China. In 2017 and 2018, the US Food and Drug Administration (FDA) approved nivolumab and pembrolizumab as second-line therapy for HCC, respectively, thus paving the way to a new era of immunotherapy use.

Second-line therapy for HCC emerged after 2017, regorafenib was approved in China for use in cases of sorafenib-resistant advanced HCC, and cabozantinib and ramucirumab were approved by the US FDA as second-line therapy for HCC. In 2019, IMbrave150 (immunotherapy + anti-angiogenesis targeted therapy) achieved the primary endpoints of progression-free survival (PFS) and overall survival (OS), breaking the pattern of exclusive molecular targeted therapy use in the first-line treatment of advanced HCC. In March 2020, camrelizumab was approved for marketing as the first programmed death protein 1 (PD-1)/PD-L1 monoclonal antibody approved for HCC in China. HCC pathogenesis exploration and treatment development are shown in Fig. 31.1.

J. Dong (✉) · L. Zhang
Beijing Tsinghua Changgung Hospital,
Beijing, China
e-mail: dongjiahong@mail.tsinghua.edu.cn

X. Chen (ed.), *Diagnosis and Treatment of Liver Cancer in China*,
https://doi.org/10.1007/978-981-97-7969-7_31

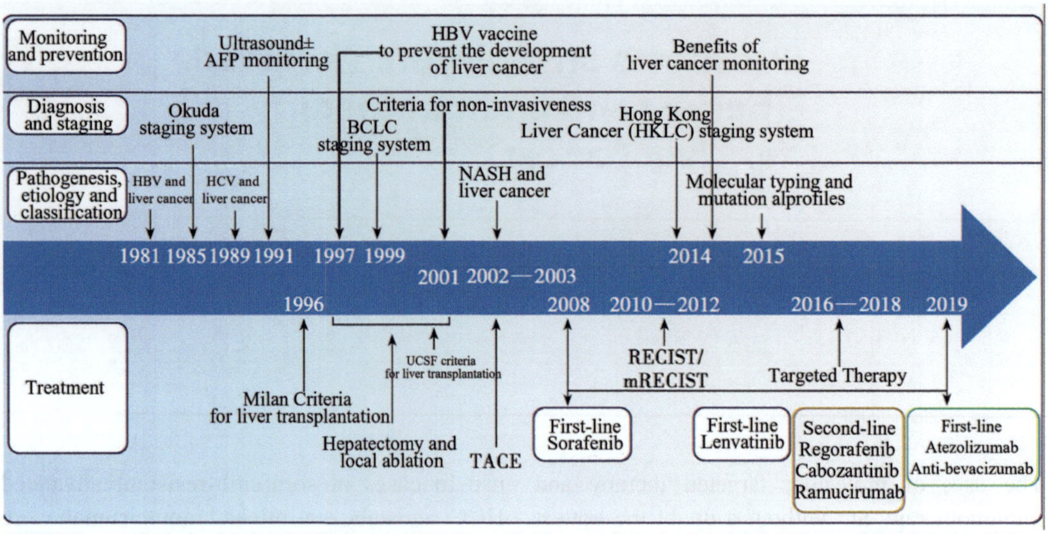

Fig. 31.1 HCC pathogenesis exploration and treatment development

31.1 HCC Molecular Targeted Drugs

31.1.1 Progress in First-Line Therapy with Molecular Targeted Drugs

1. Sorafenib: Sorafenib is an oral multi-targeted tyrosine kinase inhibitor (TKI) with anti-proliferation and anti-angiogenic effects on tumor cells. Based on the results of the 2007 SHARP trial, the US FDA approved sorafenib for the treatment of unresectable HCC, which is the first molecular targeted drug approved for the treatment of unresectable HCC. Within 10 years after the approval of sorafenib, despite the vigorous development of molecular targeted therapy, studies comparing various molecular targeted drugs with sorafenib have ended in failure. Five global phase III clinical studies (sunitinib, brinib, linifanib, or erotinib combined with sorafenib, sorafenib combined with doxorubicin versus sorafenib) failed to confirm either the non-inferiority or superiority of these drugs' OS in comparison with that of sorafenib. The recent TACTICS trial showed that TACE combined with sorafenib significantly prolonged PFS compared with TACE alone (25.2 months vs. 13.5 months, HR = 0.59, 95% confidence interval (CI): 0.41–0.87). The study design was the administration of 400 mg/day sorafenib for 2–3 weeks before TACE, with a 4-day peri-operative pause. Sorafenib may be orally administered at 400 mg twice a day in well-tolerated patients. TACE was performed on demand. The two study endpoints were PFS and OS. The key point of this trial was to not use the response evaluation criteria in solid tumors (RECIST) evaluation criteria and new intrahepatic lesions were not assessed as progressive disease (PD), thus prolonging the duration of sorafenib use. Preoperative use of sorafenib before TACE can help normalize tumor vessels and improve the efficacy of TACE. The combined use of sorafenib and TACE reduced the frequency of TACE treatment, protected liver function, and prolonged the time to progression (TTP) of patients. This study is the first study in the world in which the use of sorafenib combined with TACE achieved positive results. Meanwhile, this study proposed the use of time to TACE progression (TTTP) as TACE-related TTP, and

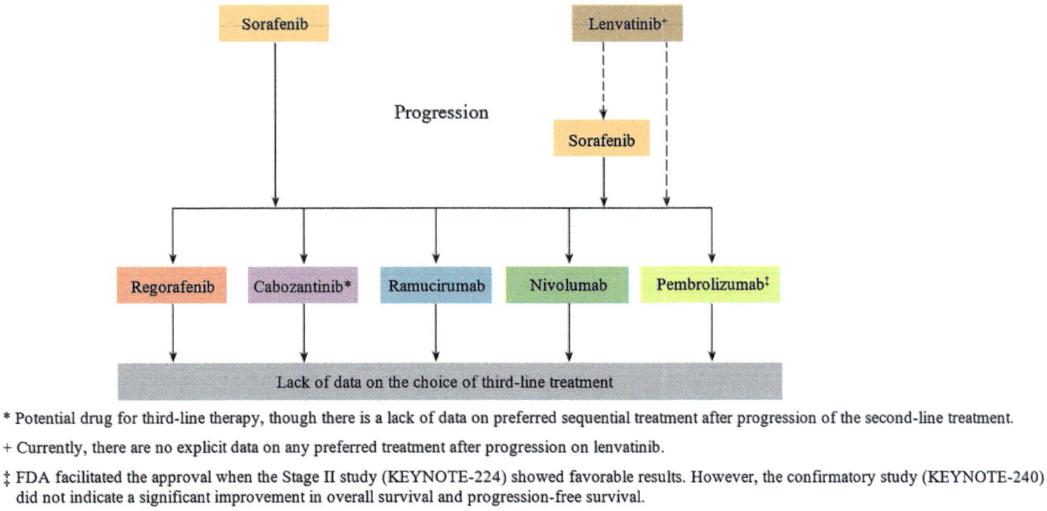

Fig. 31.2 Progress made in the selection of first-line molecular targeted drugs for advanced HCC

TACE-related PFS and TTTP as alternative indicators of OS, which are reasonable designs for this type of study. In addition, sorafenib can be a postoperative adjuvant therapy for patients with risk factors for microvascular invasion and recurrence of portal vein tumor thrombosis. A meta-analysis of 589 HCC patients published by ESMO Asia in 2019 showed that postoperative sorafenib treatment significantly reduced tumor recurrence rate and extended OS of patients compared with the surgery arm. Sorafenib is currently recommended for stage IIb–IIIb HCC patients and is ranked as the top first-line systematic treatment in the Guidelines for Diagnosis and Treatment of Primary Liver Cancer (2019 Edition). As a first-line drug for progressive HCC, sorafenib remains undefeatable after 10 years of history.

2. Lenvatinib: Lenvatinib, another multi-targeted TKI with anti-angiogenic activity, is an oral inhibitor of vascular endothelial growth factor receptors (VEGFRs) 1–3, fibroblast growth factor receptors (FGFRs) 1–4, platelet-derived growth factor receptor (PDGF-R) α, rearranged during transfection (RET), and KIT (Fig. 31.2). Lenvatinib is approved for the treatment of unresectable HCC, including patients with advanced HCC or PD following locoregional therapy. The Randomized, multicenter, open-label, Phase 3 trial to compare the Efficacy and safety of Lenvatinib versus sorafenib in First-line treatment of patients with unresectable hepatocellular carcinoma study is the first phase III global randomized open-label non-inferiority study which yielded positive results in the span of 10 years. The final results of the study showed that the median survival was 13.6 months (95% CI: 12.1–14.9) in the lenvatinib arm and 12.3 months (95% CI: 10.4–13.9) in the sorafenib arm, reaching the non-inferiority endpoint (HR = 0.92, 95% CI: 0.79–1.06). Consistent results were observed in subgroup analysis.

31.1.2 Progress Made in Second-Line Therapy Using Molecular Targeted Drugs

1. Regorafenib: Regorafenib is an oral multitargeted TKI that inhibits angiogenic kinases such as VEGFRs, PDGF-Rβ, and FGFR1, as well as mutated oncokinases such as KIT, RET, and B-Raf proto-oncogene, serine/threonine kinase (B-RAF). The global phase III Regorafenib for patients with hepatocellular carcinoma who progressed on sorafenib treatment (RESORCE) clinical study showed that

regorafenib significantly improved the OS of HCC patients who progressed after sorafenib treatment (mOS 10.6 months vs. 7.8 months, $P < 0.0001$). Compared with the control arm, the risk of death was significantly reduced by 38% in the regorafenib arm with a good safety profile. Median OS from the beginning of sorafenib treatment in the sorafenib/regorafenib arm was superior to that of the sorafenib/placebo arm (26.0 months vs. 19.2 months), suggesting that the median survival can exceed 2 years in patients receiving first- and second-line systemic treatment. Regorafenib is the first approved second-line therapy that significantly improves the OS of unresectable HCC patients with radiographic progression during sorafenib treatment.

2. Cabozantinib: Cabozantinib is a small molecule TKI that targets c-Met, VEGFR2, and AXL (Fig. 31.2). Results from the CELESTIAL trial showed that cabozantinib can significantly improve patient OS, and the drug has been approved by the US FDA for use in HCC patients who are unable to tolerate sorafenib use or whose disease is progressively exacerbated during sorafenib treatment.
3. Ramucirumab: Ramucirumab is an anti-VEGF monoclonal immunoglobulin G (IgG) antibody. It is also the first approved systemic therapy for HCC patients selected based on biomarkers, with a survival benefit for unresectable HCC patients with alpha-fetoprotein (AFP) ≥400 ng/mL and sorafenib intolerance/radiographic progression. Ramucirumab has a good adverse event profile and low incidences of dose reduction and discontinuation. Ramucirumab has been approved by the US FDA for use in HCC patients with AFP ≥400 ng/mL after sorafenib treatment. This is also the first biomarker-driven therapy for HCC approved by the US FDA. The median OS was 7.8 months for patients with AFP ≥400 ng/mL and 4.2 months for the control arm. In contrast, the median OS of patients with AFP <400 ng/mL was 10.1 months in the ramucirumab arm versus 11.8 months in the placebo arm.

31.1.3 Individualized Efficacy Evaluation and Prediction of Molecular Targeted Drugs

The proportion of the AFP response was higher in the regorafenib arm than in the placebo arm (46% vs. 11%), and the AFP response was associated with longer OS (HR = 0.72) in the regorafenib arm. The radiographic objective response rate (ORR) was similar in patients with and without an AFP response in the regorafenib arm, but the proportion of PD was higher in patients without any AFP response. The use of an AFP response as a potential predictor for HCC treatment outcome still needs to be further studied.

In addition, pharmacogenetic studies of molecular targeted drugs showed that gene polymorphism is closely associated with the efficacy and side effects of molecular targeted drugs, which needs further research and clinical transformation.

31.1.4 Prospects in Molecular Targeted Drugs for HCC

Transforming growth factor β (TGF-β) inhibitors and TGF-β signaling pathways have different or even opposite mechanisms of action in HCC. They mainly inhibit the proliferation of tumor cells in the early stage. However, in advanced stages, they are shown to promote tumor cell invasion, angiogenesis, epithelial–mesenchymal transition (EMT) transformation, and drug resistance. Moreover, the TGF-β signaling pathway reduces the efficacy of immune checkpoint inhibitors (ICIs) by T cell rejection. The phase I–II studies of galunisertib (LY2157299, TGF-β receptor 1 inhibitor) used alone and combined with sorafenib in HCC are currently ongoing.

There are also exploratory studies for the application of the MET inhibitors tepotinib and capmatinib in HCC. A phase I study of BLU9931, an fibroblast growth factor receptor 4 (FGFR4) inhibitor blocking the Recombinant Fibroblast Growth Factor 19/FGFR4 signaling pathways, is currently being carried out in HCC patients with high FGF19 expression. It is believed that with comprehensive basic and clinical research, more molecular targeted drugs will become available for HCC patients in the near future (Fig. 31.2).

31.2 ICIs for HCC

Bypassing the immune system is one of the most basic characteristics of tumor cells. Immune checkpoints on the surface of T cells are the main pathways of evasion, among which PD-1 and cytotoxic T lymphocyte-associated antigen 4 (CTLA-4) are popular topics of current research. The liver is an "immune privileged" organ and various antigens from the intestine are pooled in the portal vein and must be metabolized by the liver. In order to avoid excessive immune response, immune cells in the liver are less active than those in other tissues and organs, and chronic viral hepatitis induces tolerance in the liver immune system, which provides a natural environment for immune evasion by HCC cells.

31.2.1 Progress Made in Second-Line ICI Therapy for HCC

1. Nivolumab: Nivolumab was officially approved by the US FDA as the second-line therapy for advanced HCC in September 2017. The approval was based on the phase I/II CheckMate 040 trial, in which the ORR of 154 patients treated with sorafenib was 14.3%, according to the RECIST 1.1 criteria, with a duration of response (DOR) of 3.2–38.2 months. Follow-up studies are still ongoing. The mOS was 15.6 months in the extended arm and 15 months in the dose ascending arm.

   CheckMate 459 is the first published phase III study of immune checkpoints as the first-line treatment for advanced HCC. The study did not meet the predetermined statistically significant primary endpoint (OS); however, the data showed that first-line therapy with nivolumab tended to improve the OS of patients with advanced HCC, with a high ORR and complete response (CR) rate. The mOS was 16.4 months in the nivolumab arm and 14.7 months in the sorafenib arm (HR = 0.85, 95% CI: 0.72–1.02, P = 0.0752). Consistent OS benefits were observed in subgroups with different PD-L1 expression and other predefined subgroups. The quality of life was improved in patients treated with nivolumab.
2. Pembrolizumab: Based on the results of the phase II KEYNOTE-224 trial, pembrolizumab was approved by the US FDA in November 2018 for HCC patients whose sorafenib treatment failed.

   Subsequently, a randomized, controlled phase III KEYNOTE-240 study investigated the efficacy and safety of pembrolizumab and best supportive care in progressive HCC patients who had received treatment. The results showed that when compared with the placebo, the pembrolizumab arm had a prolonged OS of 3 months (13.9 months vs. 10.6 months, HR = 0.78, 95% CI: 0.611–0.998, P = 0.0238) and an improved PFS (3 months vs. 2.8 months, HR = 0.718, 95% CI: 0.570–0.904, P = 0.0022). Unfortunately, the difference in OS and PFS was not statistically significant (0.0174 and 0.002, respectively). The ORR was 18.3% in the pembrolizumab arm and 4.4% in the placebo arm (P = 0.00007). Pembrolizumab had sustained efficacy and a median DOR of 13.8 months (1.5–23.6 months). Pembrolizumab also had a good safety profile and comparable incidences of hepatitis and other immune-related adverse events (irAEs) as seen in previous pembrolizumab studies. Analysis of OS in different regions showed that Asian patients received greater benefits than European and American patients. KEYNOTE-394 is a randomized, double-blind phase III study of pembrolizumab plus BSC versus placebo plus BSC as second-line therapy in Asian subjects with advanced HCC who have previously received systemic therapy. The results are expected to be reported later.
3. Camrelizumab: Camrelizumab has been officially approved by the National Medical Products Administration for the treatment of advanced HCC patients who have received sorafenib therapy and/or systemic chemother-

apy containing oxaliplatin, serving as a safer and more effective alternative treatment for previously treated advanced HCC patients in China. It is also the first PD-1 immunotherapy approved for HCC in China.

The approval of camrelizumab as a second-line treatment for HCC was based on the results of a phase II clinical study. The baseline condition of enrolled patients was found to be poor: AFP ≥400 ng/mL (51%), extrahepatic metastases (82%), HBV infection (83%), and prior second- or subsequent-line systemic therapies (23%). This is far more consistent with the characteristics and national conditions of HCC patients in China. According to the results of the blind independent center review, the ORR was 14.7% (95% CI: 10.3–20.2), DCR was 44.2% (95% CI: 37.5–51.1), and the 12-month OS was 55.9% (95% CI: 48.9–62.2). Further subgroup analysis showed that in the 158 patients treated with sorafenib, the ORR was 17.1% (95% CI: 11.6–23.9) and the 6-month OS was 75.8% (95% CI: 68.3–81.7). In terms of safety, camrelizumab was found to be well tolerated in patients, with only 15% of patients requiring drug interruption and only 4% requiring drug discontinuation due to treatment-related adverse events (TRAEs). The most common TRAE was reactive cutaneous capillary endothelial proliferation (RCCEP, 67%), which was either grade 1 or 2. The analysis showed that the incidence of RCCEP was closely correlated with anti-tumor efficacy, and therefore, RCCEP may be a biomarker related to efficacy.

4. Sintilimab: Sintilimab is a recombinant fully human IgG4 monoclonal antibody targeting PD-1. Preclinical studies have shown that sintilimab binds to PD-1 with a high affinity and slow dissociation rate and that high occupancy of PD-1 leads to a better anti-tumor immune response. Clinical pharmacodynamic tests showed that the continuous PD-1 occupancy rate of sintilimab in patients with advanced solid tumors was on average over 95%. Taken together, the presence of low valence in anti-drug antibodies and low incidences of anti-drug antibodies and neutralizing antibodies indicates that sintilimab has a low immunogenicity risk. The phase II/III studies of sintilimab combined with bevacizumab biosimilar versus sorafenib as first-line therapy for advanced HCC (ORIENT-32 and CTR20182545) are currently ongoing and patient enrollment has been completed.
5. Tislelizumab: Tislelizumab is a proprietary humanized IgG4 anti-PD-1 monoclonal antibody developed by BeiGene, of which multiple clinical studies have been performed of tislelizumab injection in HCC. Preliminary results of two studies involving multiple tumor types, including HCC, have confirmed the efficacy and safety of using tislelizumab injections in advanced HCC.

At present, pembrolizumab and nivolumab have been approved as second-line treatments for HCC abroad. Compared with other second-line therapies for HCC, such as regorafenib, cabozantinib, and ramucirumab, pembrolizumab and nivolumab have demonstrated higher ORR (about 20%), longer OS, and better safety profiles in clinical studies. However, the predefined primary study endpoint was not met in the KEYNOTE-240 study. This further suggests that more effective and safe combination treatments should be explored to continue to increase the ICI values in the treatment of HCC.

31.2.2 Progress Made in First-Line ICI Therapy for HCC

The CheckMate-459 study showed that the OS (primary endpoint) of patients was not statistically significant when comparing that of sorafenib and nivolumab (HR = 0.85, 95% CI: 0.72–1.02, P = 0.0752). This indicates that nivolumab did not significantly improve the OS of patients in comparison with sorafenib. HCC is a highly heterogeneous tumor with a complex immune microenvironment, which is the main cause of ICI monotherapy failure. Therefore, combination immunotherapy should be considered as the way forward (Table 31.1).

Table 31.1 A summary of first-line combination immunotherapy regimens for HCC

Immunotherapy + anti-VEGF		
Atezolizumab + bevacizumab (IMbrave 150; phase III) anti-PD-L1 + anti-VEGF	Nivolumab + lenvatinib (phase Ib) anti-PD-L1 + TKI	Sintilimab + bevacizumab biosimilar (ORIENT-32; phase II/III) anti-PD-L1 + anti-VEGF
Atezolizumab + cabozantinib (COSMIC-312; phase III) anti-PD-L1 + TKI	Nivolumab + sorafenib (phase II) anti-PD-L1 + TKI	Avelumab + axitinib (VEGF liver 100; phase Ib) anti-PD-L1 + TKI
Pembrolizumab + lenvatinib (LEAP-002; phase III) anti-PD-L1 + TKI	Pembrolizumab + regorafenib (KN-743; phase Ib) anti-PD-L1 + TKI	Spartalizumab + sorafenib (phase Ib) anti-PD-L1 + TKI
Camrelizumab + apatinib (phase III) anti-PD-L1 + TKI	Sorafenib + pembrolizumab (phase II) anti-PD-L1 + TKI	Avelumab + regorafenib (phase I/II) anti-PD-L1 + TKI
Combination of two ICIs		
Nivolumab + ipilimumab (CheckMate-9DW; phase III) Anti-PD-L1 + anti-CTLA-4	Durvalumab ± tremelimumab (HIMALAYA; phase III) Anti-PD-L1 + anti-CTLA-4	Relatlimab ± nivolumab (phase I/II) Anti-LAG3 ± anti-PD-L1
Other combination therapy regimens		
Camrelizumab + FOLFOX (phase III) Anti-PD-L1 + chemotherapy	Durvalumab ± bevacizumab + TACE (EMERALD 1; phase III) Anti-PD-L1 + anti-VEGF+TACE	Nivolumab + TACE (phase I) Anti-PD-L1 + TACE

Note: *VEGF* vascular endothelial growth factor, *PD-1* programmed cell death receptor-1, *PD-L1* programmed cell death ligand 1, *CTLA-4* cytotoxic T lymphocyte-associated protein 4, *TKI* tyrosine kinase inhibitor, *TACE* transcatheter arterial chemoembolization, *LAG3* lymphocyte activation gene 3

31.2.3 Individualized ICI Efficacy Evaluation and Predictions

HCC arises from the accumulation of somatic, genomic, and epigenetic changes. Extensive application of whole-exome sequencing and single-nucleotide polymorphism allows for a progressively clearer and more comprehensive full picture of HCC genes to be obtained. In accordance with the major genetic changes seen in HCC, HCC can be divided into two distinct international molecular subtypes, namely, those that are either proliferative or non-proliferative. The genetic characteristics of the proliferative subtype include a clear correlation between gene characteristics and poor prognosis, TP53-gene mutations, and chromosome instability. Its clinical features include HBV infection, poorly differentiated tumor cells, high AFP expression, and poor prognosis. The genetic characteristics of the non-proliferative subtype are CTNNB1 mutations, immune rejection, and similar gene expression as normal hepatocytes. Its clinical features include HCV infection and alcoholic cirrhosis, well-differentiated tumor cells, rare occurrence of vascular invasion, and good prognosis. Therefore, most HCC patients in China are classified as the proliferative type. The immune response is characterized by increased M2 cell infiltration and immune depletion. According to immune classification, the immune status of the HCC microenvironment can be divided into immune response, immune transition, and immune rejection (Figs. 31.3 and 31.4). The correlation between different immune states and the efficacy of ICIs remains to be further explored.

1. Tumor microenvironment: In HCC, mesenchymal cells (Kupffer cells, dendritic cells (DCs), hepatic endothelial cells, and hepatic stellate cells) and immunosuppressive cytokines (such as IL-10 or TGF-β) may contribute to the immunosuppressive environment, and the PD-1/PD-L1 pathway plays an important role in the development of the immunosuppressive HCC microenvironment. HCC tumor microenvironment has extremely complex cell composition and corresponding differential protein expression, such as PD-L1 protein expression, tumor mutation burden (TMB), IFN-γ mRNA expression, microsatellite instability (MSI), tumor-associated antigen

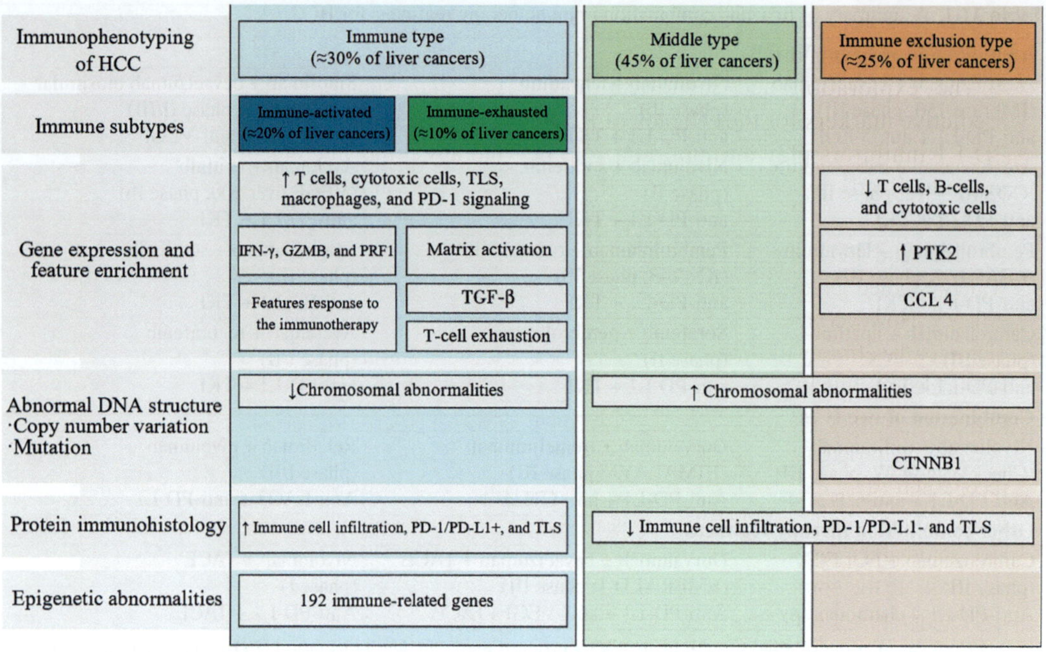

IFN-γ: interferon γ; GZMB: granzyme B; CCL: chemokine C-C motif ligand; PD-1: programmed cell death receptor-1; PD-L1: programmed cell death ligand-1; TLS: tertiary lymphoid structures; TGF-β: transforming growth factor; PKT: protein tyrosine kinase

Fig. 31.3 Classification based on the immune status of HCC microenvironment

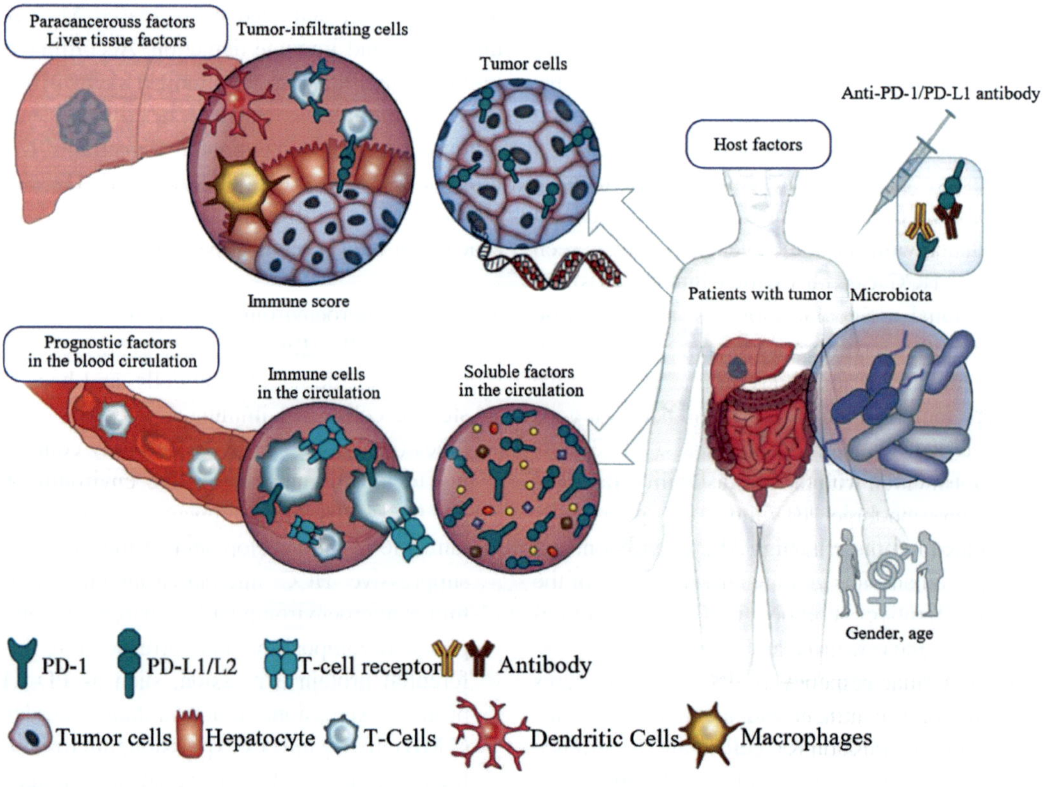

Fig. 31.4 Overview of possible markers for predicting efficacy of PD-1/PD-L1 inhibitors in HCC

(TAA)-specific cytotoxic T lymphocytes (CTLs), and tumor-infiltrating lymphocytes.

The exploration and identification of predictive markers for the efficacy of PD-1/PD-L1 inhibitors play an important role in individualized precision immunotherapy for HCC.

TMB and PD-L1 expression are the most widely studied predictive biomarkers for ICI efficacy. However, the value of TMB as a predictor for the efficacy of ICI treatment in HCC is still unclear. While PD-L1 expression is a useful predictive marker as a continuous variable, it does not help determine which patients should receive anti-PD-1 therapy. In the era of immune-based combination therapy, more comprehensive biomarker approaches are required to demonstrate the complex interactions of immunomodulatory networks in the tumor microenvironment and the efficacy of individual drugs with different immunomodulatory effects.

2. Serological/circulating factors: In order to reduce the reliance on tumor biopsy pathology, liquid biopsy techniques and CTCs or ct-DNA and ct-mRNA analysis are also very promising markers for predicting efficacy. Further understanding of the relationship between the signaling pathways and immune status such as increased PTK2 signaling is closely related to reduced T cell infiltration in tumors, and the activation of β-catenin (CTNNB1) signaling is closely related to T cell rejection, also helps with the exploration and clinical transformation of predictive markers for the efficacy of PD-1/PD-L1 inhibitors.
3. Pseudoprogression: Pseudoprogression is a type of immunotherapy response manifested as the enlargement of the primary lesion or the appearance of new lesions, which may be judged as PD. However, with the continuation of immunotherapy, the target lesion and new lesions may shrink, and the patient may experience remission. When lymphocytes infiltrate a tumor, the mass may appear enlarged or new lesions may appear. Since it takes time to develop an adaptive immune response, pseudoprogression may manifest as continued tumor growth until some degree of remission is achieved.

31.2.4 Research Progress in irAEs

Our understanding of irAE management is still evolving alongside the extensive use of immunotherapy drugs in clinical practice. The effects of cirrhosis and modified Child-Pugh scoring in HCC merit further study, as the results of early clinical trials suggest that HCC patients may experience increased liver-related adverse events when treated with ICI-based combination therapy compared with patients with other tumor types. Retrospective observations found that patients experiencing irAE had better anti-tumor effects, suggesting the existence of a common mechanism for inducing anti-tumor and autoimmune responses. Blocking an immune checkpoint pathway reduces the inhibitory effect on the immune system and activates the anti-tumor immune response, which reduces self-tolerance and thus leads to the development of irAEs. Such irAEs are usually low-grade adverse reactions, but serious or life-threatening irAEs have also been observed, which resulted in death in 1–2% of patients.

The most commonly targeted organs of irAEs include the skin, gastrointestinal tract, liver, lungs, and endocrine organs, while irAEs of the heart, kidneys, nerve, and eyes are relatively rare. Although irAEs have different onset times, they generally occur within 1–6 months, and most are reversible. The incidence of toxicity is higher in combination therapy (immunotherapy, chemotherapy, and anti-angiogenic treatment) than in monotherapy. Long half-life results in sustained inhibition and occupancy of the target, which may lead to irAEs of ICIs. The development of ICIs with short half-life and desirable anti-tumor activity is an effective strategy for better management of irAEs. Most irAEs can be controlled and reversed by dose interruption ± corticosteroids. The incidence of liver side effects is not high, but hepatitis caused by immunotherapy is usually asymptomatic immune-related hepatitis that manifests as elevated alanine aminotransferase, elevated glutamic-oxaloacetic transferase, fever, and with or without elevated bilirubin. The median onset time of elevated transaminase is 6–14 weeks after immunotherapy. In KEYNOTE-001, patients with a history of chest radiation therapy were more likely to have treatment-related lung injury after receiving pembrolizumab than patients without a history of chest radiation therapy (13% vs. 1%). Other potential risk factors may include underlying lung disease and smoking. The incidence of grade 5 pneumonia was 0.1%. The incidence of immune cardiotoxicity was 6/10,000, and 46 of 101 patients displaying severe myocarditis resulted in death. The median onset time was 27 days; 76% of cases were observed within 6 weeks, and the shortest was 5 days. RCCEP is an immune-related adverse reaction commonly seen in patients treated with camrelizumab monotherapy. RCCEP was mild and self-limiting, with an incidence of 74.1% for any grade and only 0.6% for grade 3 or greater. Grade 1 RCCEP accounted for the majority (60.1%) of RCCEP cases, which was controllable and did not affect the safety of life. The median onset time of RCCEP was 0.9 months, and the median duration was 4.6 months. After 6 months of medication, some patients may experience spontaneous remission and resolution without leaving obvious scars. Camrelizumab has a unique PD-1 binding epitope, which may be associated with triggering a unique cutaneous immune response. In addition to inhibiting immune escape, camrelizumab may activate $CD4^+$ T cells to release IL-4, stimulate the differentiation of angiogenic M2 macrophages, and ultimately cause abnormal proliferation of vascular endothelial cells. Camrelizumab combined with chemotherapy or apatinib can significantly reduce the incidence of RCCEP.

31.2.5 Prospects for the Development of HCC Immunotherapy

With further research in this field, more HCC immunotherapy drugs will become available in the future (Fig. 31.5).

HCC cells can produce a variety of TAAs. Tumor immunity is initiated by antigen-presenting cells, such as DCs that acquire TAAs and other tumor antigens and migrate to regional lymph nodes. DCs then present the processed antigens to $CD4^+$ T cells and thereby activate $CD4^+$ T proliferation and induce IFN-γ, IL-12, and type I IFN production. Cross-presentation of the relevant antigens by DCs also promotes the proliferation and activation of antigen-specific $CD8^+$ CTLs. When CTLs accumulate in HCC tumor tissues, these antigen-specific CTLs exert anti-tumor effects by secreting granzyme B and perforin. Local therapy and systemic chemotherapy can induce tumor necrosis to expose and release tumor antigens and TAA. Tumor vaccines can promote antigen presentation. Anti-CTLA-4 antibodies mainly promote Th1 polarization and activate $CD8^+$ T cells in the initial stage. Chimeric antigen receptor T-cell (CAR-T) immunotherapy can increase the number of anti-tumor immune cells in peripheral blood.

From the etiological perspective of HCC immunotherapy, different immunotherapy strategies should be adopted based on the different etiologies of HCC. Differences in immune cells in the local microenvironment of HCC with different etiologies are the basis for adopting different immunotherapies. Nonetheless, there are still many unknowns in this field that warrant further exploration (Fig. 31.6).

Exploring immunotherapy strategies according to the pathological immunotype of HCC is also an important direction of research. Recent tumor-wide immunogenomic analyses have revealed six immune profiles within tumors that are associated with specific immune escape mechanisms. The authors analyzed the distribution of the six immune profiles in HCC samples (Fig. 31.7). Clusters 1 and 2 are uncommon in HCC. Cluster 1 was associated with elevated expression of angiogenic genes, supporting the use of angiogenic inhibitors in these patients. Cluster 3 was significantly associated with a better survival rate compared to other subtypes. Cluster 4 was the most common and had no significant adverse prognostic effect. On the contrary, clusters 5 and 6 were weakly represented in HCC. Interestingly, the number of predicted

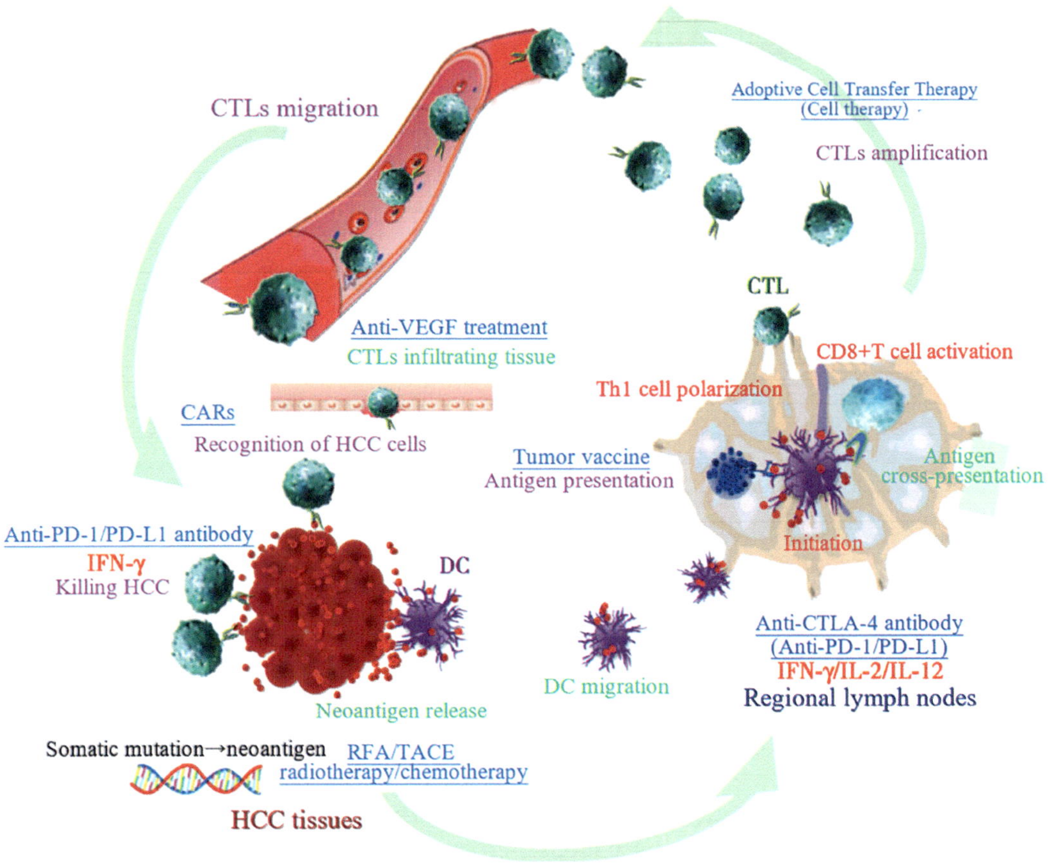

Fig. 31.5 Tumor immune circulation and immunotherapy targets

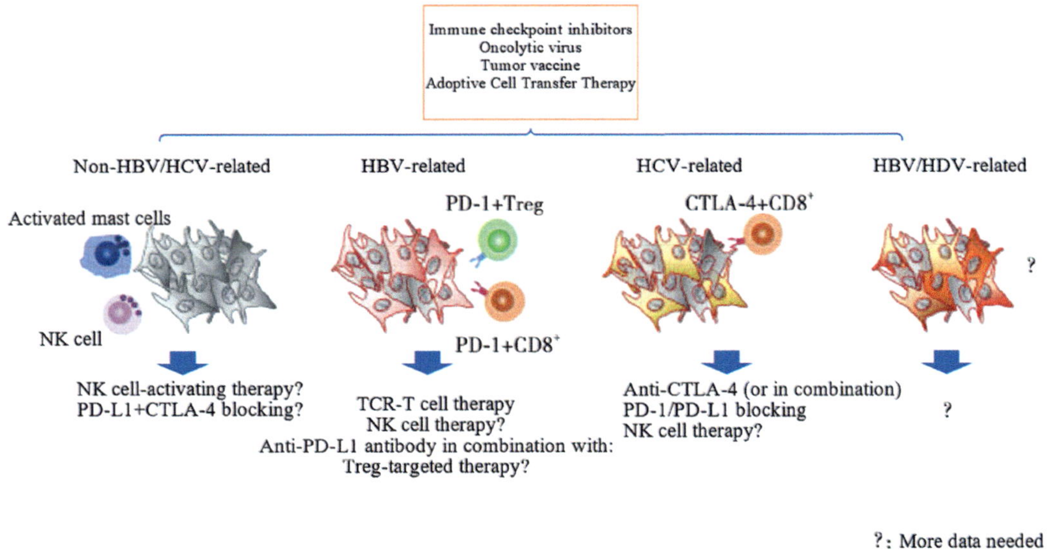

Fig. 31.6 Future development strategies for HCC immunotherapy—etiological perspective

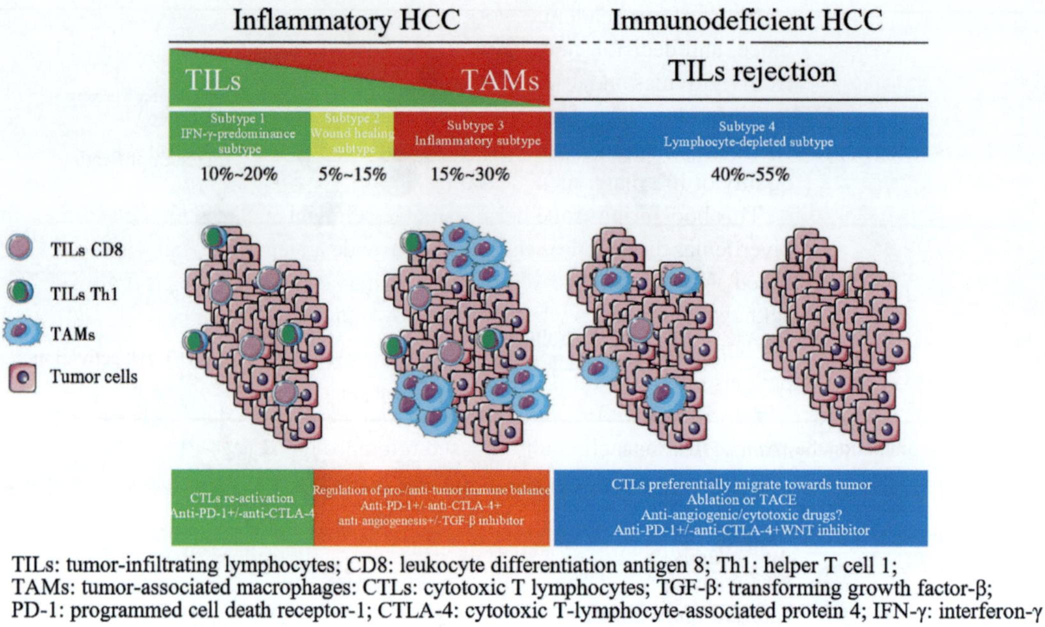

Fig. 31.7 Future development strategy for combined HCC immunotherapy—based on immunotyping

neoantigens was positively correlated with the number of $CD8^+$ T cells. High neoantigen levels were more common in clusters 2 and 3, and the CD8/T regulatory (Treg) ratio was higher than in other clusters.

31.3 Progress in and Prospects for ICI Combination Therapy in HCC

Combination therapy with ICIs is currently at the forefront of HCC research. Currently, there are various combination regimens, including the use of a combination of immunotherapy and local treatment, such as radiotherapy, surgery, and interventional therapy; a combination of immunotherapy and systemic therapy, such as systemic chemotherapy and targeted anti-angiogenic therapy; and a combination with other ICIs. In particular, immunotherapy combined with molecular targeted therapy is under active research (Fig. 31.8).

31.3.1 Progress in and Prospects for the Application of Molecular Targeted Drugs Plus ICIs in HCC

There is no doubt that using molecular targeted drugs with ICIs is currently the most promising combination therapy with the most clinical research underway. In recent years, the number of studies on this combination therapy has been rapidly increasing every year, and more combination therapy regimens are believed to be applied as first-line and second-line treatments for HCC in the future (Fig. 31.9).

31.3.2 Molecular Mechanism of Molecular Targeted Drugs Plus ICIs in HCC

Shigeta K et al. revealed the mechanism of action of immune targeted and molecular targeted combination therapy using the orthotopic

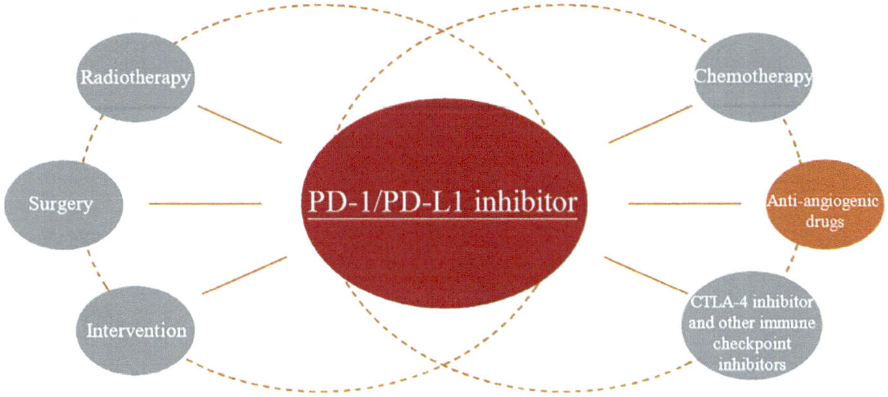

Fig. 31.8 Combination therapy with ICIs for HCC

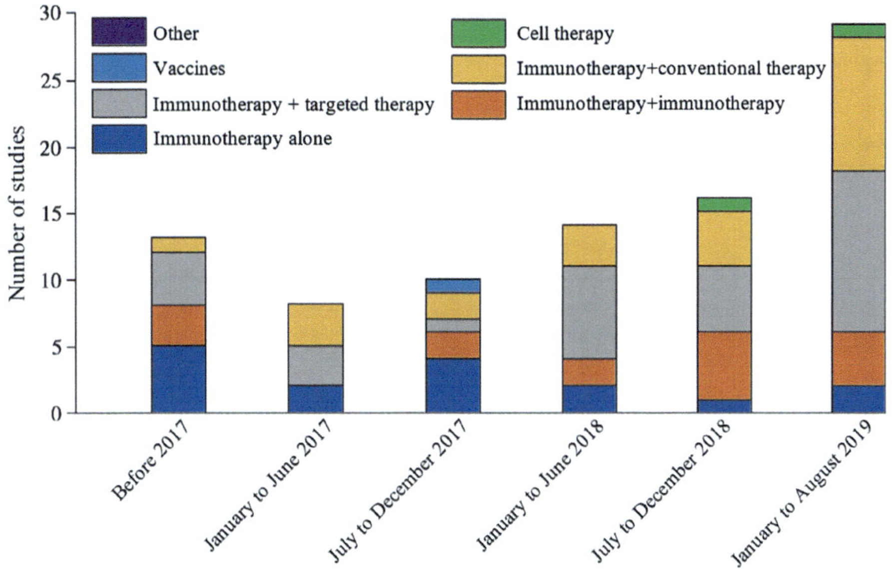

Fig. 31.9 Number of clinical studies on ICIs plus targeted therapy for HCC

transplantation model or the induced mouse model for HCC. The authors showed that dual PD-1 and VEGFR-2 blockade not only promotes vascular normalization but also enhances anti-tumor immune responses in HCC. The combination of immunotherapy and targeted therapy reprogrammed the immune microenvironment by increasing $CD8^+$ cytotoxic T cell infiltration and activation, altering the M1/M2 ratio of tumor-associated macrophages, and reducing Treg cells and $CCR2^+$ monocyte infiltration in HCC tissues. In these models, VEGFR-2 is selectively expressed in tumor endothelial cells. The study found that when VEGFR-2 is blocked on endothelial cells, PD-L1 expression is induced by HCC cells through a paracrine manner, and part of the expression is induced by interferon-γ. VEGFR-2 blockade also increases PD-1 expression on tumor-infiltrating $CD4^+$ cells.

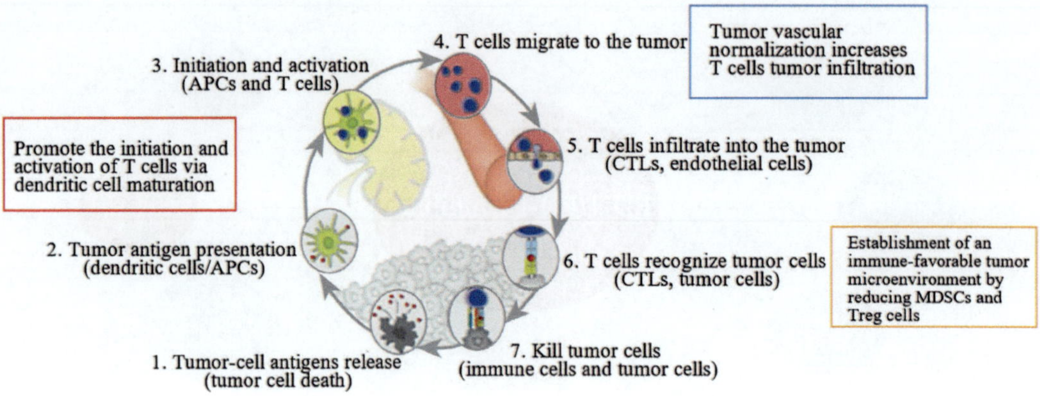

Fig. 31.10 Effect of anti-angiogenic agents on tumor immune microenvironment

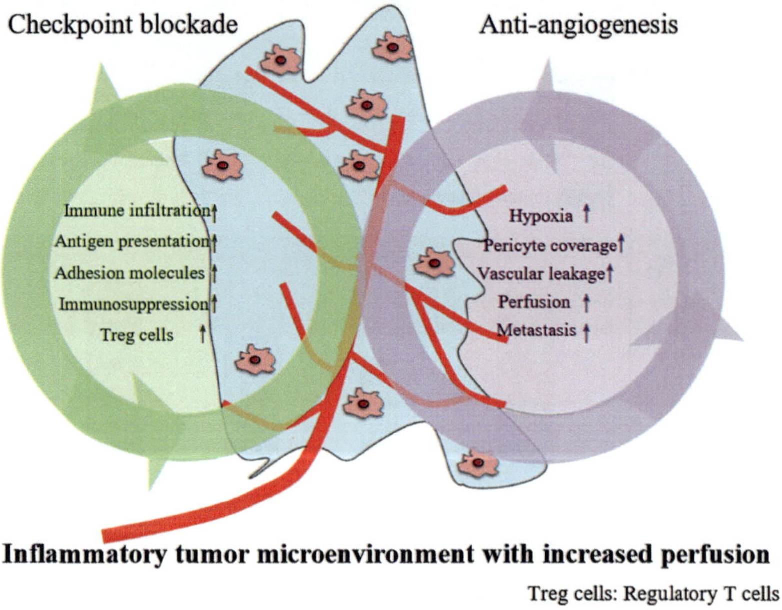

Fig. 31.11 Tumor microenvironment remodeling by the combination of ICIs and anti-angiogenic agents

Furthermore, the addition of anti-PD-1 therapy to anti-angiogenic therapy with anti-VEGFR-2 antibodies can induce $CD4^+$ cells to promote normal angiogenesis. Dual inhibition of the PD-1 and VEGFR-2 pathways resulted in a doubling of survival time. Cells in the tumor microenvironment exert systemic immunosuppressive effect by releasing VEGFs, TGF-β, and prostaglandin E2 into the circulation. Cytokines reduce the ability of antigen-presenting cells to activate T cells and thereby dampen the antitumor response of effector T cells and increase the number of myeloid-derived suppressor cells (MDSCs) and Treg cells (Figs. 31.10, 31.11, 31.12 and 31.13).

As a small molecule cytokine, VEGF release can cause changes in the immunosuppressive state of the tumor microenvironment. VEGF-A can induce MDSC expansion and Treg cell proliferation and differentiation, inhibit the maturation of dendritic precursor cells, and ultimately lead to declined NK cell and T cell functions. Numerous studies have shown that the immunomodulatory effect is related to the dose of anti-angiogenic drugs, and lower doses are more effective in inducing local activation.

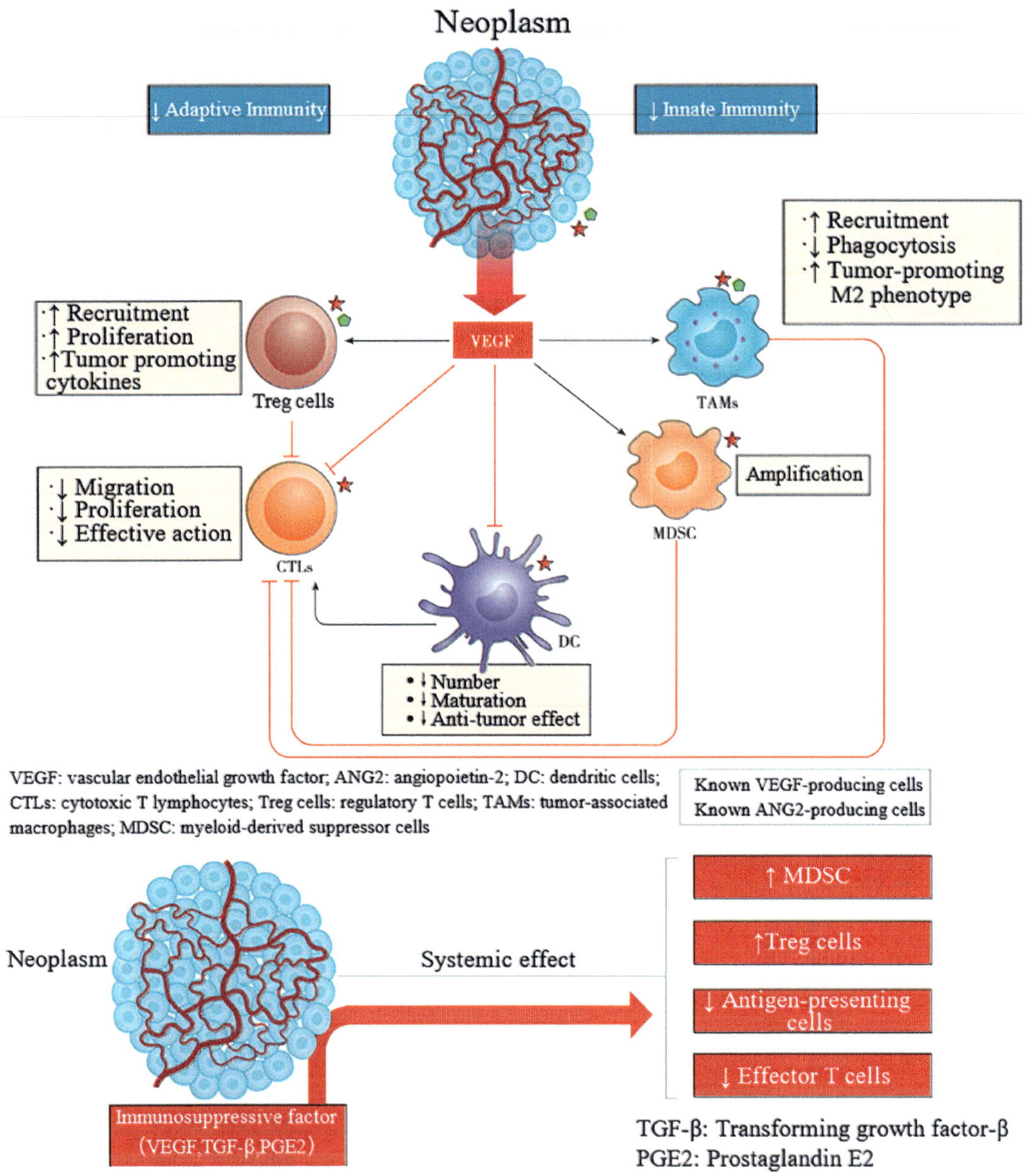

Fig. 31.12 Combined molecular mechanisms of ICIs and anti-angiogenic agents

31.3.3 Exploration of Molecular Targeted Drugs in Combination with ICI Treatment Modalities in HCC

Different molecular-targeted anti-angiogenic agents have different mechanisms of action, as well as different regulatory and molecular mechanisms in the immune microenvironment. Therefore, how to adopt a reasonable combination treatment remains to be further discussed (Fig. 31.14). For ICIs combined with small molecule TKI, attention should be paid to the following:

1. Targeted inhibition of different pathways has different effects on immune cells.

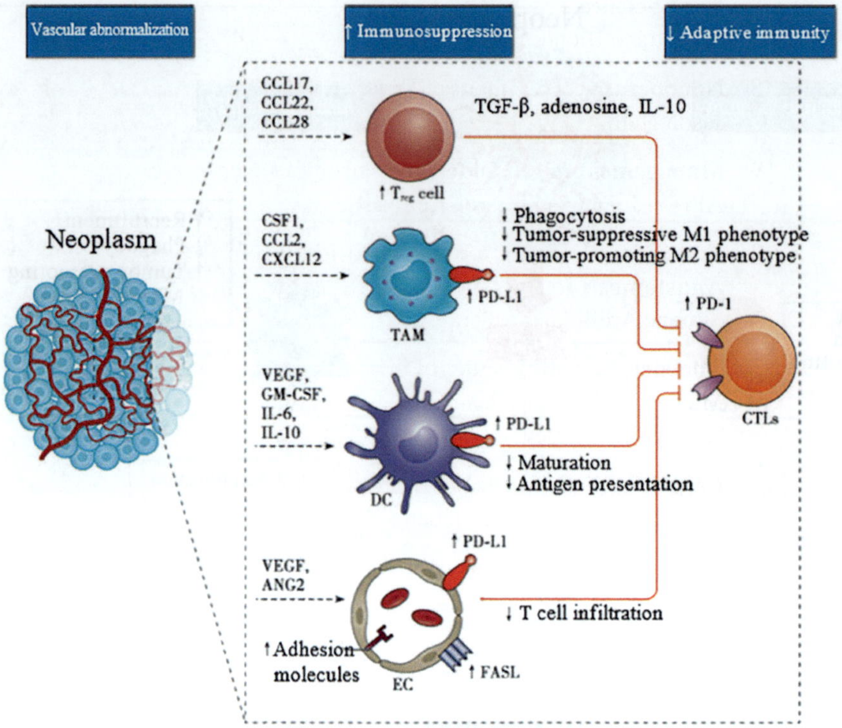

CCL: chemokine C-C motif ligand; CSF1: macrophage colony-stimulating factor 1; CXCL12: chemokine C-X-C motif ligand 12; VEGF: vascular endothelial growth factor; GM-CSF: granulocyte-macrophage colony stimulating factor; IL: interleukin; ANG2: angiopoietin-2; DC: dendritic cells; CTLs: cytotoxic T lymphocytes; EC: endothelial cells; TGF-β: transforming growth factor-β;PD-1: programmed death-1; PD-L1: programmed death ligand-1; Treg cell: regulatory T cells; TAM: tumor-associated macrophages; FASL: Fas ligand

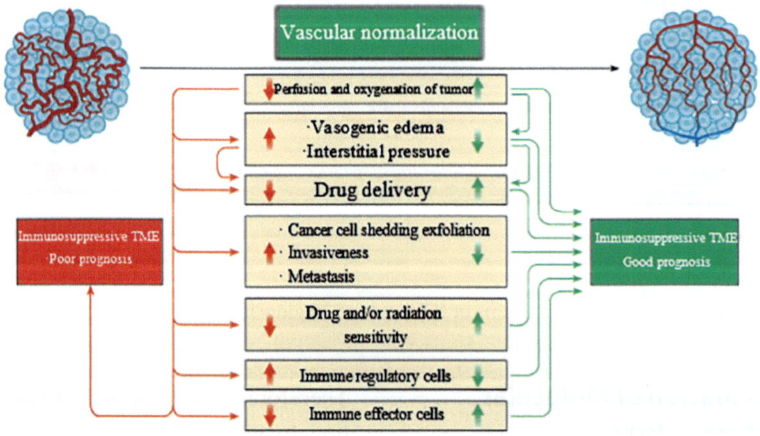

TME: Tumor microenvironment

Fig. 31.13 Vascular abnormalization mediates an immunosuppressive microenvironment—vascular normalization transforms an immunosuppressive environment into an immunosupportive environment

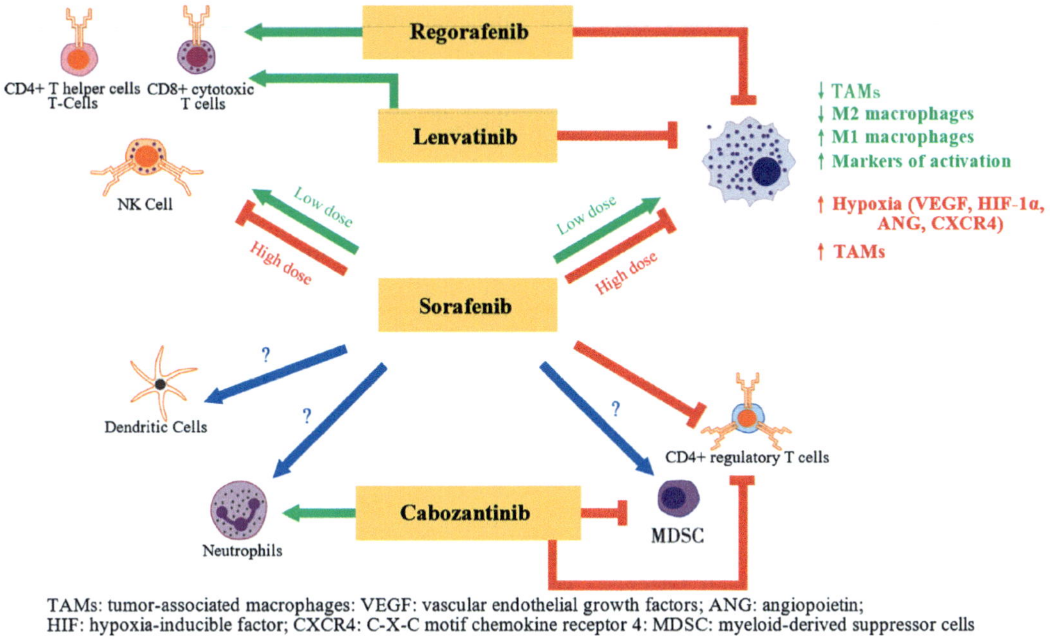

Fig. 31.14 Molecular regulatory mechanism of different molecular-targeted anti-angiogenic agents in the immune microenvironment

2. Different doses have different effects on immune cells, and the effect of sorafenib may be dose-dependent. Lower doses are more likely to induce normalization of blood vessels, reduce hypoxia, and enhance anti-tumor immunity (beneficial effects). In contrast, higher doses may perversely enhance hypoxia and promote immunosuppression (harmful effects). The dose effects of other multikinase inhibitors (regorafenib, lenvatinib, and cabozantinib) deserve further investigation.
3. How to adopt a sequential, intermittent, and continuous combination pattern for ICIs.
4. To elucidate the role of TKI in combination immunotherapy, the immune-related anti-tumor mechanism of TKI in addition to the anti-VEGFR effect needs to be clarified, and the immune effective dose of TKI needs to be optimized.
5. The isolation and identification of other key immune mediators are essential for more comprehensive use of a rational combination treatment mode.

31.3.4 Prospects for Application of Molecular Targeted Drugs + ICIs in HCC

In some early studies, immunotherapy combined with anti-angiogenic agents has led to further improvements in ORR. In the recent 2 years, breakthroughs have been achieved in a number of studies in this field, which show that the organic combination of the two is promising. In July 2018, the combined application of atezolizumab and bevacizumab was granted breakthrough therapy designation (BTD) by the US FDA for the initial treatment of advanced or metastatic HCC. The approval was mainly based on data from the GO30140 phase Ib study. The study compared the efficacy of atezolizumab plus bevacizumab versus atezolizumab alone and demonstrated that combination therapy reduced the risk of disease aggravation or death by 45% (HR = 0.55, 80%CI: 0.40–0.74, *P* = 0.0108). The IMbrave150 study, published in November 2019, is a global, randomized, multicenter, open-label phase III study that has achieved positive results in both primary endpoints of OS and PFS. The results confirmed that atezolizumab combined with bevacizumab significantly improved OS and PFS compared to the current standard sorafenib treatment. The ORR identified in the study reached 27%. With regard to safety, the co-administration of atezolizumab and bevacizumab was safe and well tolerated. The analysis of the Chinese population in the IMbrave150 study showed that the atezolizumab plus bevacizumab arm had better mOS and mPFS than the sorafenib arm, which was consistent with the main study results. IMbrave150 is the first phase III study showing positive results in the first-line therapy for HCC and confirming superiority over sorafenib. In the Chinese population, atezolizumab combined with bevacizumab resulted in a significant delay in patient-reported deterioration of quality of life compared with sorafenib, which was consistent with the findings in the global population.

In July 2019, the US FDA awarded the BTD to pembrolizumab plus lenvatinib combination therapy as the first-line treatment for advanced unresectable HCC patients. This approval was based on the results of KEYNOTE-524, an open-label, single-arm, phase Ib clinical trial of using lenvatinib combined with pembrolizumab in advanced HCC. Data recently updated at the ESMO meeting included 67 patients as of June 30, 2019. After the combined application of the two drugs, the ORR was 46.3%, PFS was 9.7 months, and mOS was 20 months as assessed by an independent radiographic evaluation center based on the mRECIST criteria. Unexpected adverse reactions were not observed in the combination regimen, and the patients' serious adverse reactions were controllable and tolerable. This study displays an unprecedented breakthrough in the field of HCC treatment, demonstrating the superior anti-tumor efficacy of lenvatinib combined with pembrolizumab in HCC. A randomized, double-blind, multicenter, phase III clinical study (LEAP-002) of lenvatinib plus pembrolizumab versus lenvatinib as first-line treatment for advanced HCC patients is being conducted across 102 centers worldwide. This study plans to enroll 750 HCC patients and is designed to evaluate the safety and efficacy of lenvatinib plus pembrolizumab versus placebo plus lenvatinib as first-line therapy for advanced HCC patients. The primary endpoints of the trial are OS and PFS, and the secondary endpoints are ORR, DOR, DCR, TTP, and safety. The trial is expected to end in 2022, and we are looking forward to the results. The phase III, multicenter, randomized, double-blinded, controlled trial (LEAP-012) of lenvatinib combined with pembrolizumab and TACE versus TACE is also ongoing. The study plans to enroll 950 unresectable advanced HCC patients without metastases, and the results are also worth looking forward to.

Camrelizumab (SHR-1210) combined with apatinib for advanced HCC, gastric cancer, or gastroesophageal junction carcinoma: In an open-label dose-escalation and extension study of 16 assessable HCC patients (n = 4 for 125 mg, n = 11 for 250 mg, and n = 1 for 500 mg), ORR and DCR were 50% (8/16) and 93.8% (15/16), respectively, and 62.5% (10/16) of patients had shrunken target lesion during treatment. ORR reached 53.8% (7/13) in the 250 mg dose arm. The study of camrelizumab plus apatinib versus sorafenib as first-line therapy for advanced HCC is the first randomized, controlled, open-label, international multi-center phase III clinical trial of PD-1 inhibitor in China. Subjects in the trial were randomized into the camrelizumab (200 mg, Q2W) plus apatinib (250 mg/day) arm and sorafenib (400 mg/day) arm. The primary endpoints were OS and PFS. The study was officially launched in Shanghai in April 2019, and we hope that the results will bring high-quality survival benefits for more HCC patients.

It is believed that more clinical study results will be published in this field in the future, and we are expecting more "combination therapies" that will bring safer and longer survival benefits for HCC patients.

31.3.5 Prospect for Combined Application of ICIs in HCC

A combined application of ICIs is also one of the hot topics of current research. The combination of dual ICIs (PD-1 + CTLA-4, CheckMate 040 study): The combination of nivolumab (NIVO) and ipilimumab (IPI) is used for the second-line treatment of HCC, and the US FDA has granted breakthrough drug designation to the combination of Opdivo and Yervoy immunotherapy (referred to as "OY" combination) for the treatment of advanced HCC patients previously treated with sorafenib. The supplemental Biologic License Application was based on the OY cohort results of the phase I/II CheckMate 040 (NCT01658878) study. This is an ongoing open-label, multi-cohort study investigating the efficacy and safety of NIVO monotherapy or NIVO combination therapy in advanced HCC patients who have not previously received sorafenib therapy (initial sorafenib treatment), or were either intolerant to or have progressed after sorafenib, with or without previous hepatitis virus infection.

The NIVO + IPI combination therapy resulted in potent and sustained responses in HCC patients previously treated with sorafenib. The ORR was higher in the combination therapy arm (ORR >30% in each group) than in the NIVO monotherapy arm (14%), and the response was achieved regardless of baseline PD-L1 status. The sustained tumor response and controllable safety of NIVO + IPI in the CheckMate040 study suggest that NIVO + IPI may be used as a novel treatment option for progressive HCC previously treated with sorafenib. Based on the good efficacy and safety profile of NIVO + IPI, the combination therapy can be further explored in HCC patients.

31.4 Prospects for Local and Systemic Treatments in HCC

Although surgery remains the preferred treatment for HCC, only 20–30% of HCC patients have the chance to undergo surgery because most have underlying liver disease with insidious onset and no typical symptoms or signs at the early stage, and were already in the intermediate to advanced stages at the time of diagnosis.

Downstaging conversion therapy for HCC refers to the conversion of unresectable intermediate to advanced HCC into surgically resectable early to intermediate HCC through downstaging such as local or combined systemic therapy, or transformation of palliative resection into radical resection through relevant treatment options. A large number of studies have shown that successful downstaging shall meet the Milan criteria, and the success rate of transplantation is 55–78%. Patients not meeting the Milan criteria who were successfully downstaged to meet the Milan criteria had comparable 5-year survival and recurrence after liver transplantation as those who met the Milan criteria and underwent liver transplantation. Studies have shown that HCC patients undergoing second-stage resection after local treatment had a 1-year survival rate of 77.0–91.4%, 3-year survival rate of 55.0–77.1%, and 5-year survival rate of 52.0–69.6%.

With the rapid development of interventional technology and radiotherapy technology, the current, most commonly used downstaging methods such as cTACE, DEB-TACE, HAIC, RFA, TARE, internal beam radiotherapy, external beam radiotherapy, and other local treatment options or combined applications can restore the chance of liver transplantation or surgical resection for patients who exceed the criteria for liver transplantation or resection by reducing tumor load and the stage of tumor.

Many studies have shown that tumor necrosis caused by local treatment is favorable for enhancing the treatment efficacy of combination immunotherapy. The release of tumor antigens and induction of immunogenic cell death by damage-related molecules can promote anti-tumor immunity. TACE-induced liver tumor necrosis enhances AFP-specific $CD4^+$ T cell response. A clinical study of 21 HCC patients showed that AFP-specific $CD4^+$ T cells increased after TACE and patients with clinical response to TACE all had higher frequency of AFP-specific $CD4^+$ T cells. Studies have shown that TACE can significantly improve the response of TAA-specific $CD8^+$ T cells. The combination of TACE and CPI is reasonable: (1) reduces tumor load; (2) CPI plays a role in the tumor microenvironment with high immunogenicity to enhance the efficacy of tumor immunotherapy; and (3) combined application activates anti-tumor immunity. RFA enhances the response of HCC-associated antigen-specific T cells. Some studies showed that 62.3% of patients had increased TAA-specific T cells, and changes in T cell phenotypes were observed after RFA. Brachytherapy combined with immunotherapy reduces the local aggregation of MDSCs and changes the immunosuppressive microenvironment.

In a randomized, open-label, perioperative phase II study of nivolumab monotherapy versus nivolumab + ipilimumab combination therapy in patients with resectable HCC, new irAEs were not observed, and grade ≤ 3 toxic reactions were observed in six patients (about 27% in the combination treatment arm). Surgical resection was safe without delay or complications, and pathological CR (pCR) was achieved in 25% of the patients.

The initiation of immunotherapy before local treatment was explored using tremelimumab, a CTLA-4 antibody. This is a feasibility study of interventional combination immunotherapy which was performed at 36 weeks after treatment. The primary endpoint was the feasibility of combination therapy. The median total TTP was 7.4 months, 6-month PFS was 57.1%, 12-month PFS was 33.1%, and mOS was 12.3 months. Safety was good without dose-limiting toxicity. The phase II clinical study of nivolumab + DEB-TACE for the treatment of intermediate HCC (NCT03143270) was initiated in May 2017 and is still in the recruitment process, pending further result announcement.

The study of combination immunotherapy in the prevention of postoperative recurrence in patients with resectable HCC is currently ongoing. This is a phase II randomized controlled trial of perioperative immunotherapy combined with surgical resection (NCT03222076), in which nivolumab plus ipilimumab was used preoperatively for resectable HCC. pCR was obtained in three of the nine enrolled patients, and pathological findings confirmed that pCR was significantly correlated with local $CD8^+$ T cell infiltration. Immunotherapy combined with other therapies not only significantly increased the OS of patients but also brought long-term survival benefits compared with molecular targeted therapy. Trials of pembrolizumab in early HCC have also been carried out. For example, KEYNOTE-937 is a phase III, double-blinded, parallel controlled trial evaluating the safety and efficacy of pembrolizumab adjuvant treatment after surgery or radiofrequency ablation in HCC patients who received up to 1 year of postoperative adjuvant treatment. This trial plans to enroll 950 patients and enrollment is currently ongoing (Fig. 31.15).

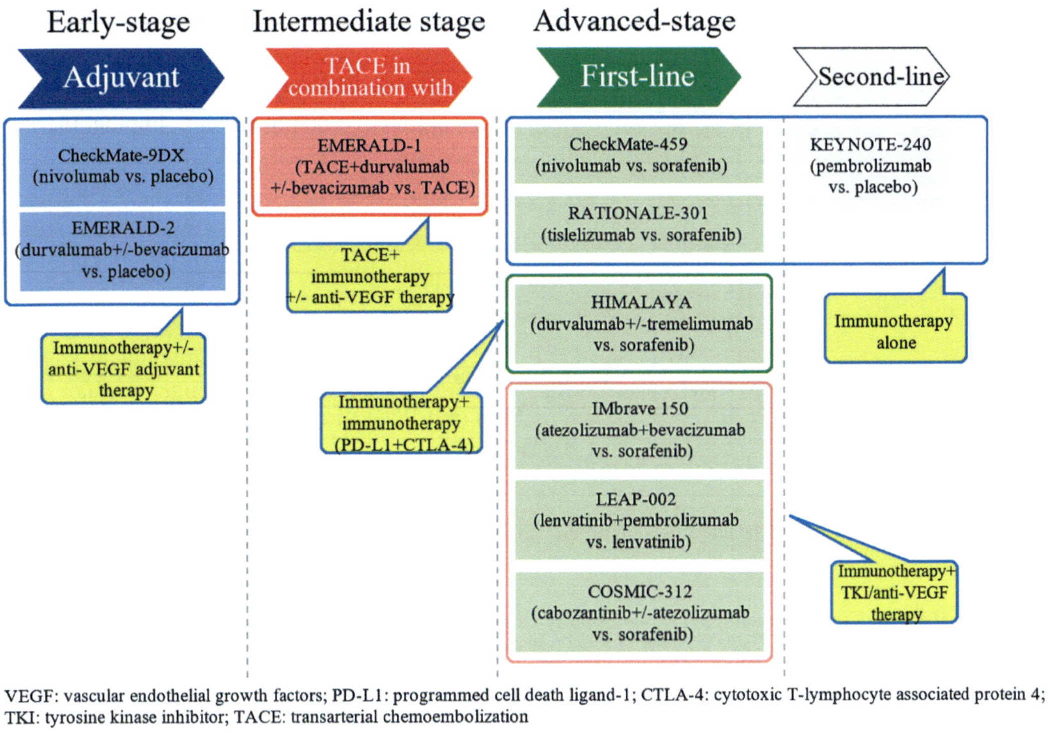

Fig. 31.15 Summary of phase III clinical studies of combination immunotherapy for early, intermediate, and advanced HCC

31.5 Summary

With the rapid development of molecular targeted drugs and ICIs, local plus systemic treatment for HCC has gradually been integrated into clinical practice. In-depth multiomics studies of HCC should be conducted to identify different molecular types and immunophenotypes of HCC in order to achieve individualized precision diagnosis and treatment. Clinical studies of biomarker-driven combination therapy, including PD-L1, TMB, MSI, and TIL, should also be carried out to actively explore the molecular markers for efficacy and safety, guide clinical studies, and hence develop individualized overall treatment regimen. Innovation and optimization of new precision surgery-centered multimodality treatments and rapid improvement of the 5-year OS of HCC in China are required to transform our dreams into reality (Fig. 31.16).

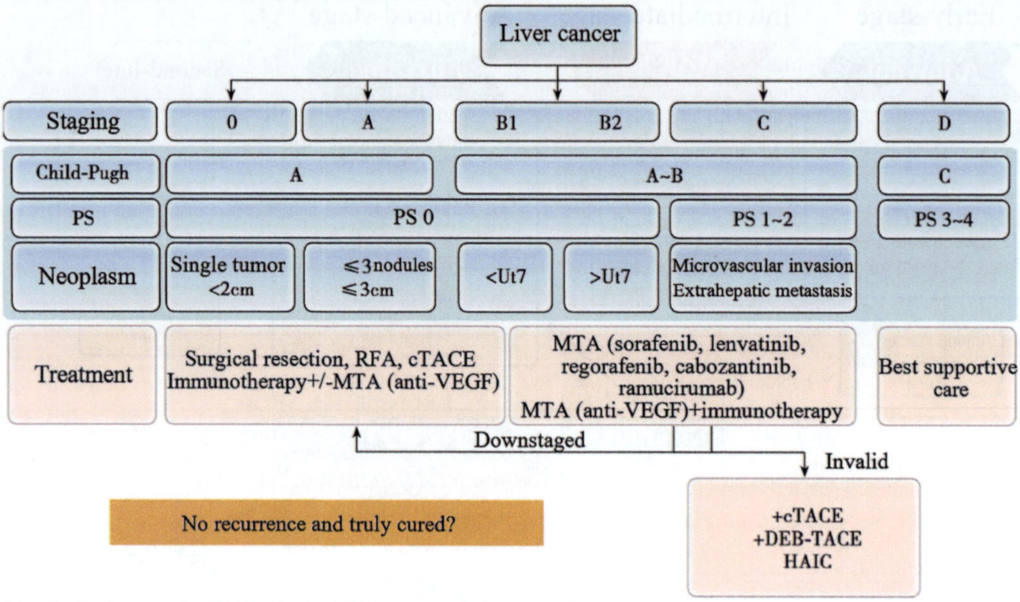

PS: physical status; Ut: Up7 criteria; MTA: molecularly targeted agents; VEGF: vascular endothelial growth factors; RFA: radiofrequency ablation; CTACE: conventional transarterial chemoembolization; DEB-TACEP: drug-eluting bead transarterial chemoembolization; HAIC: hepatic arterial infusion chemotherapy

Fig. 31.16 Future blueprint for HCC treatments

Suggested Reading

1. Nault JC, Cheng AL, Sangro B, et al. Milestones in the pathogenesis and management of primary liver cancer. J Hepatol. 2020;72(2):209–14.
2. Cheng AL, Kang YK, Lin DY, et al. Sunitinib versus sorafenib in advanced hepatocellular cancer: results of a randomized phase III trial. J Clin Oncol. 2013;31(32):4067–75.
3. Johnson PJ, Qin S, Park JW, et al. Brivanib versus sorafenib as first-line therapy in patients with unresectable, advanced hepatocellular carcinoma: results from the randomized phase III BRISK-FL study. J Clin Oncol. 2013;31(28):3517–24.
4. Cainap C, Qin S, Huang WT, et al. Linifanib versus Sorafenib in patients with advanced hepatocellular carcinoma: results of a randomized phase III trial. J Clin Oncol. 2015;33(2):172–9.
5. Zhu AX, Rosmorduc O, Evans TR, et al. SEARCH: a phase III, randomized, double-blind, placebo-controlled trial of sorafenib plus erlotinib in patients with advanced hepatocellular carcinoma. J Clin Oncol. 2015;33(6):559–66.
6. Abou-Alfa GK, Shi Q, Knox JJ, et al. Assessment of treatment with sorafenib plus doxorubicin vs sorafenib alone in patients with advanced hepatocellular carcinoma: phase 3 calgb 80802 randomized clinical trial. JAMA Oncol. 2019;5(11):1582–8.
7. Kudo M. Proposal of primary endpoints for tace combination trials with systemic therapy: lessons learned from 5 negative trials and the positive tactics trial. Liver Cancer. 2018;7(3):225–34.
8. Kudo M, Finn RS, Qin S, et al. Lenvatinib versus sorafenib in first-line treatment of patients with unresectable hepatocellular carcinoma: a randomised phase 3 non-inferiority trial. Lancet. 2018;391(10126):1163–73.
9. Duffy AG, Ulahannan SV, Makorova-Rusher O, et al. Tremelimumab in combination with ablation in patients with advanced hepatocellular carcinoma. J Hepatol. 2017;66(3):545–51.
10. Kudo M. Immuno-oncology therapy for hepatocellular carcinoma: current status and ongoing trials. Liver Cancer. 2019;8(4):221–38.
11. Tada T, Kumada T, Hiraoka A, et al. Safety and efficacy of lenvatinib in elderly patients with unresectable hepatocellular carcinoma: a multicenter analysis with propensity score matching. Hepatol Res. 2020;50(1):75–83.
12. Hiraoka A, Kumada T, Kariyama K, et al. Clinical features of lenvatinib for unresectable hepatocellular carcinoma in real-world conditions: multicenter analysis. Cancer Med. 2019;8(1):137–46.
13. Tsuchiya K, Kurosaki M, Kaneko S, et al. A nationwide multicenter study in patients with unresectable hepatocellular carcinoma treated with lenvatinib in real world practice in Japan. J Clin Oncol. 2019;37(4_suppl):364.

14. Chen S, Chao Y, Chen M, et al. Lenvatinib for the treatment of HCC: a single institute experience. J Clin Oncol. 2019;37(suppl):e15611.
15. Kudo M, Ueshima K, Chan S, et al. Lenvatinib as an initial treatment in patients with intermediate-stage hepatocellular carcinoma beyond up-to-seven criteria and Child-Pugh A liver function: a proof-of-concept study. Cancers (Basel). 2019;11(8):1084.
16. Zhu AX, Kang YK, Yen CJ, et al. Ramucirumab after sorafenib in patients with advanced hepatocellular carcinoma and increased alpha-fetoprotein concentrations (REACH-2): a randomised, double-blind, placebo-controlled, phase 3 trial. Lancet Oncol. 2019;20(2):282–96.
17. Josep ML, Chia-Jui Y, Richard SF, et al. Ramucirumab (RAM) for sorafenib intolerant patients with hepatocellular carcinoma (HCC) and elevated baseline alpha fetoprotein (AFP): outcomes from two randomized phase 3 studies (REACH, REACH2). J Clin Oncol. 2019;37(15):4073.
18. Qiu L, Qin SK, Shanzhi G, et al. Apatinib in Chinese patients with advanced hepatocellular carcinoma: a phase II randomized, open-label trial. J Clin Oncol. 2014;32(15_suppl):4019.
19. Sun HC, Zhu XD, Zhou J, et al. Effect of postoperative apatinib treatment after resection of hepatocellular carcinoma with portal vein invasion: a phase II study. J Clin Oncol. 2020;38:514.
20. Bruix J, Reig M, Merle P, et al. Alpha-fetoprotein (AFP) response in patients with unresectable hepatocellular carcinoma (HCC) in the phase 3 RESORCE trial. Ann Oncol. 2019;30(suppl_5):v253–324.
21. de Mattia E, Cecchin E, Guardascione M, et al. Pharmacogenetics of the systemic treatment in advanced hepatocellular carcinoma. World J Gastroenterol. 2019;25(29):3870–96.
22. Faivre S, Rimassa L, Finn RS. Molecular therapies for HCC: looking outside the box. J Hepatol. 2020;72(2):342–52.
23. Li D, Sedano S, Allen R, et al. Current treatment landscape for advanced hepatocellular carcinoma: patient outcomes and the impact on quality of life. Cancers. 2019;11(6):841.
24. Yau T, Park JW, Finn RS, et al. CheckMate 459: a randomized, multi-center phase 3 study of nivolumab (NIVO) vs sorafenib (SOR) as first-line (1L) treatment in patients (pts) with advanced hepatocellular carcinoma (aHCC). Ann Oncol. 2019;30(suppl_5):v851–934.
25. Finn RS, Ryoo BY, Merle P, et al. Pembrolizumab as second-line therapy in patients with advanced hepatocellular carcinoma in keynote-240: a randomized, double-blind, phase III trial. J Clin Oncol. 2020;38(3):193–202.
26. Deng L, Liang H, Burnette B, et al. Irradiation and anti-PD-L1 treatment synergistically promote antitumor immunity in mice. J Clin Invest. 2014;124(2):687–95.
27. Kudo M, Lim HY, Cheng AL, et al. Phase III study of pembrolizumab (pembro) versus best supportive care (BSC) for second-line therapy in advanced hepatocellular carcinoma (aHCC): KEYNOTE-240 Asian subgroup. J Clin Oncol. 2020;38(4_suppl):526.
28. Qin S, Ren Z, Meng Z, et al. Camrelizumab in patients with previously treated advanced hepatocellular carcinoma: a multicentre, open-label, parallel-group, randomised, phase 2 trial. Lancet Oncol. 2020;21(4):571–80.
29. Wang J, Fei K, Jing H, et al. Durable blockade of PD-1 signaling links preclinical efficacy of sintilimab to its clinical benefit. MAbs. 2019;11(8):1443–51.
30. Andrew X, Richard S, Julien E, et al. Pembrolizumab in patients with advanced hepatocellular carcinoma previously treated with sorafenib (KEYNOTE-224): a non-randomised, open-label phase 2 trial. Lancet Oncol. 2018;19(7):940–52.
31. Todd S. Nivolumab (nivo) in sorafenib (sor)-naive andexperienced pts with advanced hepatocellular carcinoma (HCC): CheckMate 040 study. J Clin Oncol. 2017;5(15_suppl):4013.
32. Villanueva A. Hepatocellular carcinoma. N Engl J Med. 2019;380(15):1450–62.
33. Sia D, Jiao Y, Martinez-Quetglas I, et al. Identification of an immune-specific class of hepatocellular carcinoma, based on molecular features. Gastroenterology. 2017;153(3):812–26.
34. Jilkova ZM, Aspord C, Decaens T. Aspord and t.decaens, predictive factors for response to PD-1/PD-11 checkpoint inhibition in the field of hepatocellular carcinoma: current status and challenges. Cancers. 2019;11(10):1554.
35. Nishino M, Ramaiya NH, Hatabu H, et al. Monitoring immune-checkpoint blockade: response evaluation and biomarker development. Nat Rev Clin Oncol. 2017;14(11):655–68.
36. Llovet JM, Montal R, Sia D, et al. Molecular therapies and precision medicine for hepatocellular carcinoma. Nat Rev Clin Oncol. 2018;15(10):599–616.
37. Wang Q, Gao J, Wu X. Pseudoprogression and hyperprogression after checkpoint blockade. Int Immunopharmacol. 2018;58:125–35.
38. Weinmann H. Cancer immunotherapy: selected targets and small-molecule modulators. Chem Med Chem. 2016;11(5):450–66.
39. Sasikumar P, Shrimali R, Adurthi S, et al. A novel peptide therapeutic targeting PD1 immune checkpoint with equipotent antagonism of both ligands and a potential for better management of immune-related adverse events. J Immunother Cancer. 2013;1(Suppl 1):24.
40. Shaverdian N, Lisberg AE, Bornazyan K, et al. Previous radiotherapy and the clinical activity and toxicity of pembrolizumab in the treatment of non-small-cell lung cancer: a secondary analysis of the KEYNOTE-001 phase 1 trial. Lancet Oncol. 2017;18(7):895–903.
41. Moslehi JJ, Salem JE, Sosman JA, et al. Increased reporting of fatal immune checkpoint inhibitor-associated myocarditis. Lancet. 2018;391(10124):933.

42. Joo-Ho L, Soo YO, Jin YK, et al. Cancer immunotherapy for hepatocellular carcinoma. Hepatoma Res. 2018;4:51.
43. Mizukoshi E, Yamashita T, Arai K, et al. Enhancement of tumor-associatedantigen-specific T cell responses by radiofrequency ablation of hepatocellular carcinoma. Hepatology. 2013;57(4):1448–57.
44. Hilmi M, Neuzillet C, Calderaro J, et al. Angiogenesis and immune checkpoint inhibitors as therapies for hepatocellular carcinoma: current knowledge and future research directions. J Immunother Cancer. 2019;7(1):1–13.
45. Cheng A, Hsu C, Chan SL, et al. Challenges of combination therapy with immune checkpoint inhibitors for hepatocellular carcinoma. J Hepatol. 2020;72(2):307–19.
46. Shigeta K, Datta M, Hato T, et al. Dual programmed death receptor-1 and vascular endothelial growth factor receptor-2 blockade promotes vascular normalization and enhances antitumor immune responses in hepatocellular carcinoma. Hepatology. 2020;71(4):1247–61.
47. Motzer RJ, Powles T, Atkins MB, et al. IMmotion151: a randomized phase iii study of atezolizumab plus bevacizumab vs sunitinib in untreated metastatic renal cell carcinoma (mRCC). J Clin Oncol. 2018;36(6_suppl):578.
48. Andreas P, Dominik W, Axel H, et al. Synergies of targeting tumor angiogenesis and immune checkpoints in non-small-cell lung cancer and renal cell cancer: from basic concepts to clinical reality. Int J Mol Sci. 2017;18(11):2291.
49. Fukumura D, Kloepper J, Amoozgar A, et al. Enhancing cancer immunotherapy using antiangiogenics: opportunities and challenges. Nat Rev Clin Oncol. 2018;15(5):325–40.
50. Chen D, Mellman I. Oncology meets immunology: the cancer-immunity cycle. Immunity. 2013;39(1):1–10.
51. Lin YY, Tan CT, Chen CW, et al. Immunomodulatory effects of current targeted therapies on hepatocellular carcinoma: implication for the future of immunotherapy. Semin Liver Dis. 2018;38(4):379.
52. Ayaru L, Pereira SP, Alisa A, et al. Unmasking of alpha-fetoprotein-specific CD4(+) T cell responses in hepatocellular carcinoma patients undergoing embolization. J Immunol. 2007;178(3):1914–22.
53. Xu J, Zhang Y, Jia R, et al. Anti-PD-1 antibody SHR-1210 combined with apatinib for advanced hepatocellular carcinoma, gastric, or esophagogastric junction cancer: an open-label, dose escalation and expansion study. Clin Cancer Res. 2019;25(2):515–23.
54. Kaseb AO, Vence L, Blando J, et al. Immunologic correlates of pathologic complete response to preoperative immunotherapy in hepatocellular carcinoma. Cancer Immunol Res. 2019;7(9):1390–5.

32 Prospects on the Whole-Course Management of Liver Cancer Based on the Big Data

Xiaobin Feng and Jiahong Dong

32.1 China Has High Numbers of Liver Cancer Cases, Which Lays a Reliable Foundation for the Development of Big Data on Liver Cancer

There are 854,000 new cases of liver cancer worldwide each year, among which 466,000 cases are observed in China, accounting for 55% of all global cases. Liver cancer is the second and sixth global leading cause of cancer in men and women, respectively. There is a high degree of heterogeneity in the etiology, epidemiological characteristics, clinical manifestations and staging, molecular biological behavior, and therapeutic strategies of liver cancer, and this is evident in the fact that primary liver cancer in China is very different from cases seen in Europe and the United States. In China, liver cancer is most prevalent in Qidong of Jiangsu Province and Fusui of Guangxi Province. Comparatively, the incidence of liver cancer abroad is found to be relatively high in sub-Saharan Africa and the Pacific Coast of Asia. The age of onset is mainly 40–49 years, and the ratio of male to female is 2–5:1. Viral hepatitis and/or alcohol consumption are the main pathogenic factors (accounting for 70–80% of cases), among which hepatitis B virus (HBV) infection plays a dominant role. Hepatobiliary diseases impart tremendous social and economic pressure to our country and will continue to increase for some time to come.

With the development of big data and artificial intelligence (AI) technology, intelligent applications have begun to take shape in hepatobiliary tumor diagnosis and treatment, and thus medical treatment is expected to fully enter the era of big data in the near future. Recently, renowned medical journals such as Nature, JAMA, and Science have published a series of articles on solving medical problems by AI. In particular, in January 2019, Nature Medicine published an unprecedented eight concurrent papers, which pushed for the application of big data and AI to a new level in the medical field. Predictably, AI-assisted medical services will be a promising solution for medicine in the future for liver tumor diagnosis and treatment, convolutional neural networks, and other AI technologies that have played active roles in foci detection, lesion identification and evaluation, liver sectioning and reconstruction, diffuse liver disease evaluation and classification, diagnosis and treatment planning, and efficacy prediction. For example, Konda et al. examined the ultrasound characteristics of liver cancer patients using a support vector machine, and the accuracy of the diagnostic model for distinguishing benign hepatic space-occupying lesions, liver cancer, and metastatic liver cancer reached 84.4%, 87.7%, and 85.7%, respectively.

X. Feng · J. Dong (✉)
Beijing Tsinghua Changgung Hospital,
Beijing, China
e-mail: dongjiahong@mail.tsinghua.edu.cn

X. Chen (ed.), *Diagnosis and Treatment of Liver Cancer in China*,
https://doi.org/10.1007/978-981-97-7969-7_32

Despite our efforts, we continue to face many unfavorable factors in the development of liver cancer big data. While there are large numbers of liver cancer patients in China, there is still a lamentable lack of usable, effective data, and a comprehensive understanding of clinical diagnosis and treatment. As such, we are still behind international levels when it comes to the standardization, normalization, and specialization of diagnosis and treatment. In addition, the accuracy of liver cancer clinical staging and the reliability of classification directly affect the short-term efficacy and long-term survival of hepatocellular carcinoma (HCC) patients. At present, there are different liver cancer staging systems at home and abroad, all of which have different shortcomings, such as a small sample size for model construction and a small number of indicators. Therefore, it is difficult to precisely evaluate the prognosis of HCC patients based on a few non-standardized samples and a few parameters. Only by establishing a diversified and standardized sample database and multi-modal indicators that fully account for the above factors, the overall picture of the disease can be fully and precisely reflected and the outcome of the disease and patient survival be quantitatively assessed. Therefore, the development of an intelligent classification system for liver cancer that takes into account multiple factors and has strong operability remains an urgent task in liver cancer diagnosis and treatment.

32.2 Construction and Application of Primary Liver Cancer Database in China

From very early on, a large number of multicenter foreign medical research databases were established. For example, American society of clinical oncology (ASCO) CancerLinQ has over one million cancer cases, while Flatiron Health database has information on over 1.5 million. Because these databases are completely shared, there are numerous data sources and a large amount of data, which are of great significance for clinical reference or the exploration of the pattern of disease development. Health and medical-related big data have become increasingly attractive as an excellent strategic resource for national innovation and development. A series of important policies have been issued at the national level, including the *Action Plan for Further Improving Medical Services* (2018–2020), *Notice on Further Promoting the Informatization Construction of Medical Institutions with Electronic Medical Records*, and *Administrative Measures for National Health and Medical Big Data Standards, Safety and Services (Trial)*. The large population of liver cancer patients and liver diseases in China makes it highly favorable for the development of liver cancer big data. So far, a variety of big data platforms, including comprehensive, specialized, and thematic platforms, have been established by the government, academic institutions, enterprises, experts, and scholars. Some of these are for the purpose of management, while others are for the purpose of research. The contents of such platforms include electronic medical records, tissue samples, imaging data, and gene databases. All of these platforms have effectively promoted progress in liver cancer diagnosis and treatment in China.

32.2.1 Database Construction

1. Hospital Quality Monitoring System (HQMS): The HQMS data reporting system is a database developed by the former Department of Medical Management of the Ministry of Health for the purpose of medical service supervision. It is an early application of computer and network technology in China to report and review medical information, especially medical quality indicators, generated in hospitals. Data sources include inpatient death, re-admission, nosocomial infection, surgical complications, patient safety, rational drug use in medical institutions, and hospital operation management indicators. The early focus of the system is to automatically connect the data on the first

page of medical records, requiring each center to achieve automatic data acquisition to ensure the authenticity of hospital review and evaluation data. The HQMS study center is responsible for providing data docking to national tertiary hospitals and assisting in the completion of data docking. The unique advantages of this database are automatic, timely, complete, authentic, continuous completion of data docking without human intervention, and inclusion of system docking situations into tertiary hospital evaluation indicators. Since 2019, HQMS has gradually begun integrating relevant text, testing, and examination information as well as improving the integrity of the database information, which may still be used as a disease database through further development. However, there are still some problems with the quality of the database, such as inconsistent data across different areas and data loss. Furthermore, although over 2000 tertiary hospitals are connected, a data reporting network covering all areas at the village, town, county, and prefecture levels and above is still not available. The lack of data representation limits its range of application.

2. Chinese Primary Liver Cancer Clinical Survey (CLCS): This database focuses on real-world liver cancer research. Previous evidence-based medicine emphasizes randomized controlled trial (RCT) research, which requires strict inclusion and exclusion criteria. The sample size is generally small, and therefore it is difficult for the research conclusions to be widely applied. In contrast, real-world research of primary liver cancer based on big data can be used to better guide clinical practices. CLCS is an extensive sample disease database that was established for purposes which includes demographic information, diagnosis and treatment measures, efficacy, and safety. A total of 49 clinical centers have participated in this survey, including 14,478 primary liver cancer patients. CLCS is expected to cover more than 200 hospitals in the Asia-Pacific region by 2021. An interim analysis has shown that HBV infection is the most common cause of liver cancer and HCC is the most common pathologic type, with most patients being in the intermediate and advanced stages at the time of hospitalization. Surgical treatment is the most commonly used regimen in the diagnosis and treatment of liver cancer, while Trans-arterial chemoembolisation (TACE) is the most common combination treatment. The study suggests that in the current cancer diagnosis and treatment process, more emphasis should be placed on multidisciplinary involvement in addition to multimodality treatment, reinforcement of the integration of disciplines and interdisciplinary communication and cooperation, and active participation of more clinicians, experts, and scholars in order to provide the optimal systemic treatment for patients.
3. Primary Liver Cancer Big Data (PLCBD) and National Liver Cancer Sample Database: The PLCBD system was jointly established by the Third Affiliated Hospital of People's Liberation Army (PLA) Navy Military Medical University, Mengchao Hepatobiliary Hospital of Fujian Medical University, and 92 Liver Disease Medical Consortium units. The sources for this data include electronic medical record systems, hospital information systems, laboratory information management systems, medical image archiving and communication systems, sample banks, and other recorded clinical data of liver cancer. The database preliminarily includes a total of 33,709 patients with primary liver cancer comprising of 17 sub-databases containing demographic information, medical history and diagnosis, and 1421 dimensions. A total of 31,571 patients had treatment records, including surgery, local treatment (radiofrequency ablation, interventional therapy, or radiotherapy), and systematic therapy (molecular targeted therapy, chemotherapy, traditional Chinese medicine, or immunotherapy). The system also has complete follow-up data, with a follow-up time of up to 18 years. In addition, PLCBD provided the simulation image data of 11,000 liver cancer cases for the national competition "Big Data Medical

Treatment—Artificial Intelligence Diagnosis of Liver Cancer Image." The liver cancer sample bank was jointly initiated by the National Liver Cancer Science Center, the Third Affiliated Hospital of PLA Navy Military Medical University, Nanfang Hospital of Southern University of Medical Science and Technology, and member enterprises of Berry Genetics. This was used as a prospective national multi-centered, 10,000-person cohort, preemptive liver cancer warning marker screening project in China. The preliminary study showed that the detection sensitivity for liver cancer was over 97% under the condition of 100% specificity. This result indicated that the liver cancer early screening project has successfully constructed a cirrhosis and liver cancer classification model based on second-generation sequencing (next-generation sequencing (NGS)), which can accurately identify hepatic cirrhosis patients developing cancer, and is expected to be applied to the early screening of liver cancer.

4. Database of Zhongshan Hospital, Fudan University: The liver cancer gene clinical study database is constructed based on the large number of liver cancer cases seen at Zhongshan Hospital and the collection of a substantial amount of public data. This database uses single-sample data interpretation algorithms and unified information standardization and data storage to achieve data integration. At present, the database has accumulated the public expression data of more than 3500 liver cancer patients and control populations. The liver cancer gene clinical study database aims to further the current understanding of the relationship between genes and the development, progression, and drug interaction of liver cancer, thus playing an important role in promoting the early intervention and prevention of liver cancer, as well as individualized diagnosis and treatment.
5. Multi-dimensional multidisciplinary team (MDT) big data platform for hepatobiliary tumors: This big data platform is committed to the creation of the most influential collaborative systems for hepatobiliary cancer treatment and research in China, and serving experts and managers in the field of hepatobiliary cancer. The decision-making knowledge base of the MDT big data platform primarily originates from clinical guidelines and references, while the largest part of underlying data comes from hospital databases, including those from 35 national hospitals and over 20,000 liver cancer patients, which serve as the cornerstone of the platform. Using patient clinical data, 16S sequencing data, bile acid, and inflammatory factor data from this integrated hepatobiliary tumor database, has allowed a number of high-quality studies on tumor markers for intrahepatic cholangiocarcinoma (ICC) to be published on Hepatology. This has provided new insights for the further study of the pathogenesis of ICC and the finding of effective therapeutic targets, greatly improving the clinical diagnostic efficiency of ICC. This big data platform includes a clinical decision support system and MDT consultation platform, which allow for grassroots hospitals to acquire 80% of the diagnostic and treatment capabilities of large hospitals. It can also help create new drug clinical trial bases, improve the mode of new drug clinical trials, and shorten the research and development cycle of new drugs.
6. LinkDoc Technology Tumor Database: This big data platform includes more than 50 real-world tumor databases, covering lung cancer, gastric cancer, liver cancer, and breast cancer. This platform has standardized and structured clinical medical records of well-defined high-quality data taken based on dimensions of standardization, interconnection, enhancement, and richness, reforming the methods of medical record processing in the traditional electronic data capture system, establishing a Hubble intelligent follow-up system, and providing whole-course management for 400,000 cancer patients. In 2016, the big data platform released "China's first medical migration map of cancer patients," which for the first time enabled the Chinese people to visualize the medical migration routes of hundreds of thousands of cancer patients on a map of China.

Both the First Affiliated Hospital of Guangzhou Medical University and Fuzhou University have collaboratively conducted big data research using this system, and as a result, were awarded the ASCO Merit Award for structured analysis of medical records and identification of liver and gallbladder lesions as well as the subdivision first place of the 2019 Digital China Innovation Competition. The focus of future development is to cover the whole-course management of single disease diagnosis and treatment, including early screening, auxiliary diagnosis, treatment and regimen recommendation, efficacy evaluation, risk prediction, prognostic analysis, and patient follow-up.

7. Hubei Data Center for Hepatobiliary and Pancreatic Malignancies: The data center was initiated and established by Professor Xiaoping CHEN of Tongji Hospital affiliated with Tongji Medical College of Huazhong University of Science and Technology in 2017. This data center is a hepatobiliary and pancreatic cancer sample database covering over 60 million people in the Hubei province and surrounding provinces. It is expected to achieve information sharing and mutual recognition for the treatment of hepatobiliary and pancreatic cancers within the province. With the Liver Surgery Center of Tongji Hospital as its main headquarters, the big data center will connect with over 200 medical institutions at the county level and above in the provinces to collect relevant data of patients with hepatobiliary and pancreatic cancers in each medical institution. Medical institutions can use the interconnected big data information platform to share and recognize information, provide health services such as electronic medical records, health records, and telemedicine, and thus improve the overall diagnosis and treatment of hepatobiliary and pancreatic surgery in Hubei Province. On this basis, the China Hepatobiliary and Pancreatic Specialty Alliance was established on May 25, 2018, to fully promote medical informatization construction for hepatobiliary and pancreatic diseases, aiming to achieve the interconnection of medical and health data resources for hepatobiliary and pancreatic tumors. In the future, we will standardize the industry standards for hepatobiliary and pancreatic medicine, achieve information interconnection through the transmission of new developments at home and abroad, promote resource sharing and resource allocation, and establish a national big data center for hepatobiliary and pancreatic diseases in order to improve the overall level of scientific research on hepatobiliary and pancreatic diseases in China.
8. Human Digital Liver Database: The Human Digital Liver Database is the world's first and largest human digital liver open platform database that is the collaborative effort of over 16 Chinese hospitals, including the Affiliated Hospital of Qingdao University, the Children's Hospital of Fudan University, Shengjing Hospital of China Medical University, the Children's Hospital of Zhejiang University School of Medicine, the Children's Hospital of Capital Institute of Pediatrics, Xinhua Hospital Affiliated to Shanghai Jiaotong University School of Medicine, and Tongji Hospital of Tongji Medical College of Huazhong University of Science and Technology. The data platform collects original enhanced CT DICOM files of 1260 normal human livers of all age groups from the cooperating hospitals, importing them into the computer-assisted surgery system (Hisense CAS) which was developed by Professor Qian DONG from the Affiliated Hospital of Qingdao University and Hisense Group in order to obtain digital liver models for 3D reconstruction. The platform displays 3D digital models of normal human livers and major hepatobiliary and pancreatic diseases constructed based on the substantial amount of data in different age groups. By combining the case details and annotation of liver data, the digital liver is clearly and completely displayed in the database open platform by means of all-round static digital liver pictures and analog animation. The human digital liver database has met the preliminary access requirements for digital liver data and is open

to doctors, medical students, and ordinary Internet users for free. It will gradually develop into an open platform for medical image data in the future.

9. National Health Commission (NHC) standard hepatobiliary database: The construction of China's first standardized big database of systemic diseases was officially launched in December 2019 with Beijing Tsinghua Changgung Hospital in charge of the construction of the NHC standard hepatobiliary database. There are plans that include creating a clinical imaging database for major hepatobiliary diseases, such as cholangiocarcinoma and liver cancer and carry out electronic medical records-based intelligent classification of liver cancer and multimodal radiomics research on liver segment structure, function, and pathological features. Based on the clinical big data center of the Institute of Precision Medicine of Tsinghua University, the database has included 51 large grade A centers, aiming to build the largest and most representative standard data-sharing platform for hepatobiliary diseases in China. The project will strengthen the research on basic platforms and core technologies and focus on establishing regulations for robust health and medical big data quality specifications, open sharing and data security, driving precision medicine, drug R&D, and R&D and evaluation of AI medical devices, thus promoting the innovative development of smart medical care, digital medical care, medical insurance payment, and commercial insurance.

32.2.2 Problems in the Construction and Application of Liver Cancer Big Data

Although liver cancer big data has great potential, its development is relatively slow. There are still many bottleneck problems that have to be resolved in the implementation of interconnection and scientific application of health and medical data.

1. Database development mode and research support mode: At present, most of the liver cancer databases in China are developed independently of one another, leading to a lack of national databases such as the United States surveillance, epidemiology, and results databases. In addition, the process of database and data construction lacks transparency, existing mostly as handwritten records, and lacks traceability and credibility. Therefore, the construction of a nationwide pan-representative PLCBD that spans the whole course of diagnosis, treatment, and the entire lifecycle is urgently needed.

   In terms of research-related application support, there is an urgent need and huge market present in both academia and industry, including a large number of drug clinical trials, investigator-initiated clinical studies, as well as a large number of medical device registration studies for medical engineering AI products. Regardless of the type of research, a case report form (CRF) is always required, which includes information on inclusion screening, eligibility criteria, exclusion criteria, regular follow-up visits, and outcomes. CRF should be strictly filled, retained for a long time, and traceable on demand. At present, most of the work is carried out by a relevant professional team through manual recording, double-check procedures, and regular entry of follow-up data. This mode has some defects including low efficiency, insufficient "source" data, and obvious artificial errors and is far from meeting the requirements of high-quality clinical research and the degree of medical informatization.

2. Data standards and data sharing: The format of electronic medical records for specialized diseases and specialties has not been unified in China, which causes many problems such as a large number of medical records, unstructured data, lack of unified standards in the industry, and difficult follow-up. This in turn leads to inadequate mining and application of value, and only a small amount of data being qualified for application to clinical studies. Different regions, different centers, and even

different departments in the same center may have information incompatibility and data fusion problems. In addition, China is a vast country with different language habits and thinking patterns across many regions, which results in the non-standardization of medical record descriptions and the inability to make clinical data "ready for use."

In terms of data sharing technology, there is currently no designated health and medical data network and transmission encryption technology, which causes great difficulties in data security management, sharing, and interconnection. In addition, the efficient operation of the data platform and the method of data sharing based on authorization need to be explored. The establishment of national standards and national standard datasets for liver cancer electronic medical records can provide not only clinical data that meet a uniform quality standard but also uniform testing for the R&D of liver cancer AI products, which is expected to break the current dilemma in big data and AI development.

3. Information specification and data privacy: The people and regulatory authorities at home and abroad are taking data privacy seriously. For example, Google's "Project Nightingale" collected the health data of millions of American patients without their knowledge, causing a public outcry over whether patient privacy is protected, despite the fact that there is no evidence of misuse of data. Medical information security is highly emphasized and regarded as the "top leading" project in all hospitals; however, due to the lack of national and authoritative specifications on "de-privacy and de-labeling" and medical data ethics, hospitals "dare not" and "cannot" practice "interconnection." Therefore, with regard to the establishment of laws and regulations, we also need to set up corresponding standards and safety boundaries for the use of liver cancer big data to solve the "dare not" issue in the use of medical big data, and the application of special encrypted channels and intelligent means to solve the "cannot" issue for safe use, so as to revolutionize the access security and application efficiency of health and medical data.

32.3 Mutual Promotion of Liver Cancer Big Data and Whole-Course Management of Liver Cancer Diagnosis and Treatment

In recent years, rapid progress has been achieved in liver cancer surgery, molecular targeted therapy, and immunotherapy in China. Many new advances have also been included in the *Guidelines for Diagnosis and Treatment of Primary Liver Cancer* (2019 Edition), including new techniques for early diagnosis and support for TCM treatments to reduce recurrence and prolong survival. As the overall survival of liver cancer patients increases, the survival of advanced-stage patients can also be prolonged from the previous 7 or 8 months to over 20 months now. With the increase of the aforementioned treatment methods, the improvement of multimodality treatment efficacy, and the prolongation of survival time, whole-course management of liver cancer becomes increasingly important, which is also emphasized in the *Guidelines for Diagnosis and Treatment of Primary Liver Cancer* (2019 Edition). Health and medical big data can play an important role in the supply side of the "whole-course and whole-chain" medical service system for liver cancer that affects all dimensions of patients' health, including monitoring and screening of high-risk populations, early diagnosis and treatment, and rehabilitation guidance. The concept of whole-course management was first proposed by the United States in the late 1980s, which emphasizes care and management of the whole process from the onset of illness to recovery. Prolonged survival also means a shift in cancer treatment options and strategies. The objective of cancer treatment is to not only completely remove the tumor but also improve the quality of life of patients as much as possible while reducing unnecessary deaths and other complications.

For patients with primary liver cancer, the prioritized meaning of "the whole course" should be the "whole course of disease," in other words, the patient's entire diagnosis and treatment process. Like other tumors, liver cancer is also considered a systemic disease, and hence surgery-centered multidisciplinary multimodality treatments are being increasingly emphasized. Surgery also includes preoperative assessment, diagnosis and treatment strategy formulation, treatment method selection, surgical skills, intraoperative plan adjustment, postoperative management, prevention and treatment of complications, control of drug side effects, recurrence prevention, and even adjustment of patients' nutritional status and mental state and many other management details. The multidisciplinary diagnosis and treatment model also puts forward higher requirements for doctors in the diagnosis and treatment of liver cancer while maximizing the benefit of cancer patients. Doctors should pay attention to not only the diagnosis and treatment process but also the patients' quality of life, treatment-related side effects, and a large amount of medical data. Therefore, efficient big data management is essential for the implementation of the whole-course management strategy.

The whole-course management of liver cancer also requires that medical service providers provide both "seamless" and "continuous" health services. There are many specific goals and requirements for liver cancer prevention and control in China and abroad. For example, the World Health Organization has proposed the goal of eliminating hepatitis as a hazard by 2030, which has become the "No.1 Subject" in the field of liver disease prevention and control worldwide. In 1992, China included the HBV vaccine in the national immunization program. The current HBV infection rate in individuals who are 18 years and under is less than 1%, indicating a remarkable improvement. The current situation of liver disease prevention and control in China plays an important role in realizing this goal, which requires us to actively explore a full-chain service model integrating medical treatment, rehabilitation, health care, and prevention. Big data of liver cancer will play an important role in this stage of prevention and control. At present, describing disease characteristics and classification (including clinical features, molecular features, and overall features), elucidating the biological mechanisms of disease (expression networks, transcriptome, proteome, genome, drug metabolome), and screening biological markers of diseases and disease subtypes (multi-gene and multi-feature biomarkers) are the main directions of medical big data application.

As for the treatment of liver cancer, although hepatectomy is the preferred regimen for liver cancer, the early recurrence rate is high, and the long-term prognosis is poor after resection. Nowadays, the treatment of liver cancer has fully entered into the era of multi-modality treatment, including a series of means such as precise preoperative prediction, precise surgical procedure, precise postoperative evaluation, and precise molecular targeted therapy, all of which are of great significance to improve the overall prognosis of patients. The development and application of a clinical decision support system is also one of the important application directions of big data medical treatment. For example, postoperative pathological features can be matched and fused with preoperative imaging features using big data and AI technology to achieve precise imaging predictions, which will be invaluable for guiding the surgical planning, precise diagnosis, and treatment of liver cancer. For first-time patients diagnosed with unresectable liver cancer, quality of life, economic-physical-mental-social burden, and improvement of efficacy should be comprehensively considered while emphasizing life prolongation and maximizing the survival benefit of patients. Through multidisciplinary diagnosis and treatment, we can promote the collaboration of various subspecialties, accelerate the development of multi-modality treatments with radiotherapy, targeted therapy, and immunotherapy for intermediate to advanced liver cancer, and help patients with intermediate and advanced liver cancer gain more chances to survive. First-line molecular targeted therapy drugs for liver cancer include sorafenib and lenvatinib, and second-line molecular targeted therapy drugs include regorafenib and cabozantinib. In recent years, TACE combined with sorafenib and TACE combined with lenvatinib have been reported to downstage and transform liver cancer into resectable tumor, thereby facilitating successful radical resection. Tumor immunotherapy is expected to transform immune-privileged "cold tumors" into the more susceptible "hot tumors," which is also the most promising new concept in the field of tumor treatment, and may change the treatment outcome of patients with intermediate and advanced liver cancer. In the MDT diagnosis and treatment process mentioned above, the essence of big data medical care lies in the application of massive medical data information and medical big data platforms to analyze the data characteristics of each patient, so as to provide patients with the optimal diagnostic opinions and treatment standards without increasing medical costs. In addition, big data will also be an ideal tool for monitoring side effects and evaluating real-world efficacy.

Whole-course management also requires the continuous provision of health care services without interruption. We have always been focused on "in-patient treatment" and not so much on the whereabouts of patients after the treatment. For example, patients undergoing surgery in hospital A may go to hospital B for re-examination, and then receive follow-up treatment after detection of recurrence in hospital C. This mobile medical treatment mode means that patients receive fragmented health services, where patients often move between different departments, experts, and medical institutions and even receive different therapies. This may lead to unnecessary and repeated examination, declined treatment, and reduced overall medical quality, all of which are unfavorable for the rehabilitation and continuous monitoring of patient conditions. The tracing of the "interval" process between visits and details of diagnosis and treatment between different hospitals makes conventional record management systems seem inadequate. Thus, it is of great importance to establish a standardized and shared liver cancer big data platform.

32.4 Prospects for Use of Big Data Liver Cancer

Liver cancer big data originates from a wide range of sources involving clinical diagnosis, treatment and medication, efficacy observation, image acquisition parameters, and laboratory testing data and can include thousands of kinds of complex and diverse data from many fields. Therefore, we need to develop a national scientific research platform for health and medical data to achieve multi-centered, diversified, multi-source liver cancer data collection, cleaning, tagging, management, and traceability for the national vertical alliance of hepatobiliary specialties; in addition to establishing a large scale database of medical terminology and basic knowledge base of liver cancer using advanced technologies, such as medical natural language recognition and deep learning-based multi-modal image recognition. Finally, we hope to realize a data knowledge system that integrates free text and multimodal images based on the understanding of the context and the unstructured text information of the noumenon's electronic medical records, and the identification and screening of new image feature spectrum, so as to build a large-scale and nationally representative big data sharing platform for primary cancer of liver through the new secure multi-party interconnection technology and computer technology and support the prevention, screening and early diagnosis, standardized diagnosis and treatment, precision medicine, and clinical research of primary liver cancer in China. This will be our main development direction in the future. It should also be pointed out that the construction of liver cancer big data cannot be completed by just one institution, but requires guidance and support from all relevant ministries and commissions of the state, the full cooperation of multiple centers across the country, and the coordination and cooperation of interdisciplinary and multidisciplinary experts in clinical medicine, preventive medicine, big data, and AI. It is only through this cooperation that China's liver cancer big data project is built into a world-leading health science and technology innovation platform integrating medical research and enterprises, serving the whole-course management of primary liver cancer, and ultimately realizing maximized benefits for liver cancer patients!

Suggested Reading

1. Siegel RL, Jemal A, Wender RC, et al. An assessment of progress in cancer control. CA Cancer J Clin. 2018;68(5):329–39.
2. Tanaka M, Katayama F, Kato H, et al. Hepatitis B and C virus infection and hepatocellular carcinoma in China: a review of epidemiology and control measures. J Epidemiol. 2011;21(6):401–16.
3. Liu Z, Wang S, Dong D, et al. The applications of radiomics in precision diagnosis and treatment of oncology: opportunities and challenges. Theranostics. 2019;9(5):1303–22.
4. Zhou M, Wang H, Zeng X, et al. Mortality, morbidity, and risk factors in China and its provinces, 1990-2017: a systematic analysis for the Global Burden of Disease Study 2017. Lancet. 2019;396(10243):26.
5. Docherty AB, Lone NI. Exploiting big data for critical care research. Curr Opin Crit Care. 2015;21(5):467–72.
6. Yau T, Tang VY, Yao TJ, et al. Development of Hong Kong Liver Cancer staging system with treatment stratification for patients with hepatocellular carcinoma. Gastroenterology. 2014;146(7):1691–700, e3.
7. Bruix J, Reig M, Sherman M. Evidence-based diagnosis, staging, and treatment of patients with hepatocellular carcinoma. Gastroenterology. 2016;150(4):835–53.
8. Wang LN, Zhang Z. Mendelian randomization approach, used for causal inferences. Zhonghua Liu Xing Bing Xue Za Zhi. 2017;38(4):547–52.
9. American Society of Clinical Oncology. The state of cancer care in America, 2017: a report by the American Society of Clinical Oncology. J Oncol Pract. 2017;13(4):e353–94.
10. Towle EL, Barr TR, Senese JL. The National Practice Benchmark for oncology, 2014 report on 2013 data. J Oncol Pract. 2014;10(6):385–406.
11. Wang L, Guo PF, Yang Y, et al. Preliminary exploration of the construction of primary liver cancer big data. Chin J Hepatobiliary Surg. 2019;25(9):695–8.
12. Chen FQ, Zhou JQ, Liu YM, et al. Information security management of liver cancer sample bank. China Digit Med. 2015;10(3):86–8.
13. Jia X, Lu S, Zeng Z, et al. Characterization of gut microbiota, bile acid metabolism, and cytokines in intrahepatic cholangiocarcinoma. Hepatology. 2019;71(3):893–906.
14. Liang X, Bi S, Yang W, et al. Epidemiological serosurvey of hepatitis B in China—declining HBV prevalence due to hepatitis B vaccination. Vaccine. 2009;27(47):6550–7.
15. Zeng Y, Liao MH. Study on the whole-course management of liver cancer from the perspectives of accelerated rehabilitation and multidisciplinary collaboration. Chin J Digest Surg. 2019;18(4):316–20.
16. Jiang XF. Application status of medical big data in clinical medicine. Chin J Clin (Electronic Edition). 2018;12(8):427–31.
17. Lu CJ, Li JL, Guo JJ, et al. Medical artificial intelligence and clinical medical terminology standards. J Med Inform. 2018;39(5):8–11, 24.